Postharvest Biology and Technology for Preserving Fruit Quality

Daniel Valero and María Serrano

CRC Press
Taylor & Francis Group
Boca Raton London New York

CRC Press is an imprint of the
Taylor & Francis Group, an **informa** business

CRC Press
Taylor & Francis Group
6000 Broken Sound Parkway NW, Suite 300
Boca Raton, FL 33487-2742

International Standard Book Number: 978-1-4398-0266-3 (Hardback)

Library of Congress Cataloging-in-Publication Data

Valero, Daniel.
Postharvest biology and technology for preserving fruit quality / Daniel Valero and Maria Serrano.
p. cm.
Includes bibliographical references and index.
ISBN 978-1-4398-0266-3 (alk. paper)
1. Fruit--Postharvest technology. 2. Fruit--Ripening. 3. Fruit--Storage. 4. Fruit--Quality. I. Serrano, María, 1963- II. Title.

SB360.5.V35 2010
634'.0468--dc22 2009048483

Visit the Taylor & Francis Web site at
http://www.taylorandfrancis.com

and the CRC Press Web site at
http://www.crcpress.com

Dedication

To our families, for their unconditional support.

Contents

Preface

Postharvest Biology and Technology for Preserving Fruit Quality will be an extremely useful book to anyone concerned with the storage life of fresh fruits. It presents both physiological and technological approaches to fruits within a single cover offering a general vision of the different postharvest technologies during fruit storage. Teachers, students, and researchers, as well as the fruit industry, can read about the scientific principles that govern the ripening process of fruits as well the major technologies that maintain fruit quality during postharvest storage. In this sense, this book will provide a comprehensive view of this subject, offering a firm background in basic knowledge and its technological and practical applications.

The book contains 11 chapters, and although each chapter constitutes a separate unit, the order and continuity of the chapters are relevant to a better understanding of the whole subject.

The introductory chapter (Chapter 1, "Introduction and Overview") contains a brief history of the changes in the postharvest discipline over the past three decades. It is clear that technological advances are possible only because of knowledge about the postharvest physiology of the raw produce.

Chapter 2, "Fruit Ripening," contains updated reviews of the fruit-ripening process, with special focus on the parameters related to organoleptic (color, texture, and aroma) and nutritive (soluble solids and organic acids) quality. The changes occurring on the bioactive compounds with antioxidant properties during on-plant fruit growth and ripening are provided together with the physiological changes.

Chapter 3, "Changes in Fruit Quality Attributes During Handling, Processing, and Storage," includes topics on the postharvest produce quality changes during handling and storage, with special emphasis on decay and preharvest factors that affect the postharvest life of fresh fruits. A detailed section is focused on mechanical damage and its effect on fruit postharvest physiology, one of the less common types of stress studied.

The effect of cold storage on fruit quality parameters is addressed in Chapter 4, "Cold Storage and Fruit Quality," with a description of the main precooling systems followed by the study of chilling injury, its physiological implications, and the ways to minimize its occurrence.

The next chapters cover the main technologies to maintain or improve the postharvest quality of fresh fruits, with special emphasis on the physiological basis by which these technologies are successful in the areas of harvest, handling, and storage. All of them contain information about the physiological and biochemical changes induced by these postharvest treatments, as well as their repercussion on fruit quality parameters. Among them, the discussion of the effects of the several technologies on the bioactive compounds with antioxidant properties (phenolics, anthocyanins, carotenoids, and antioxidant vitamins) is quite innovative and could not be found in similar books. Some of them are currently being applied in the industry, but others have scientific fundamentals to be used in a near future. Chapter 5, "Heat Treatments," reflects the wide interest in heat treatments for controlling fruit decay and maintenance of postharvest quality. Heat treatments include hot water dips, hot air, and vapor heat, which have been adapted to fruit commodities to achieve direct benefits without causing damage. This chapter discusses some of the effects that high temperatures have on harvested commodities, both beneficial and detrimental, on the fruit ripening process and the parameters related to quality. The chapter ends with the application of heat treatments on alleviating chilling injury and fruit decay.

Chapter 6, "Calcium Treatments," deals with the use of calcium, at either preharvest or postharvest, as a safe and potentially effective way to increase the quality and storage life of fruit commodities. Calcium, as a physiological cation, is able to induce benefits in terms of fruit size and related quality parameters. In addition, calcium has shown its role in reducing chilling injury symptoms and postharvest decay by modifications in the physiological status of the fresh fruits.

A new and updated chapter about polyamines and fruit is presented in Chapter 7, "Polyamine Treatments." Polyamines, as organic cations found in all plant cells, are intimately involved in, and required for, distinct biological functions. In the specific case of fruits, the considerable progress in the knowledge of polyamine physiological roles makes them a new postharvest technology to be applied in the horticultural industries. The recent and significant findings provide a fundamental basis to establish the role of polyamines in fruit physiology: from fruit development on tree, which justifies the polyamine as preharvest treatment, to postharvest storage by improving some parameters related to quality and minimizing some stresses such as chilling injury and mechanical damage.

1-Methylcyclopropene (1-MCP), the revolutionary inhibitor of ethylene action, which binds irreversibly with the ethylene receptors, is covered in Chapter 8, "1-Methylcyclopropene Treatments." During the last decade, much evidence on the positive effects of 1-MCP on fresh fruits and the classification as a nontoxic mode of action, the low concentrations needed to achieve its biological effects, and its low or undetectable residue levels has resulted in its relatively quick registration by a large number of countries worldwide. Thus, the major impact of 1-MCP has been on climacteric fruits. The interaction of 1-MCP and the ethylene receptor and the benefits in delaying the ripening process and the associated fruit quality parameters are addressed in depth. The incipient preharvest application of 1-MCP, its role in some physiological disorders, and the application in nonclimacteric fruits is also provided.

Chapter 9, "Storage in Modified Atmosphere Packaging," describes the technology of modified atmosphere packaging (MAP). MAP has become an essential technology for preserving fruits and vegetables and has been increasingly introduced worldwide. In MAP packages, the gaseous environment is modified affecting the concentrations of oxygen and carbon dioxide to create an optimum gas mixture to extend the shelf life and quality of fresh commodities. To achieve this system, plastic films with different permeabilities to gases are necessary. The effects of MAP on the parameters related to fruit quality are updated. In addition, MAP can serve as a basis for active packaging of fruits, which is addressed in Chapter 10, "Active Packaging." In modern societies, innovative packaging with enhanced functions is constantly sought in response to consumer demands for minimally processed foods with fewer preservatives, increased regulatory requirements, market globalization, and concern for food safety. In this chapter, the latest advances in ethylene adsorbers and antimicrobial packaging with natural compounds are discussed, and it ends with a discussion of the development and use of novel edible coatings.

The book concludes with current topics about some emerging technologies (Chapter 11, "Emerging Technologies"), such as atmospheres with high O_2, biological control, and the use of UV light. These technologies, with promising introduction in the horticultural sector, are encouraged to develop new preservation systems that will maintain the quality and extend the shelf life of fruits without compromising their safety, appearance, or sensory properties.

This book brings together original illustrations on a broad range of approaches after many years of research on postharvest physiology and technology by the authors to address some of the fundamental issues of the postharvest biology and technology of fresh fruits.

Daniel Valero & María Serrano

Acknowledgments

The authors wish to gratefully acknowledge the special collaboration and contributions of the members of the Postharvest Group of Fruits and Vegetables at the University Miguel Hernández, Orihuela, Alicante, Spain. Much appreciation is expressed to our colleagues Dr. Domingo Martínez-Romero, Dr. Salvador Castillo, Dr. Fabián Guillén, and Dr. Pedro J. Zapata. Each of them has offered considerable and valuable information that was employed extensively throughout the preparation of this book. The authors also would like to express appreciation to many graduate and PhD students, visiting scientists, and collaborators for their contributions to our research programs. The financial support by the Spanish Ministry of Science and Technology, Generalitat Valenciana and European Union, are deeply appreciated. Finally, the authors would like to thank David Fausel and Stephen Zollo (CRC/Taylor & Francis) for their support and encouragement in the preparation of the book proposal and manuscript.

About the Authors

The authors have joined efforts and knowledge for the last 15 years, working hand in hand. During this period they have developed together several research actions through national and international projects, and contracts for regional, national, and international companies. This collaborative background led them to coauthor the present book.

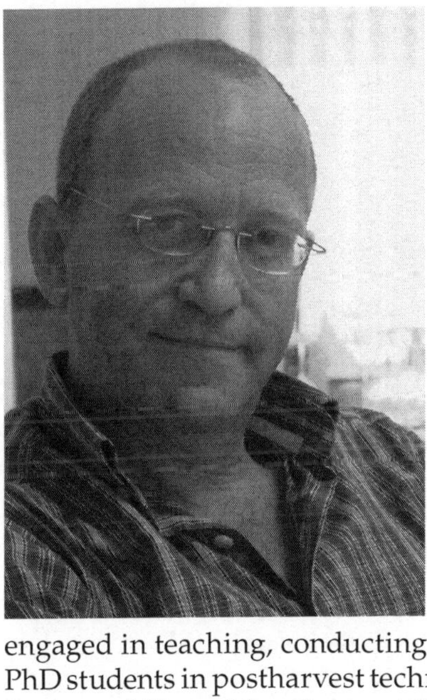

Daniel Valero is currently professor in the Department of Food Technology at the University Miguel Hernández (UMH), Alicante, Spain. Dr. Valero received his BSc in 1997 and MSc with Honor from the Faculty of Pharmacy at the University of Granada, Spain, in 1988. He received a PhD Fellowship at the Centro de Edafología y Biología Aplicada del Segura (CEBAS-CSIC) and graduated with a PhD in plant biology at the University of Granada, Spain, with qualification "Apto cum laude" in 1993. He received a postdoctoral position at the Long Ashton Research Station, University of Bristol, 1994–1995. At his present position at Universidad Miguel Hernández, he is engaged in teaching, conducting research, and supervising graduate and PhD students in postharvest technology. He is the leader of the Postharvest Fruits and Vegetables Group at the UMH. Dr. Valero has a broad research background with more than 70 peer-reviewed papers in the last 20 years as a specialist in the postharvest technology of fruits and vegetables, holding one patent. He is also the author of many chapters in books edited by Spanish and international editors and serves as Reviewer of Research Projects for the Spanish Ministry of Science and Technology, the European Commission (VI Frame work), the International Foundation for

Science (Sweden), Agencia Nacional de Promoción Científica y Tecnológica (Argentina), and Binational Agricultural Research and Development Fund (BARD, USA-Israel). Dr. Valero is reviewer for more than 35 international journals within the areas of food science and technology, agriculture and plant biology of the JCR. He is a member of the editorial board of the following journals: *Postharvest Biology & Technology, Spanish Journal of Agricultural Research* (Associate Editor, Section Postharvest), *Journal of Applied Horticulture*, and *Journal of Food Agriculture & Environment*.

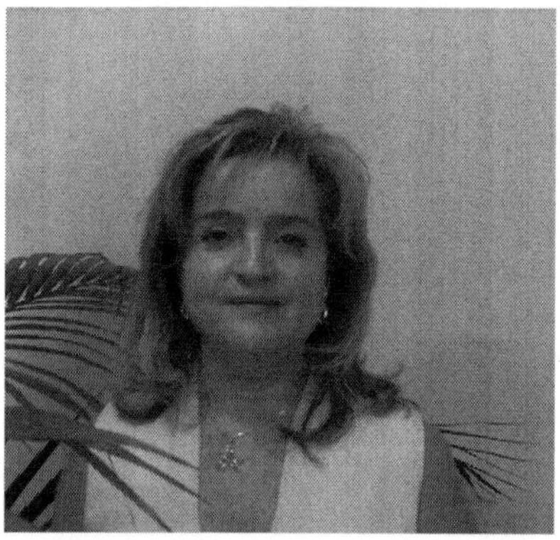

María Serrano is currently a professor in the Department of Applied Biology at the University Miguel Hernández, Alicante, Spain. Dr. Serrano obtained a BSc in 1986 and MSc with Honor in biology at the University of Murcia, Spain, in 1987. She received a PhD Fellowship at the Centro de Edafología y Biología Aplicada del Segura (CEBAS-CSIC) and graduated with a PhD in plant physiology from the University of Murcia, Spain, with qualification "Apto cum laude" in 1990. Dr. Serrano has a wide research background with more than 90 peer-reviewed papers in the last 20 years as a specialist in preharvest and postharvest physiology of fruits, vegetables, and cut flowers. She holds two patents and is the author of many chapters in books edited by Spanish and international editors in this area. In her current position at Universidad Miguel Hernández, she is in charge of teaching plant biology and plant physiology. Dr. Serrano is conducting research and supervising graduate and PhD students in postharvest physiology and technology. She acts as Reviewer of Research Projects for the Spanish Ministry of Science and Technology, and is a reviewer for more than 20 international journals within the areas of food science and technology, agriculture and plant biology of the JCR.

List of Abbreviations

ABN	Arabinase
ACC	1-Aminocyclopropane-1-carboxylic acid
ACO	ACC oxidase
ACS	ACC synthase
ADC	Arginine decarboxylase
AG	Arabinogalactan
AIH	Agmatine iminohydrolase
CA	Controlled atmosphere
CAT	Catalase
CI	Chilling injury
DAO	Diamine oxidases
DCSAM	Decarboxylated S-adenosylmethionine
DFMA	DL-α-difluoromethylarginine
DFMO	DL-α-difluoromethylornithine
EGases	Endo-β-1,4-glucanases
EXPs	Expansins
α-GAL	α-Galactosidase
β-GAL	β-Galactosidase
HGA	Homogalacturonan
HSPs	Heat shock proteins
H-TAA	Hydrophilic total antioxidant activity
IW	Intermittent warming
LDPE	Low density polyethylene
L-TAA	Lipophilic total antioxidant activity
MA	Modified atmosphere
MAP	Modified atmosphere packaging
1-MCP	1-Methylcyclopropene
MGBG	Methylglyoxal-bis-guanylhydrazone
MRL	Minimum residue limit

ODC	Ornithine decarboxylase
PAL	Phenylalanine ammonia lyase
PAs	Polyamines
PAO	Polyamine oxidase
PE	Polyethylene
PG	Polygalacturonase
PL	Pectate lyase
PME	Pectin methylesterase
POX	Peroxidase
PP	Polypropylene
PPO	Polyphenoloxidase
Put	Putrescine
PVC	Polyvinyl chloride
RGase	Rhamnogalacturonase
RGI	Rhamnogalacturonan I
RGII	Rhamnogalacturonan II
RH	Relative humidity
ROS	Reactive oxygen species
RQ	Respiration quotient
SAM	S-Adenosylmethionine
SAMDC	S-Adenosylmethionine decarboxylase
SOD	Superoxide dismutase
Spd	Spermidine
SpdS	Spermidine synthase
Spm	Spermine
SpmS	Spermine synthase
TA	Total acidity
TAA	Total antioxidant activity
TSS	Total soluble solids
UV	Ultraviolet
WPTR	Water vapor transmission rate
XET	Xyloglycan endotransglycosylase
XGA	Xylogalacturonan

chapter one

Introduction and overview

Research into the postharvest behavior of fruits and vegetables has a long history. In the 1930s most of the physiological effects of ethylene on plants had already been described (Pech et al., 1992), and after this period ethylene became the object of numerous studies due to commercial interest related to its action on the ripening and conservation of fruit. After a long time using ethylene in growth and development manipulations, it was presupposed that this gas was an endogenous growth regulator. The ethylene biosynthesis pathway has now been completely elucidated due to advances in molecular biology and signaling receptors (Binder, 2008; Cara and Giovannoni, 2008) based on the Yang cycle (Yang and Hoffman, 1984). The discovery of the ethylene biosynthesis pathway has been a crucial step in the isolation of the two main regulatory enzymes from the precursor S-adenosylmethionine (SAM) to form 1-aminocyclopropane-1-carboxylic acid (ACC) by ACC synthase (ACS) and the conversion of ACC to ethylene by ACC oxidase (ACO) and their encoding genes.

Ripening is regulated by both internal and external stimuli, including temperature, light, plant nutrient status, water availability, and hormones. Many fruits, in particular the so-called climacteric fruits, require ethylene for ripening, resulting in the targeting of this hormone as a means of ripening control. Although nonclimacteric fruits typically produce little ethylene during ripening, many have still been shown to be affected by exogenous ethylene during ripening, making ethylene control a target for shelf-life manipulation even in species whose fruit do not require ethylene to ripen (Giovanonni, 2004). The inheritance of the climacteric character and the discrimination between ethylene-dependent and -independent regulation has been recently reviewed (Pech et al., 2008), and the understanding of ripening processes continues to increase rapidly at the molecular level.

The field of postharvest physiology has traditionally focused on the integrated functional processes that are involved in handling, storage, and marketing of fruit organs that ensures quality in the markets. The field has increasingly diversified to include the area of fresh-cut products. Initially the research was focused on the control of ripening through the plant hormone ethylene and its influence on softening and color development. Currently involvement of nutrition and sensory metabolism in ripening and senescence are subjects of new investigation. Lately the antioxidant potential of fruits has being intensively studied to evaluate their effects on health. The increased understanding of the developmental physiology and biochemistry during growth and ripening of fruits has led to the development of new postharvest technologies to maintain the shelf life and quality of fruits.

The fruit market is very important worldwide, and the quality of organoleptic attributes represents a key role at the consumer level. This quality is related to many attributes, such as sweetness, acidity, aroma, color, and firmness, all of which are associated with specific metabolic pathways that are typically coordinated during the ripening process. The development of these quality attributes depends on many factors, such as cultivar, growing conditions, ripening stage at harvest, and storage environments. During ripening, many changes in fruit composition occur; these include increase in size during development by both cell division and cell expansion, and the synthesis and degradation of pigments, changes in the concentrations of organic acids and sugars, and the accumulation of volatile compounds. In this sense, the importance of preharvest factors that influence the postharvest quality of fresh produce is increasing.

Postharvest management of fruit quality has always been challenged by the paradox that quality can be maximized only when the product is harvested more mature or ripe, whereas shelf and storage life are generally extended if it is harvested less mature or unripe. Much of the efforts of past and current postharvest physiology-based research have focused on finding such a compromise. In many cases, produce is harvested as mature as commercially feasible while ensuring that the fruit is not overripe or senescent, resulting in as much storage and shelf life as is possible (Toivonen, 2007).

Fruits deteriorate rapidly after harvest and in some cases do not reach consumers at optimal quality after transport and marketing. The main causes of fruit deterioration are dehydration, with the subsequent weight loss, color changes, softening, surface pitting, browning, loss of acidity, and microbial spoilage, among others. However, deterioration rate is affected by different factors, such as intrinsic characteristics of the product and storage conditions in terms of temperature, relative humidity, storage atmosphere composition, etc. The main objective of postharvest technology is quality optimization and reduction of losses along the postharvest chain, in which existing technologies are being complemented with revolutionary new ones such as 1-methylcyclopropene (1-MCP) or active packaging, as well as some emerging technologies. Among the classical technologies, low temperature storage, heat treatments, and modification of the stored atmosphere are the most commonly used. There are some interesting technologies at research level but with promising future, such as calcium and polyamine treatments, and some emerging technologies such as biological control, atmospheres with high O_2, and the use of UV light.

Perishable food items, such as fruits, that are exposed to variable temperature conditions during storage will experience high rates of deterioration. Storage at low temperature has been the main postharvest technology to maintain fruit quality. The rate of biochemical reactions is related to temperature, such that lower storage temperatures lead to slower degradation of foods by reduced growth of bacteria and fungi. There may also be limited bactericidal effects at very low temperatures. Typical Q_{10} values for spoilage reactions are approximately 2 for fruits, implying that spoilage rates would double for each 10°C rise, or conversely that shelf life would double for each 10°C reduction. The use of refrigerated storage is limited by the sensitivity of raw materials to low temperatures. The freezing point is a limiting factor for many fruits, as the tissues will become disrupted on thawing. Further, optimum temperature for postharvest storage varies with the product, the cultivar, and the ripening stage at harvest. For most temperate species maximum storage life is achieved at the lowest nonfreezing temperature (–1 to +2°C) and for tropical products it is achieved at 7–14°C, depending upon species. Fruits and vegetables may display physiological problems that limit their storage temperatures, probably as a result of metabolic imbalance leading to a buildup of undesirable chemical species in the tissues and eventually cell death. In addition, low temperature of storage is also limited by cost. Precooling systems to remove field heat is an effective strategy to reduce the period of high initial respiration rate in rapidly respiring produce prior to transportation and storage.

The research effort on postharvest heat treatment has been increasing steadily in recent years, with successful laboratory investigations and some scale-up development of the use of hot water, hot air, or vapor heat in disinfection, chilling injury (CI) control, and retardation of the ripening process in many types of horticultural produce. Several aspects of the mechanism of heat treatment in terms of decay control, induction of thermotolerance, and heat transfer under uniform heating media have been thoroughly evaluated. The threshold temperature and uniformity in space throughout the entire duration of the process are the two most important factors that should be taken into account during heat treatment process development on an industrial scale (Lu et al., 2007).

Calcium is an essential plant nutrient and as a divalent cation (Ca^{2+}) is required for structural roles in the cell wall and membranes of the fruits. In this sense, pre- and postharvest calcium applications have been demonstrated to produce beneficial effects on whole fruit quality, decreasing the incidence of physiological disorders and fungal decay. Infiltration methods under pressure or vacuum provide a rapid and effective postharvest method for increasing calcium content and in turn maintaining cell turgor, membrane integrity, tissue firmness and delaying membrane lipid catabolism, extending storage life of fresh fruits. Most of the studies dealing with Ca^{2+} have examined the effects of this cation on fruit firmness and decay after harvest as the main effect. Calcium salts have also been used to preserve the quality of minimally processed commodities. The ultimate objective of calcium applications, as of any other postharvest treatment, is to enhance consumer acceptance of the commodity and/or to maintain it for as long as possible (Martín-Diana et al., 2007).

Polyamines (PAs) are natural compounds involved in many growth and developmental processes with ubiquitous presence in all cells. Fruits have been the main plant organ about which comprehensive research has been developed to get a better understanding of the role of PAs, both endogenous and exogenous, especially during the ripening and senescence processes (Valero et al., 2002a). The beneficial effects of the exogenous PAs in fruits are numerous, but the commercial application is nowadays limited. PAs, applied at late fruit developmental stages and at several concentrations, resulted in marked inhibition of ethylene production, flesh softening and soluble solids accumulation, retention of titratable acidity, and inhibition of fruit drop (Torrigiani et al., 2008). In studies on PA physiology a frequently adopted approach is the treatment of detached fruit, the results having important scientific implications in clarifying the biochemical and molecular aspects of PA function during fruit development and ripening, and having a practical relevance for the control of postharvest fruit quality. The inhibition of ethylene production by PA treatment after harvest leads to similar effects in terms of delaying the parameters related to ripening (Martínez-Romero et al., 2007a). Additionally, PAs reduce some type of stresses such as CI and mechanical damage. From these postharvest studies, some of the suggested treatments may be suitable for large-scale application.

The recent registration of 1-MCP to inhibit ethylene perception in horticultural products has resulted in an exciting era for postharvest scientists. 1-MCP is being used not only as a tool to increase understanding of the involvement of ethylene in ripening and senescence processes, but also as the basis of a new technology for horticultural industries (Watkins, 2008). 1-MCP is used in most cases as a supplement to proper temperature and relative humidity management, and can replace or be utilized in combination with controlled atmosphere (CA). Potential success of fruit response to 1-MCP treatment depends on six main factors or sets of factors: (1) genotype (species and cultivar) and ripening physiology, (2) preharvest environmental conditions and practices, (3) harvest date (physiological age of fruit), (4) treatment conditions, (5) effect on susceptibility to pathological disorders, and (6) the postharvest environment (Sozzi and Beaudry, 2007).

As fruits and vegetables are still alive after harvesting it is necessary to restrain their respiratory activity and metabolism in order to delay ripening and senescence. Their physiological activity is mainly noticed as a sequence of color, flavor, aroma, and softening changes that happen as a result of the biochemical reactions that take place among their components. An energy contribution is needed to set the reactions that determine normal ripening. This energy is obtained from respiration, which consists of biological oxidation of organic substrates with energy production (Artés et al., 2006) resulting in O_2 consumption and CO_2 production. Conventional cold storage can be optimized by acting on these gases that take part in the respiration. In this sense, the principle of the storage of fruits and vegetables under modified atmosphere packaging (MAP) consists of changes of the quantitative relation of the normal ambient air components by decreasing O_2 or increasing CO_2 in a refrigerated and gastight area with the aid of plastic films with selective permeability to the gases. Advances in MAP of fresh produce are centered on matching appropriate films to specific products. The commercial application of MAP for storage and transport of fresh whole produce has been limited to a few horticultural products for the reason that produce requires a diversity of packaging films.

However, a rapid expansion of MAP has occurred for minimally processed (fresh-cut) fruits and vegetables. The market for fresh-cut fruits and vegetables increased during the 1990s due to consumer demand for fresh, healthy, and convenient products. However, commercial development of fresh-cut fruit and vegetable products is still hampered by the reduced shelf life of minimally processed products. Fresh-cut processing and subsequent packaging generates stress for fruit and vegetable tissues, generally leading to a shorter shelf life for fresh-cut products as compared with intact fruits and vegetables. It results in increased respiration rates and ethylene production depending on the physiological status of the raw product, as well as processing, storage, temperature, and MAP conditions. Mechanical cutting operations remove the natural protection of the epidermis and destroy the internal compartmentation that separates enzymes and substrates, leading to metabolic activation of biochemical reactions, potentially affecting color, flavor, texture, and nutritional quality (Oms-Oliu et al., 2009).

Based on MAP technology, active packaging technologies offer new opportunities for the food industry in the preservation of foods. Current important active packaging systems include oxygen scavengers, carbon dioxide emitters/absorbers, moisture absorbers, ethylene absorbers, ethanol emitters, flavor releasing/absorbing systems, time-temperature indicators, and antimicrobial containing films (Ozdemir and Floros, 2004). *Active packaging* is defined as an intelligent or smart system that involves interactions between package or package components and food or internal gas atmosphere and complies with consumer demands for high quality, freshness, and safety. The creation of innovative technological developments by using an active packaging based on the combination of MAP with natural antimicrobial compounds (essential oils) has been recently reported (Serrano et al., 2008a). This active packaging was effective on the delay of fruit ripening and the extension of shelf life based on safety and the preservation of sensory attributes and bioactive compounds with functional properties.

Emerging technologies, such as the use of biological control and UV light to counteract the postharvest fungal decay, are currently being developed. However, in many cases these tools are less effective than synthetic fungicides, especially in large-scale tests, and these technologies should be combined with existing strategies. Novel high O_2 MAP has the potential to maintain quality and ensure the microbial safety of fresh-cut products.

In summary, fruit consumers are not only looking for traditional quality attributes such as sugar, acidity, firmness, and color, but also value other attributes, including nutrients and bioactive compounds availability, antioxidants, and aroma. Therefore, a major goal for growing fruits should emphasize on a good balance among the quality attributes already mentioned and the use of appropriate postharvest technologies considered to be safe and environmentally friendly.

In the following chapters, the fruit ripening process and all of the postharvest technologies to preserve fruit quality from harvesting to consumers mentioned in this chapter will be treated in detail.

chapter two

Fruit ripening

2.1 Introduction

Fruit is considered as a commercially important and nutritionally essential food commodity due to the provision of nutrients such as sugars, organic acids, vitamins, and minerals, as well as other non-nutrient constituents including dietary fiber and secondary metabolites with health-beneficial effects. From the botanical point of view, fruits are highly diverse ranging from dry seed capsules (both dehiscent and nondehiscent) to relatively large complex fleshy fruits that have developed bright color and complex aromas to attract animals for seed dispersion. In most cases, fruits are formed from a fertilized ovary although other parts of the flower or inflorescence may also contribute to fruit formation, such as receptacle tissues and sepals for strawberry and pineapple, respectively. However, in a few species fruits are set and mature without fertilization and without seed development. Such fruits are called *parthenocarpic* fruits and are known in some fig, pear, apple, peach, cherry, table grape, banana, and citrus species. In some species of fruit trees, such as cherry and peach, the parthenocarpic fruit requires pollination and fertilization and then seedlessness may occur because the embryo aborts before the fruit matures. In other species, pollination stimulates fruit development, but fruits mature without the pollen reaching the ovule, and in the species with the most commercial interest, such as citrus and banana, fruit development may occur without pollination.

Fruit ripening is a highly coordinated, genetically programmed process occurring at the later stages of maturation and involving a series of physiological, biochemical, and sensory changes leading to the development of an edible ripe fruit with desirable quality parameters (Brady, 1987). Maturation refers to the processes that lead to ripening, and in many cases maturation and ripening overlap in time (Giovannoni, 2001). Specific biochemical and physiological changes vary among species although generally include altered sugar metabolism, softening, color changes, synthesis of aroma volatiles, and increased susceptibility to pathogen infection, suggesting that the underlying genetic mechanisms that regulate fruit ripening are well conserved between fruits of different species (Adams-Philips et al., 2004; Giovannoni, 2004).

From the physiology point of view two major classifications of fruit ripening have been classically accepted: climacteric and nonclimacteric. In this sense, climacteric fruits are characterized by their increased respiration and ethylene biosynthesis rates during ripening, while in nonclimacteric fruits a gradual decrease in both respiration rate and ethylene production occurs (Barry and Giovannoni, 2007). This physiological behavior of the fruits has a great importance in the postharvest biology and technology of these commodities (Martínez-Romero et al., 2007a). Table 2.1 shows some examples of both types of fruit that are mostly used in ripening and postharvest studies.

In this chapter, a detailed study about the physiological and biochemical changes related to physical, chemical, nutritive, and functional properties during fruit ripening on plants is provided, taking into account fresh fruit with both climacteric and nonclimacteric pattern.

2.2 Fruit growth

The time required for fruit growth, anthesis to ripening, varies widely among species and genotypes, ranging from 3 weeks in strawberry to 60 weeks in Valencia orange, but in fruits of many species this interval is about 15 weeks. However, it should be taken into account that fruit growth rate varies greatly among seasons, environmental conditions, cultural practices, and even different fruit in the same crop.

Fruit growth involves various degrees of cell division and cell expansion. During fruit set, when a flower has been successfully pollinated (and exceptionality in parthenocarpic fruits), the fruit becomes an active

Table 2.1 Some Examples of Fruit Having a Climacteric or Nonclimacteric Ripening Pattern

Climacteric fruit	Nonclimacteric fruit
Tomato	Pomegranate
Peach	Grape
Nectarine	Pepper
Plum	Blackberry
Apricot	Sweet cherry
Apple	Strawberry
Pear	Orange
Banana	Lemon
Watermelon	Cucumber
Kiwifruit	Cranberry
Mango	Loquat
Cherimoya	Blueberry

carbohydrate sink, and many of its tissues become meristematic. In some fruits, such as currants and blackberries, cell division is completed by the time of pollination, although in most of them cell division occurs for a short time after pollination and in still others, such as avocado, cell division continues throughout the life of the fruit. Thus, in most species, increase in cell size makes the greatest contribution to total fruit expansion. For example, in grape, the increase in cell number accounts for a doubling of fruit size, whereas the increase in cell volume accounts for a 300-fold size increase (Monselise, 1986).

Fruit growth on plants can be followed by physical measurements such as weight, length, width, and volume. The evolution of these parameters shows a simple or double-sigmoid curve depending of fruit type. In general, the double sigmoid type is characteristic of stone fruits such as cherry, peach, apricot, plum, and olive, as well as of some nonstone fruits such as grape and currant. In this double-sigmoid growth curve, four distinct stages (S1–S4) could be established, as can be seen in Figure 2.1 for Angeleno plum. S1 is the first exponential growth phase and is characterized by cell division and elongation. S2 shows little or null fruit growth but the endocarp hardens to form a solid stone. S3 is the second exponential growth phase due to cell enlargement, while in S4 the fruit growth rate decreases and fruit ripening occurs. In contrast, fruits containing a large number of seeds (such as apple, pear, orange, pepper, banana, avocado, strawberry, mango, and lemon) show a single-sigmoid growth

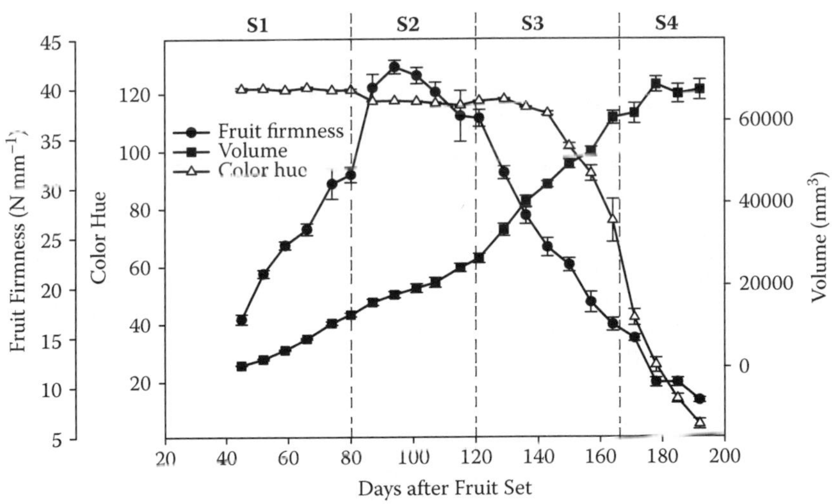

Figure 2.1 Evolution of fruit volume, firmness, and skin color (expressed as Hue angle) during Angeleno plum development on tree. S1–S4 represent the four phases of the double-sigmoid growth of this stone fruit.

curve, with a first phase of cell division and slow growth followed by a second phase of fast growth due to cell expansion and finally a third phase with reduced growth until reaching the maximum fruit size, which is displayed in Figure 2.2 for pepper fruit.

2.3 *Fruit ripening and related parameters*

Defining fruit ripening to satisfy everyone is very difficult. Consumers of fruit are interested in such aspects of ripening as taste, color, texture, aroma, and nutritional values of fruits. From this point of view ripening has been defined as the composite of processes leading to changes in color, texture, flavor, aroma, sugars, organic acids, and other nutritive components that occur from the last stages of growth through the earliest stages of senescence, rendering a fruit attractive for consumption (Tucker and Grierson, 1987). The time of ripening varies with the developmental stage of fruits. In fruits with a single-sigmoid pattern of growth, ripening usually occurs during the final phase of slow growth. As displayed in Figure 2.2 for pepper, the change in color from green (negative values of color a* parameter) to red (positive values) occurs with the beginning of phase S3. However, in fruits with a double-sigmoid growth curve, ripening begins during phase S3, along with the second phase of fast growth. Figure 2.1 shows that Hue angle in Angeleno plum starts to decrease at this phase indicating the change of skin color from green to the characteristic red-purple of this plum cultivar.

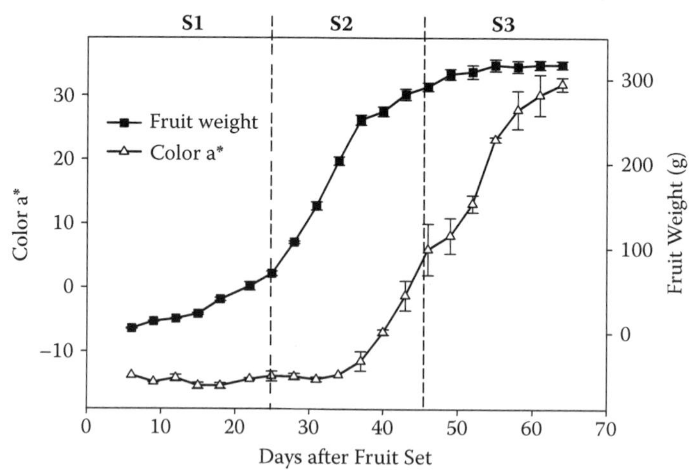

Figure 2.2 Evolution of fruit weight and color a* parameter during pepper fruit growth and ripening on plant. S1–S3 represent the three phases of the single-sigmoid growth curve of this seeded fruit.

Ripening could be also defined as a physiological process that is genetically programmed and comprises several physical, chemical, and biochemical changes that renders fruit attractive and palatable (Lelièvre et al., 1997; Giovannoni, 2001). The main changes associated with ripening include color (loss of green color and development of yellow, orange, red, and other color characteristics depending on species and cultivar), firmness (softening by cell-wall degrading activities), taste (increase in sugars and decline in organic acids), and flavor (production of volatile compounds providing the characteristic aroma).

2.3.1 Color changes

The color changes are due to loss of chlorophyll, and concomitant synthesis of the characteristic pigment for each fruit, that is anthocyanins or carotenoids. Anthocyanins are hydro-soluble pigments located in the vacuole that are responsible for the blue, red, and purple color of the fruits and classified as flavonoids with glycosilated derivatives of the 3,5,7,3′-tetrahydroxyflavylium cation (Figure 2.3). The free aglycones (anthocyanidins) are highly reactive with sugars to form the glycosides,

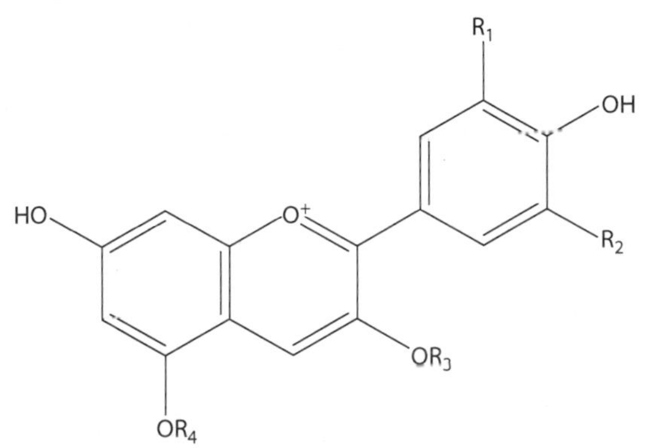

R_1	R_2	Aglycone	Abbreviation	Color
H	H	Pelargonidin	Pg	Orange
OH	H	Cyanidin	Cy	Orange-Red
OMe	H	Peonidin	Pn	Orange-Red
OH	OH	Delphinidin	Dp	Bluish-Red
OMe	OH	Petunidin	Pt	Bluish-Red
OMe	OMe	Malvidin	Mv	Purple

R_3 or R_4 could be H or sugar

Figure 2.3 General structure of anthocyanidin (tetrahydroxiflavylium cation) and the different substituent for R_1 and R_2 to form the free aglycones, which are later glycosilated to form anthocyanins.

and all anthocyanins are *O*-glycosilated. The main aglycones found in fruits are pelargonidin, cyanidin, peonidin, delphinidin, petunidin, and malvidin, while the most relevant sugars are D-glucose, L-rhamnose, D-galactose, D-xylose, and arabinose (Francis, 1989; Welch et al., 2008). Figure 2.4 shows the anthocyanin synthesis pathway from cyanidin-3-glucoside. In general, anthocyanin concentration increases during ripening in a range of pink-, red-, and purple-colored fruits, both climacteric and nonclimacteric ones, although great variations exists in the total anthocyanin content at commercial harvest among fruit species and cultivars as well as in the predominant anthocyanin (Table 2.2). Thus, strawberry has comparatively low total anthocyanin concentration, ranging from 20 to 60 mg 100 g^{-1}, depending on cultivar, the major anthocyanin

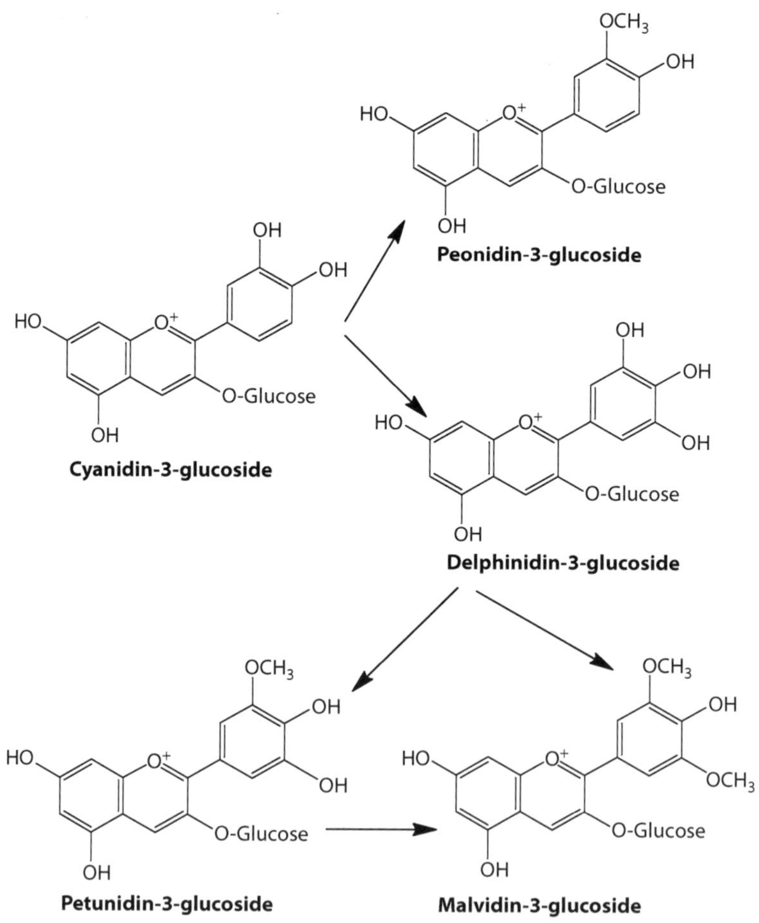

Figure 2.4 Anthocyanin biosynthesis pathway from cyanidin-3-glucoside.

Table 2.2 Major Anthocyanins in Some Fruits and Range of Total Anthocyanin Concentration by Fruit Type Depending on Cultivar, Cultural Practices, and Analytical Method

Major anthocyanin	Fruit	Total anthocyanin (mg 100 g^{-1})	Reference
Pelargonidin 3-glucoside	Strawberry	20–60	Lopes-da-Silva et al., 2002.
	Sarsaparilla		Longo and Vasapollo, 2006.
Cyanidin 3-rutinoside Cyanidin 3-glucoside	Sweet cherry	2–300	Gao and Mazza, 1995; Mozetiĉ et al., 2002; Chaovanalikit and Wrolstad, 2004; Serrano et al., 2009.
Cyanidin 3-glucoside	Plum	100–800 in skin 2–100 in flesh	Tomas-Barberán et al., 2001; Cevallos-Casals et al., 2006; Vizzotto et al., 2007; Díaz-Mula et al., 2008.
	Blackberry	70–200	Fan-Chiang and Wrolstad, 2005.
	Pomegranate	80–160	Martí et al., 2001; Mirdehghan et al., 2007c.
Peonidin 3-glucoside, Cyanidin 3-glucoside Malvidin 3-glucoside	Grapes	6–200 in juice with skin and flesh together	Carreño et al., 1997; Fernández-López et al., 1998; Cantos et al., 2002; González-Neves et al., 2004; Orak, 2007.
Malvidin 3-glucoside	Blueberry	100–300	Connor et al., 2002; Wang et al., 2008.

being pelargonidin 3-glucoside (Lopes da Silva et al., 2007). In blackberry higher concentration has been reported, from 70 to 200 mg 100 g^{-1}, depending on cultivar, in which cyanidin 3-glucoside contributed more than 70% (Fan-Chiang and Wrolstad, 2005). However, the greatest variation among cultivars has been found on sweet cherry, with variations between 2 and 300 mg 100 g^{-1}, from light-colored to dark cherry cultivars, in all of them the major being cyanidin 3-rutinoside and cyanidin 3-glucoside (Gao and Mazza, 1995; Mozetiĉ et al., 2002; Chaovanalikit and Wrolstad, 2004; Serrano et al., 2009). Great variations have also been found among table grape cultivars (6–200 mg 100 g^{-1}), and even the major anthocyanin (cyanidin 3-glucoside, peonidin 3-glucoside, or malvidin 3-glucoside) was different depending on cultivar (Carreño et al., 1997; Orak, 2007). For red-purple plum cultivars total anthocyanin concentration is higher in the skin (100–800 mg 100 g^{-1}) than in the flesh (2–100 mg 100 g^{-1}), and in both tissues cyanidin 3-glucoside has been reported as the major anthocyanin (Tomás-Barberán et al., 2001; Vizzotto et al., 2007; Díaz-Mula et al., 2008). Anthocyanins are also present in peaches at total concentration ranging from 1.5 to 260 mg 100 g^{-1} from white- to red-skin genotypes (Vizzotto et al., 2007). However, these anthocyanin levels could be considered as illustrative, since environmental conditions and cultural practices have a great effect in the anthocyanin content for a particular fruit. For instance, the total anthocyanin content of Cabernet Suavignon was determined as 108 and 194 mg 100 g^{-1} in consecutive years, 2001–2002 (González-Neves et al., 2004).

However, carotenoids are the most widespread group of pigments in nature and are present in all photosynthetic organisms and are responsible for most yellow to red color of fruits and flowers. In fruits, carotenoids are C_{40} tetraterpenoids formed from eight C5 isoprenoid units joined head to tail resulting in a symmetrical molecule located in the chromoplasts. The hydrocarbon carotenoids are known as carotenes (ß-carotene, lycopene, etc.) while xanthophylls are oxygenated derivatives containing at least one hydroxyl group and then being more polar than carotenes. However, carotenoids can be acyclic (e.g., lycopene), monocyclic (γ-carotene), or dicyclic (α- and ß-carotene). Figure 2.5 shows chemical structures of the main carotenoids found in fruits, which exist generally under the all-*trans* form (the most stable) although occurrence at much lower concentrations has been also found of *cis* isomers (Rodriguez-Amaya and Kimura, 2004). Fruit and vegetables vary qualitatively and quantitatively in their carotenoid composition, with green vegetables having a defined qualitative pattern, with lutein, ß-carotene, violaxanthin, and neoxanthin being the main carotenoids, while fruits exhibit a carotenoid composition much more complex and variable. Table 2.3 shows the predominant carotenoid in a range of fruits, both climacteric and nonclimacteric ones.

During fruit ripening, large variations have been found not only in the pigment profile but also in the concentration, with a general increase in the ripening process for all fruits and higher contents in the skin than in the flesh. However, important differences in the pigment concentration at commercial ripening stage have been found among species and cultivars, and are also affected by several factors such as environmental conditions and cultural practices.

For carotenoids, the reported levels (mg 100 g^{-1}) are in the range of 0.1–4 for apricot (Kurz et al., 2008), 2–7 for tomato (Kaur et al., 2006), 0.02–5 for *Citrus* sp. (Fanciullino et al., 2008), 1.5–3 for papaya (De Souza et al.,

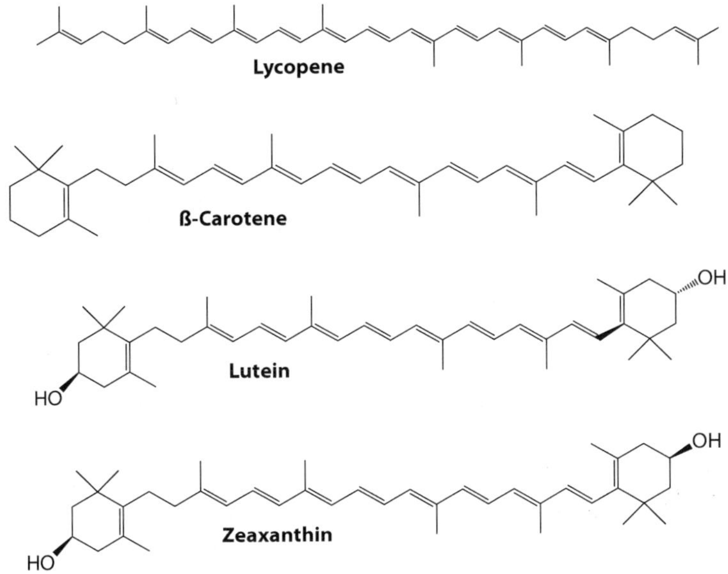

Figure 2.5 Chemical structures of the main carotenoids found in fruits.

Table 2.3 Major Carotenoids in Fruits

Major carotenoid	Fruit	Reference
Capsanthin	Red pepper	Marín et al., 2004; Topuz and Ozdemir, 2007.
Lycopene	Tomato	Raffo et al., 2006.
	Watermelon	Perkins-Veazie et al., 2001.
	Papaya	De Souza et al., 2008.
	Guava	Mercadente et al., 1999.
	Deep Red and Star Ruby pummelo	Fanciullino et al., 2008.
ß-carotene	Peach, nectarine, plum	Gil et al., 2002; Dias et al., 2009.
	Loquat	Zhou et al., 2007.
	Apricot	Kurz et al., 2008.
	Mexican lime and citron	Fanciullino et al., 2008.
ß-cryptoxanthin	Mandarin, lemon, and Rangpur lime	Fanciullino et al., 2008.
Violaxanthin	Chandler pummelo and orange	Fanciullino et al., 2008.

2008), 0.1–2 for loquat (Zhou et al., 2007), 0.2–20 for pepper (Topuz and Ozdemir, 2007), and 3–7 for watermelon (Perkins-Veazie et al., 2001).

2.3.2 Sugar and organic acids

Cell division in fleshy fruits occurs in the very early stage of fruit development but this plant organ enlarges enormously due to cell expansion. Since most of the cell volume in fruits is occupied by a large central vacuole, fruit growth and cell expansion depend on enlargement of vacuoles. The vacuole is the most important organelle for fruit quality because the compounds responsible for the taste and flavor (sugars and organic acids) are all within the vacuole at high concentrations (Shiratake and Martinola, 2007). Thus, the levels of sugars and organic acids are important factors in determining the taste of ripe fleshy fruit, and the relative content of these constituents depends on the activity and the interaction of sugar and acid metabolism (Rhodes, 1980). Sugar accumulation during fruit growth and ripening is mainly a matter of carbon import in the form of sucrose (and sorbitol in Rosaceae species) from photosynthetic leaves, leading to increase in total soluble solids (TSS). Thus, TSS increased from 40 and 80 days after fruit set in Sonata sweet cherry and Golden Japan plum, reaching values close to 18 and 11°Brix, respectively, at the end of the ripening process (Figure 2.6). However, important

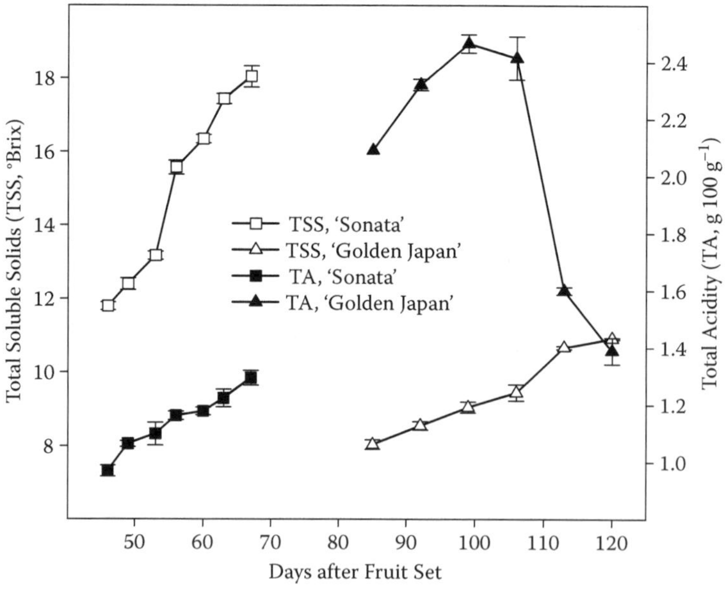

Figure 2.6 Total soluble solids (TSS) and total acidity (TA) evolution in Golden Japan plum and Sonata sweet cherry during growth and ripening on tree.

differences in sugar content at commercial harvest exist among species and cultivars. For example, in plum cultivars sugar content ranges from 11 to 16% (Crisosto et al., 2007; Díaz-Mula et al., 2008), in tomato cultivars from 4 to 7.5% (Guillén et al., 2006; Zapata et al., 2008), and in sweet cherry cultivars from 13 to 20% (Usenik et al., 2008; Serrano et al., 2009). The translocated assimilates enter in the metabolism to form fructose, glucose, and sucrose, which accumulate in the growing fruit as occurs in sweet cherry and plum. However, other fruits, such as mango, kiwifruit, and banana, among others, use the translocated sugars to form starch, the main reserve carbohydrate, which is hydrolyzed into sugars during ripening (Berüter, 2004). In addition, the hydrolysis of sucrose into fructose and glucose is also intensified during fruit ripening and the main sugar at fruit ripening stage depends on plant species as shown in Table 2.4. Thus, glucose is the major sugar in table grape, while fructose is the predominant sugar in berries, mango, and citrus species. Those fruits that accumulate fructose or glucose show very low concentrations of sucrose. However, apricot, plum, nectarine, and peach have sucrose as the main sugar, which is accumulated during stage S3 as a result of a rise in the activity of sucrose synthase [EC 2.4.1.13] (Morandi et al., 2008). Interestingly, wild type tomatoes have sucrose as the main sugar while domesticated fruits accumulate fructose followed by glucose (Kortstee et al., 2007; Zapata et al., 2008). The proportions of fructose, glucose, and sucrose are important in the perception of taste since fructose is 80%

Table 2.4 Major Sugar and Organic Acid in Some Fruits

Fruit	Sugar	Organic acid	Reference
Table grape	Glucose	Tartaric acid	Valero et al., 2006.
Strawberry, blueberry, date plum persimmon, mango, tomato (domesticated), *Citrus* spp. (lime, orange, lemon)	Fructose	Citric acid	Glew et al., 2005; Albertini et al., 2006. Kafkas et al., 2007; Wang et al., 2008; Zapata et al., 2008; Thanaraj et al., 2009.
Apricot, plum, nectarine, peach, loquat	Sucrose	Malic acid	Amorós et al., 2003; Aubert et al., 2003; Cascales et al., 2005; Aubert and Chanforan, 2007; García-Mariño et al., 2008; Morandi et al., 2008.
Tomato (wildtype)	Sucrose	Citric acid	Kortstee et al., 2007.
Pomegranate, sweet cherry	Fructose	Malic acid	Mirdehgham et al., 2006; Serrano et al., 2005a.

sweeter than sucrose, while glucose is only 60% sweeter than sucrose (Yamaguchi et al., 1970).

Developing fruits are extremely acidic due to accumulation of many organic acids, although mature fruits do not taste acidic because of the large amounts of accumulated sugars and the decrease of total acidity (TA) that usually occur during ripening. Nevertheless, as in sugar concentration, important differences are observed among fruit species and cultivars in total acidity at harvest: from 0.4 to 1.7% in tomato cultivars (Guillén et al., 2006; Zapata et al., 2008), from 1.0 to 1.5% in sweet cherry cultivars (Usenik et al., 2008; Serrano et al., 2009), and from 0.7 to 1.6% in plums (Crisosto et al., 2007; Díaz-Mula et al., 2008). Another factor determining fruit acidity is the type of organic acids, the most important being malic, citric, tartaric, quinic, oxalic, fumaric, and succinic acid, each of which has a unique taste that contributes to the overall flavor of fruits. In Table 2.4, some examples of the principal organic acid in fruit species are given. Malic acid is the main organic acid of fruits belonging to the Rosaceae family for both *Prunus* (plum, apricot, peach, nectarine, sweet cherry) and *Malus* (apple, pear) genera. For these fruits, TA is very high at the beginning of development with accumulation of malic acid during the first rapid growth phase, which takes place at the end of the cell division phase, but diminishes over the maturation and ripening processes, with the exception of sweet cherry, for which a continuous increase in acidity occurs during on-tree ripening (Serrano et al., 2005a; Díaz-Mula et al., 2009a). This different behavior between plum and sweet cherry on TA evolution can be observed in Figure 2.6, which shows a continuous increase of TA through the ripening process on the tree of Sonata sweet cherry and a decrease of TA in the Golden Japan plum in the last days before harvesting. The decline in TA in plum cultivars appears to be related to the dilution process caused by the intense water uptake that occurs during the second fast growth phase (García-Mariño et al., 2008). The enzymes involved in malic acid synthesis are phospho*enol*pyruvate carboxylase [EC 4.1.1.31] and NAD-malate dehydrogenase [EC 1.1.1.37], while NADP-malic enzyme [EC 1.1.1.37] is responsible for malic acid degradation, and all of these enzymes are located at the cytosol (Etienne et al., 2002). On the contrary, citric acid is the characteristic organic acid of *Citrus* sp. (orange, lemon, mandarin, lime, and grapefruit), which accounts for 50–80% of the total organic acids, although other fruits such as tomato, mango, and small berries also have this organic acid as predominant. During maturation of citrus fruits, citric acid generally decreases with the exception of lemon, which remains constant. *Citrus* sp. shows a single-sigmoid growth pattern (Monselise, 1986) and citric acid accumulates during the second stage of development. The enzymes responsible for citric acid synthesis are citrate synthase [EC 4.1.3.7] and aconitase [EC 4.2.1.3], which are located at the mitochondria, while the cytosolic aconitase and

NADP-isocitrate dehydrogenase [EC 1.1.1.42] are involved in citric acid catabolism (Etienne et al., 2002). Tartaric is the predominant organic acid in grapes and its diminution has been a useful parameter for checking the maturation process of this fruit (Mato et al., 2005).

For practical purposes and as an index of fruit ripening, the ratio between soluble solids and acidity (TSS/TA) is used rather than the soluble sugars content alone since it is related to the overall consumer appreciation. The proportions of individual acids are also important, since citric acid masks the perception of sucrose and fructose, while malic acid enhances sucrose perception (Lobit et al., 2003).

2.3.3 *Fruit softening*

The metabolic events responsible for the textural changes leading to fruit softening during maturation and ripening involve loss in turgor pressure (due to an accumulation of osmotic solutes in the apoplast), degradation, and other physiological changes in the composition of membranes, modifications in the symplast/apoplast relations, degradation of starch, and modifications in the cell wall structure and dynamics. The relative contribution of each event in fruit softening is not clear, and probably depends on the species, although changes in cell wall composition, especially cell wall mechanical strength and cell-to-cell adhesion, have been considered to be the most important factors (Lasbrook, 2005; Brummell, 2006; Goulao and Oliveira, 2008). Fruits can be divided into two categories according to their softening behavior: those that soften greatly to a melting texture due to swelling of the cell as they ripen (e.g., tomato, peach, strawberry, and kiwifruit), and those that soften moderately, without cell swelling, and are characterized by a crisp fracturable texture (apple or cranberry). In addition, the time of softening is different in each fruit, since softening may start after finishing fruit growth (e.g., in pome fruits) or before the fruits stop growing (e.g., avocado and strawberry). Therefore, considering the wide range of fruit types, softening may proceed via different mechanisms among fruit species and even among cultivars that belong to the same species. Nevertheless, changes in the structure of the cell wall by dissolution of the middle lamella and disruption of the primary cell wall, which will be discussed in the next section, are considered to be common to all fresh fruit species.

2.3.3.1 *Cell wall composition and structure*

Flesh of fresh fruit is composed mainly by parenchymatic cells that have a thin primary cell wall composed by cellulose microfibrils embedded in a matrix of glycan polysaccharides (formerly known as *hemicelluloses*), pectic substances, enzymatic and structural proteins, mineral ions, and some phenolics. The external rind of the primary cell wall is known as the *middle lamella* and is common to two adjacent cells and provides intercellular connections, in which the major components are pectins accompanied by proteins and the absence of cellulose microfibrils (Rose and Bennett, 1999; Carpita and McCann, 2000; Jarvis et al., 2003).

Cellulose is a chain containing 3000–5000 D-glucose residues linked via β-(1→4) linkages and 50–60 of them are grouped in long parallel arrays (associated by extensive hydrogen bonding) called *microfibrils,* which are oriented in the cell wall more or less at random. Cellulose microfibrils are rigid, insoluble, and crystalline, except in the ends where the β-(1→4) glucan chains are less ordered. Among the matrix glycans the most abundant is xyloglucan, which is a polymer of 1,4-β-D-glucose (like cellulose) but has numerous regularly spaced xylose side chains, some extended with either galactose-fructose or with arabinose, which modify the physical properties of the polymer. The two other more abundant matrix glycans are glucoarabinoxylan, a 1,4 β-D-xylan backbone with occasional single α-D-glucuronic acid and α-L-arabinose side chains, and glucomannan, which is composed of alternating regions of 1,4-β-D-glucan and 1,4-β-D-mannan, with a single galactose side chain.

Pectins are linear or branched polymers that have a high content of galacturonic acid and that may contain as many as 17 different monosaccharides. Four main types of pectins have been structurally characterized—homogalacturonan, rhamnogalacturonan I, rhamnogalacturonan II, and xylogalacturonan—which differ in both the structure of the macromolecule backbone and the presence and diversity of side chains. Homogalacturonan (HGA) is a linear homopolymer composed of long chains of (1→4)α-D-galacturonic acid highly methyl-esterified at C-6 and carrying acetyl groups on O-2 and O-3 in the primary cell wall. HGA is the main component of the middle lamella in which the level of methyl-esterification is lower than in the primary cell wall. Xylogalacturonan (XGA) is a homogalacturonan with (1,3)-β-xylopiranoside side chains, which like HGA can be methyl-esterified. Rhamnogalacturonan I (RGI) is made of alternating α-D-(1,2)rhamnose and α-D-(1,4)galacturonic acid with long side chains attached to the rhamnose residues of either unbranched (1→4)-β-D-galactan or branched (1→5)-α-L-arabinans or arabinogalactans. RGI is the major component of the primary cell wall and middle lamella of dicotyledonous plant and the primary reason for the chemical and structural diversity of pectins. Finally, the fourth type is Rhamnogalacturonan II (RGII), which is made of a backbone of (1→4) α-D-galacturonic acid (like HGA) but with complex side chains of several types of neutral sugars. RGII is invariably present as a minor component of the cell wall and is absent in the middle lamella. These three pectins have the same backbone as homogalacturonan and are referred to as *galacturonans.*

Some neutral polysaccharides, such as galactans, arabinans, and arabinogalactans, are also grouped under pectins, mainly because of their association with acidic pectins as side chains of the main galacturonan backbone, although they may also be present as free polymers. Galactans are linear chains of β(1→4) linked D-galactose residues. Arabinans are polymers of α(1→5) linked L-arabinose residues with single arabinose side chains. Arabinogalactans (AG) are heteropolymers of D-galactose and L-arabinose and two different forms are found: AGI, which is a simple polysaccharide, composed of chains of β-(1→4) D-galactose with simple L-arabinose residues; and AGII, which is a complex and branched polysaccharide that consists of β(1→3)D-galactose backbone and contains short side chains of arabinose and galactose residues, the latter of which are in turn linked to terminal L-arabinose residues. AGII is mainly associated with proteins as arabinogalactan proteins. Finally, the major structural proteins in the cell wall are glycoproteins with high content in hydroxyproline (extensions), proline or glycine, and arabinogalactan proteins. The phenolic components are principally ferulic acid and *p*-cumaric acid, which are found esterified to arabinose and galactose moieties of pectic polysaccharides.

Numerous types of bonds, both ionic and covalent, interlink the various components of the primary cell wall, and four main models have been proposed to explain the arrangement and bond interlinks of the cell wall components (reviewed by Carpita and Gibeaut, 1993; Rose and Bennett, 1999; Cosgrove, 2001; Vincken et al., 2003; Brummell, 2006). However, little information on the detailed structure of particular fruit cell walls is available, although the basic structure is probably as follows: a framework of cellulose microfibrils (which suppose 25% of the cell wall components) and matrix glycans (20% of the cell wall components), the more abundant being xyloglucan; this cellulose/matrix glycan network is imbibed in a matrix of interconnected highly hydrated pectins, which represent more than 40–50% of the cell wall. Xyloglucan are attached to the cellulose by hydrogen bonds, pairs of RGII are connected together through borate diesters, homogalacturonan molecules are attached to each other through ionic calcium bridges between carboxyl groups of two galacturonic acid residues, and ester bonds probably attach pectin molecules to other pectin, glycan, or phenolic molecules. In addition, there may be covalent links between structural proteins and between structural proteins and phenolics. There are also covalent linkages between xyloglucan and the arabinan/galactan side chains of RGI and between RGI and the structural protein extensins. Moreover, xyloglucans are interwoven into the outside layers of cellulose microfibrils and RGI side chains may go around the microfibrils, anchoring pectin and cellulose together and thus potentially interlocking the pectin network with the glycan-cellulose network within primary cell wall and between primary cell wall and middle lamella, contributing to cell-to-cell adhesion (Brummell and Harpster, 2001; Vincken et al., 2003; Brummell, 2006).

2.3.3.2 Cell wall changes during fruit softening

When examined by electron microscopy, the first change observed in a ripening fruit is dissolution of the middle lamella, leading to diminution of intercellular adhesion, followed by disruption of the ordered structure of the primary cell wall and certainly fruit cell wall becomes noticeably thinner during ripening. However, cell wall component disassembly and hydrolysis varies considerably among species and cultivars. In general, it is considered that pectin degrading enzymes are mostly implicated in fruit softening, although other enzymes acting on the glycan polysaccharides and cellulose microfibrils also contribute to the softening process as will be addressed later in this chapter (Brownleader et al., 1999; Rose and Bennett, 1999; Brummell and Harpster, 2001; Lasbrook, 2005; Brummell, 2006; Prasanna et al., 2007; Goulao and Oliveira, 2008).

Enzymes that act on pectins are mainly polygalacturonase [EC 3.2.1.15, PG], pectin methylesterase [EC 3.1.1.11, PME], β-galactosidase [EC 3.2.1.23, β-GAL], and pectate lyase [EC 4.2.2.2, PL], all of them existing in multigene families, with a subset of one or more gene family members regulating the cell wall modification processes associated to fruit ripening.

PME de-esterifies polyuronides by removing methyl groups from the C6 position of galacturonic acid residues of high-molecular-weight pectins, releasing methanol and protons and leading to changes in pH and charge in the cell wall, since negative carboxyl groups are created. This allows the aggregation of polyuronides into a calcium-linked gel structure and makes the polyuronides susceptible to degradation by PG. PME action begins in the middle lamella and spreads throughout the cell wall during ripening, which may be a prerequisite for PG activity during fruit ripening. PGs catalyze the hydrolytic cleavage of α-(1→4) galacturonide linkages and can be exo- or endo-acting types. The exo-PG removes single galacturonic acid units from the nonreducing end of polygalacturonic acid, whereas the endo-PG cleaves such polymers at random. Both exo- and endo-PG types are found in fruit, although the fruit ripening specific enzyme usually referred as PG is of the endo-acting type. The substrates for PG are HGAs, RGI, and RGII, PG being the primary contributor to pectin depolymerization and leads to loss of the cell wall structure. In addition, it is generally accepted that PG is primarily responsible for dissolution of the middle lamella during fruit ripening, although PG-independent solubilization also exists. However, HGAs are secreted to the cell wall in a high methyl-esterified form and must be de-esterified before they can become a substrate for PG.

PL also preferentially acts on de-esterified homogalacturonic acid by cleaving the α-1,4-linkages between the galacturonic acid residues of HGAs. Exo-PL acts from the nonreducing end, whereas endo-PL acts randomly on de-esterified galacturonans. Endo-PG, PL, or both are detected in most ripening fruit, and their activities lead to degradation of HGA, the main component of the middle lamella, and in turn to reduction of intercellular adhesion and firmness. β-GAL cleaves the galactan or AG side chains of RGI by hydrolyzing terminal β–D-galactosyl residues, acting as an exo-enzyme. This enzyme also acts on short chain oligomers of galactose units present as glycoproteins or glycolipid and the terminal galactosyl residues of xyloglucan side chains. Then, β-GAL causes a decrease in polymeric galactose and an increase in free galactose. α-Galactosidase [EC 3.2.1.22, α-GAL] could act on α-galacturosidic linkages of RGII, although the levels of this type of linkage are low in these structural polysaccharides.

Rhamnogalacturonase [EC 3.2.1, RGase] is an enzyme that catalyzes the hydrolysis of glycosidic bonds between galacturonic acid and rhamnose units in RG backbone, enhancing its activity when the ester group has been de-esterified and the side chains removed. Arabinases [EC 3.2.1.99, ABN] are found of two types: endo-arabinase, which hydrolyzes linear arabinan side chains of RGI and RGII in a random fashion producing oligomers of shorter lengths; and arabino furanosidase, which degrades branched arabinans to a linear chain by splitting of terminal α-1,3-linked arabinofuranosyl side chains, its substrates being arabinans, arabinogalactans, and arabinoxylans. Finally, it has been also proposed that ascorbate, copper ion, and H_2O_2, naturally produced in the cell wall, generate hydroxyl residues that can cause nonenzymatic scission of polysaccharides contributing to solubilization of fruit pectin.

Structural modifications in hemicellulose-cellulose domains are due to xyloglycan endotransglycosylase [EC 2.4.1.207] (namely, XTH, XET, or EXGT), endo-β-1,4-glucanases [EC 3.2.1.152, EGases], β-D-xylosidase [EC 3.2.1.37], endo-β-mannan transglycosylases [EC 3.2.1.25, manase), and expansins. XETs cleave internal 1,4 linkages within the β-D-glucan backbone of xyloglucans and transfer the newly formed potentially reducing end to the C-4 position of the glucose unit at the nonreducing end of another xyloglucan polymer or oligosaccharide. XETs are encoded by large gene families. High levels of XET present in young fruits are involved in cell expansion and fruit growth, but the role of XET activity in fruit softening remains unclear. However, in kiwifruit XET activity from ripening fruits possesses hydrolase activity and could contribute to xyloglucan depolimerization occurring during softening. EGases (also referred to as *cellulases*) hydrolyze internal linkages of (1→4) β-D-glucan chains adjacent to unsubstituted residues of xyloglucan, integral and peripheral regions of noncrystalline cellulose and possibly glucomanan, where sufficient consecutive (1→4) β-D-linked glucan residues occur for substrate binding, resulting in loosening of the cellulose-xyloglucan network. EGases are also encoded by multigene families and have been found in all species examined, although their activities vary considerably among them. For example, avocado has 160 times more EGase activity than peach and 770 more than tomato on a fresh weight basis.

Mannase catalyzes the hydrolysis of mannan polymers and expansins act by causing a reversible disruption of hydrogen bonding between cellulose microfibrils and matrix polysaccharides, particularly xyloglucan, resulting in a disassembling of the hemicellulose network and increasing the accessibility of other cell wall degrading enzymes to their substrates. They are also encoded by large gene families, and different types are involved in cell growth or softening, the accumulation of ripening-related expansins being a common feature of fruit ripening.

It is probable that fruit of all species have the same range of enzymatic activities, all of them acting together in a cooperative interdependent way to achieve controlled changes in softening. However, it must be remembered that important differences have been reported among species and even among cultivars, since the expression of cell wall degrading enzymes is regulated both in time and amount in each particular fruit (Brummell, 2006; Bennett and Labavitch, 2008; Goulao and Oliveira, 2008). In general, depolymerization of matrix glycans begins during early ripening, and it is followed by loss of galactan and arabinan side chains of RGI and dimethyl-esterification of polyuronides, and finally pectin depolymerization occurs by endo- or exo-PG, which starts at mid- or late ripening depending on fruit. In addition, fruits with a crisp fracturable texture at ripeness (apple, watermelon, bell pepper) have a low grade of pectin solubilization and depolymerization compared to the melting-flesh fruit, suggesting that the integrity of intercellular connections is an important component of crispness. These differences affect the extent of the modification of the polysaccharides of the cell wall and the expression and regulation of cell wall–modifying enzymes. Finally, genetic manipulation of cell wall–modifying genes has re-opened the discussion about the real effect of these enzymes in the cell wall and their role in fruit softening.

2.3.4 *Aroma compounds*

Fruit aromas are perceived by human nasal olfactory epithelium, a relatively small area of the mucous-covered inner surface of the nasal cavity. Most fruits produce a significant number of volatile compounds and their qualitative and quantitative composition determines fruit aromatic characteristic. Many of these volatile compounds are produced in trace amounts, which are below the thresholds of most analytical instruments but can be detected by human olfaction (Zhu et al., 2005; Goff and Klee, 2006; Song and Forney, 2008; Defilippi et al., 2009).

Fruit volatile composition includes an array of chemicals from various classes, such as alcohols, aldehydes, esters, ketones, and terpenes, and it plays a principal role in the market success of any fruit. In addition, the recognized flavor of a particular type of fruit is usually absent in the early stage of its development and instead is acquired during the ripening process as a consequence of volatile accumulation. Volatiles responsible for fruit aroma can be classified as primary or secondary, indicating whether they are present in intact fruit tissue or produced as a result of tissue disruption. Volatiles collected from intact fruit reflect the consumer smelling and perceiving ripening signals of the fruit, while volatiles generated after tissue disruption may better represent the flavor perception during eating.

Volatiles from intact, cut, or macerated fruit can be collected using headspace techniques and analyzed directly or after concentration using various trapping technologies. In addition, volatile compounds can be extracted from homogenized fruits using various distillation and solvent extraction techniques. Then, to identify and quantify fruit aroma compounds, the most useful technique is gas chromatography-mass spectrometry (GC-MS). However, aroma extraction methods affect the profile and concentration of the extracted volatile compounds, and important differences also occur between aroma released by intact fruit and those determined after fruit ground and extraction (Guillot et al., 2006; Aubert and Chanforan, 2007; Song and Forney, 2008; Defilippi et al., 2009). The electronic nose (e-nose) has also been utilized to study changes in aroma compounds in many fruits such as apples, peach, and apricots. This technique is based on electrochemical sensors that allow for the analysis of aroma intensity and has the advantage of being a nondestructive technique, but it cannot, however, identify particular aroma compounds (Benedetti et al., 2008). Finally, to relate the contribution of volatile compounds to fruit aroma and flavor, human olfactory analysis is required, since humans can smell volatile compounds at ppb levels or lower (Goff and Klee, 2006). Thus, the combination of sensory analysis of fruit flavor with instrumental analysis provides greater insights into the impact of volatile compounds on flavor than either alone (Baldwin et al., 2007; Song and Forney, 2008).

An overwhelming number of chemical compounds have been identified as volatile compounds in fresh fruit, based on their quantitative abundance and olfactory thresholds, although only a fraction of these compounds have been identified as fruit flavor impact compounds. In Table 2.5 some examples about aroma substances and description of their odor are shown. Due to the large number of studies characterizing the aroma profile of fruits, we have selected only some of them, based on economic importance and the amount of relevant information published, to provide an overall view of volatile composition with regard to common chemical groups.

Table 2.5 Aroma Substances in Fruits and a Description of Their Odor

Aroma substance	Odor description
Acetaldehyde	Pungent, penetrating
Acetone	Sweet, pungent
Ethyl acetate	Ether-like, pineapple, anise
Methyl butyrate	Apple
Dimethyl disulfide	Onion, cabbage
Ethyl butyrate	Fruity, pineapple
Butyl acetate	Fruity
1-Methyl-ethyl butyrate	Apple
Hexanal	Cut grass
Hexenal	Sweet, almond, green
2-Hexenal	Green leaf
Heptanone	Banana
Methyl hexanoate	Ether-like, pineapple
Butyl butyrate	Fruity, pear
Ethyl hexanoate	Fruity
Hexyl acetate	Fruity, apricot
Linalool	Fruity, floral, citrus
B-lanone-trans	Warm, woody, balsamic, rose

Citrus fruits possess unique aromas rarely found in other fruit species, mainly due to mono- and sesquiterpenes (the major components of citrus essential oils), which accumulate in specialized oil glands in the flavedo and oil bodies in the juice sacs. The monoterpene limonene normally accounts for over 90% of essential oils of the citrus fruit, although several unique sesquiterpene compounds present in small quantities have a profound effect on flavor and aroma of each particular citrus fruit species and cultivar. Thus, the sesquiterpenes valencene and α- and β-sinensal are present in minor quantities in orange fruits and play an important role in their characteristic aroma. Nootkatone, a putative derivative of valencene, has a dominant role in the flavor and aroma of pummelo and some pummelo hybrids, such as grapefruit, while the bitter flavanone neohesperidoside flavor compounds are distinctly associated with species/varieties of pummelo origin. Accumulation of valencene and nootkatone occurs at the ripening stage and seems to be ethylene dependent, even in these nonclimacteric fruits (Sharon-Asa et al., 2003).

In mango cultivars mono- and sesquiterpene hydrocarbons also dominate the compound profiles, while aldehydes occur at lower concentration, although they are responsible for the flesh, grassy and fatty-green in some mango cultivars, and they impart the characteristic smell in these fruits, even at their extremely low concentrations (Pino et al., 2005; Pandit et al.,

2009). In tomato fruits over 400 volatile compounds have been detected, the most important contributor to tomato fruit aroma being hexanal, hexenal, hexenol, 3-methylbutanal, 3-methylbutanol, methylnitrobutane, and isobutyl thiazole, and a general increase in these and other volatiles occurs during ripening (Zhu et al., 2005; Birtic et al., 2009). Accordingly, volatiles in apple also increase during ripening and the aroma profile changes from an abundance of aldehyde volatiles to a profile dominated by esters. Thus, in these fruits the ethyl, buthyl, and hexyl esters of acetic, butanoic, and hexanoic acids are often the most important contributors to their flavors at ripe stage. Specifically three esters—butyl acetate, 2-methylbutyl acetate, and hexyl acetate—are considered the major contributors to the characteristic apple-like aroma and flavor in most cultivars, although the total number and concentration of volatile compounds are cultivar specific (Dixon and Hewett, 2000; Villatoro et al., 2008).

Esters have been reported as the main components of aroma of Charentais cantaloupe melons, and among them, 2-methylpropyl acetate, ethyl butyrate, ethyl 2-methyl butyrate, butyl acetate, 2-methylbutyl acetate, benzyl acetate, and hexyl acetate were the most abundant, followed by some thioesters, all of them being at low concentration in long shelf life cultivars as compared to mid- and wildtype ones. These compounds are considered as having low odor values, while ethyl-2-methyl propanoate and ethyl-2-methyl butanoate are potent odorants (Aubert and Bourger, 2004; Pech et al., 2008). Hexyl acetate and butyl acetate have also been identified as the main contributors to apricot fruit aroma, together with ethyl acetate, linalool, α-terpineol, γ-hexalactone, and γ- and δ-decalactone (Aubert and Chanforan, 2007; Defilippi et al., 2009). Finally, in plum cultivars, low quantities of aroma compounds have been identified. For instance, Lozano and colleagues (2009) identified 40 volatile compounds in six plum cultivars, with guanidine, 3-hexen-1-ol, and the esters 4-hexen-1-ol acetate and hexyl acetate being present in all cultivars at the greatest proportions.

2.3.5 Bioactive compounds and antioxidant activity

Foods from plant origin contain hundreds of non-nutrient constituents with significant biological activity, generally called *bioactive compounds* or *phytochemicals* with antioxidant activity. The word *antioxidant* is increasingly popular in modern society, as it gains publicity through mass media coverage concerning its health benefits. According to the dictionary, the term *antioxidant* refers to a substance that opposes oxidation or inhibits reactions promoted by oxygen or peroxides, although a more biologically relevant definition is synthetic or natural substances that prevent or delay oxidation reaction in biological systems.

Free radicals are molecules with one or more unpaired electrons, such as superoxide anions ($O\bullet^{2-}$), hydroxyl radicals ($OH\bullet$), and peroxyl radicals

(ROO•), among reactive oxygen species (ROS). These free radicals are generated during normal aerobic metabolism, inflammatory processes, and macrophages action. They are short-lived and highly reactive, constantly seeking for another electron to be paired causing oxidation in other molecules such as lipids, proteins, and nucleic acids and spreading oxidation chains. Thus, free radicals are implicated as mediators in the ageing process, in degenerative and chronic deteriorative, inflammatory, and auto-immune diseases, diabetes, hypertension, cancer, arthritis, brain dysfunction, and others. In living cells there are defense systems against these free radicals. The primary defense system directly interacts with harmful free radicals by preventing their formation or by removing them as soon as they are formed and avoiding the damage of the body's cellular components. Enzymes such as catalase [EC 1.11.1.6, CAT] and superoxide dismutase [EC 1.15.1.1, SOD], and small molecules such as vitamins C and E and other minor food components, generally known as *antioxidants*, are involved in this primary defense system. The secondary defense system consists of other enzymes and antioxidants that repair the already damaged biomolecules. Thus, problems leading to cellular aging and the previously mentioned diseases arise only when the balance between free radicals and antioxidant defense systems tilts to the side of free radicals (Yeum et al., 2004; Willcox et al., 2004; Tsao and Akhtar, 2005).

In this sense, fruit and vegetable consumption has shown protective effects against several chronic diseases associated with aging—including atherosclerosis; cardiovascular diseases; cancer; cataracts; blood pressure increase; ulcerous, neurodegenerative diseases; and brain and immune dysfunction—and even against bacterial and viral diseases. The impact of this scientific inquiry has resulted in the development of many epidemiological studies to correlate the presence of these bioactive compounds with alleviating one or more of the above diseases. The protection that fruit and vegetables provide against these degenerative diseases has been attributed to several antioxidant compounds, which vary widely in chemical structure and function in plant tissues and are grouped in vitamins (C and E), carotenoids, and phenolic and thiol (SH) compounds (Kris-Etherton et al., 2002; Pennington, 2002; Scalbert et al., 2005; Nichenametla et al., 2006; Lister et al., 2007; Saura-Calixto and Goñi, 2009).

2.3.5.1 Phenolic compounds including anthocyanins

Plant tissues synthesize a large number of secondary metabolites, from which phenolic compounds are the most distributed in the plant kingdom. The chemical definition of *phenol* and *polyphenol* refers to compounds that posses an aromatic ring bearing one (phenol) or more (polyphenols) hydroxyl radicals. However, from the biological point of view, plant phenolic or polyphenolics are defined as secondary natural metabolites formed from the phenylpropanoid pathway that exhibit a very broad range of physiological roles in plants including pigmentation, growth, and resistance to pathogens, among many other functions (Daayf and Lattancio, 2008). However, special emphasis about the role of the phenolic compounds as antioxidant agents has increased in recent years, as is addressed later in this chapter. Thus, this group of substances are attractive to scientific, nutritionist, manufacturing, and consumer communities due to their putative beneficial effects on human health, especially in the last two decades. In this sense, there is growing scientific evidence that dietary antioxidants may be a critical mediator of the beneficial effects of the Mediterranean diet. A recent study has shown that the daily intake of total phenolics in the Spanish Mediterranean diet was estimated to be 1171 mg/person/day, which is considerably higher than the daily intake of other antioxidant compounds such as carotenoids (4 mg), vitamin C (126 mg), and vitamin E (13 mg) (Saura-Calixto and Goñi, 2006).

The structure of plant phenolics and polyphenols can be either very simple (phenolic acids) or highly polymerized compounds (proanthocyanindins). In nature several thousand different compounds have been identified with large variation of structures, the main phenolics in fruit and vegetables being classified according to their basic skeleton: C_6-C_1 (phenolic acids), C_6-C_3 (hydroxycinnamic acids), C_6-C_2-C_6 (stilbenes), and C_6-C_3-C_6 (flavonoids). Table 2.6 and Figure 2.7 show the phenolic groups and subgroups and the chemical structures of the phenolics most commonly found in fruits. Of all of them, flavonoids are the most important group with about 8000 different compounds already identified. The flavonoid group can be divided into five

Table 2.6 Main Phenolic Groups and Subgroups Found in Fruits

Phenolic groups	Subgroups	Compounds
Phenolic acids (C_6-C_1)		Gallic acid, ellagic acid
Hydroxycinnamic acids (C_6-C_3)		*p*-Coumaric acid, caffeic acid, ferulic acid
Stilbenes (C_6-C_2-C_6)		*Cis*-resveratrol, *trans*-resveratrol
Flavonoids (C_6-C_2-C_6)	Flavonols	Quercetin, kaempherol, myrcetin, isorhamnetin
	Flavan-3-ols	Catechin, epicathechin, gallocatechin, proanthocyanidins
	Flavones	Apigenin, luteolin, chryoeriol
	Flavanones	Naringenin, herperidin, eriodyctol
	Anthocyanindins	Cyanidin, delphinidin, malvidin, petunidin, peonidin, pelargonidin

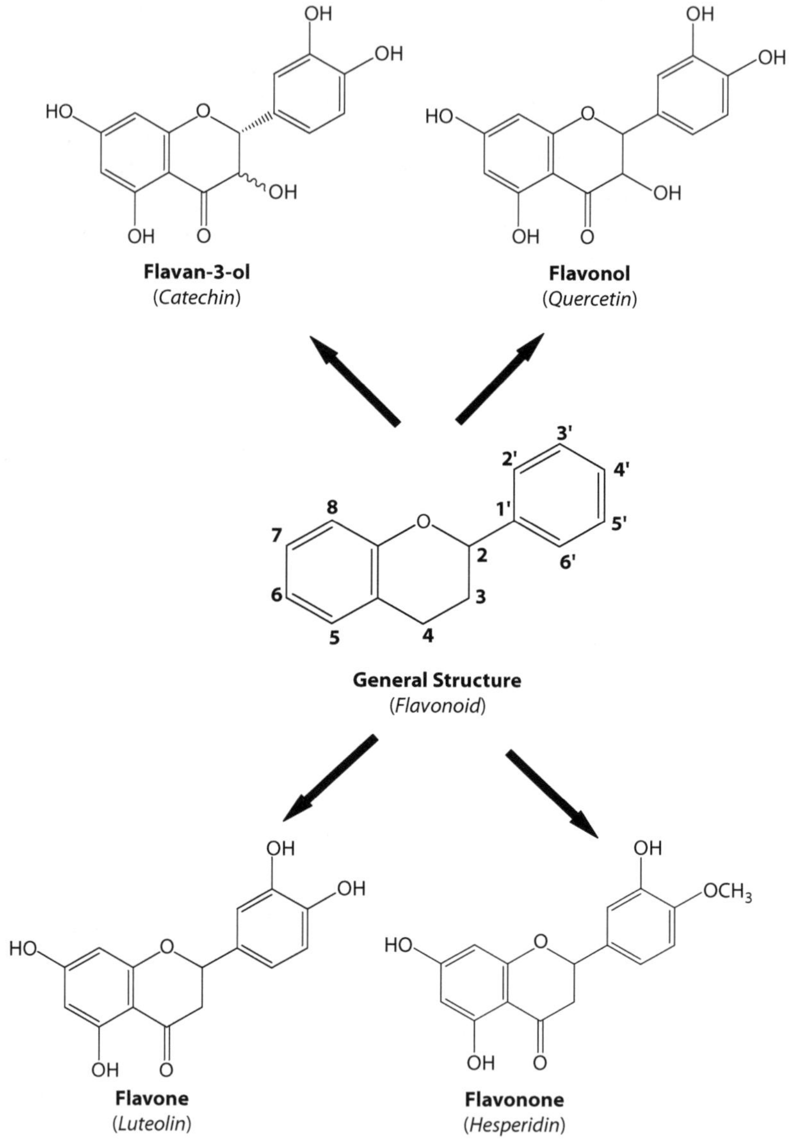

Figure 2.7 General structures of some flavonoid subgroups and other phenolic compounds.

subgroups including flavonols, flavan-3-ols, flavones, flavonones, and anthocyanindins (Figure 2.3). These are known as *aglycones* and are usually bound through glycosidic bonds to several sugar moieties to form the glycosilated derivatives, the main sugar being glucose, rhamnose, and rutinoside.

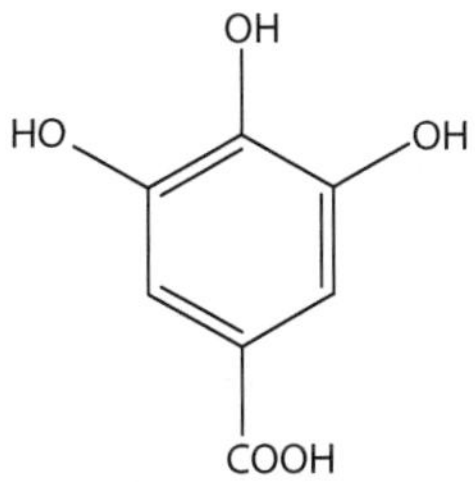

Phenolic acid
(*Gallic acid*)

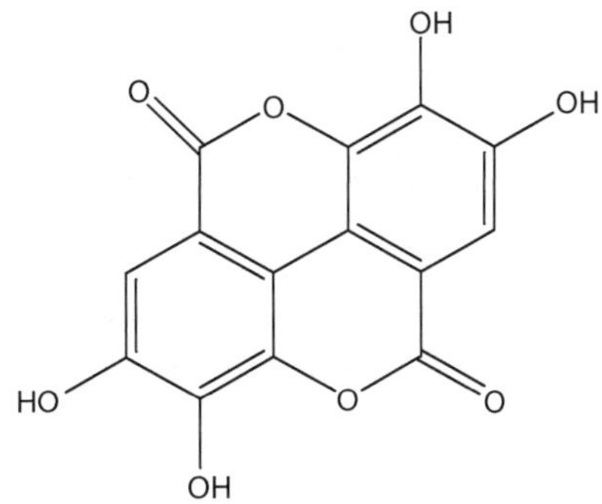

Phenolic acid
(Ellagic *acid*)

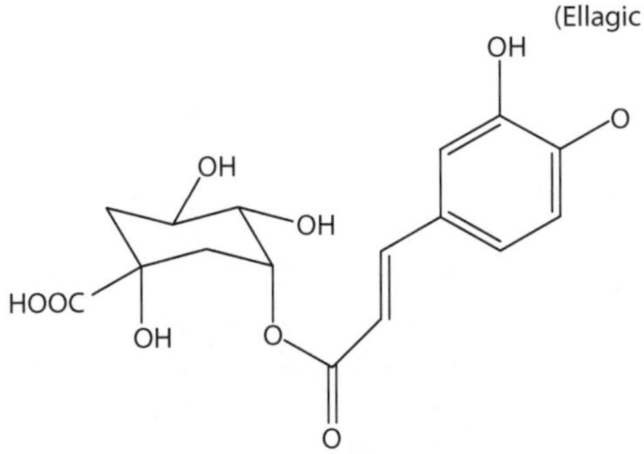

Hydroxycinnamic Acid
(3-*O*-Caffeoylquinic Acid)
(Cholorgenic *acid*)

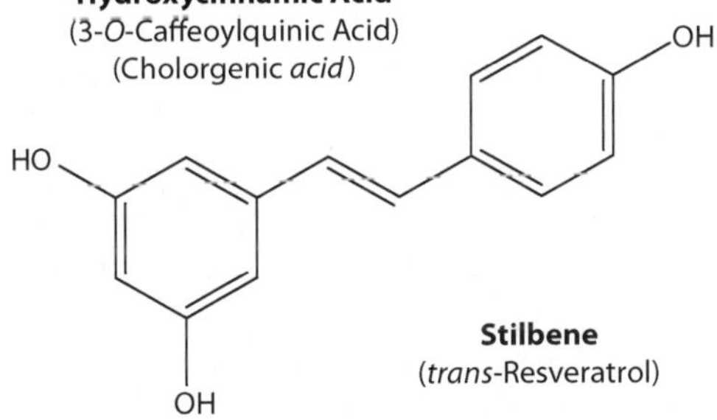

Stilbene
(*trans*-Resveratrol)

Figure 2.7 (Continued)

Phenolics as a group represent the strongest antioxidants in plant foods, although the antioxidant activity of individual phenolic compounds may vary depending on their chemical structure. This antioxidant activity of the phenolics is attributable to the electron delocalization over the aromatic ring and their high redox potential, which allow them to act as reducing agents, hydrogen donors, and singlet oxygen quenchers. In addition, they have metal-chelating potential, decreasing the lipid peroxidation, and can trap nitrate and prevent the formation of mutagenic N-nitroso compounds (Tsao and Akhtar, 2005; Fernández-Panchón et al., 2008). Therefore, the inverse relationship between fruit and vegetable intake and risk of cardiovascular and neurodegenerative diseases, cancer, diabetes, and osteoporosis has partially been ascribed to dietary phenolics (Kris-Etherton et al., 2002; Scalbert et al., 2005; Halliwell, 2007; Tucker and Robards, 2008). Accordingly, recent findings have shown that berry (blackberry, raspberry, blueberry, cranberry, and strawberry) extracts and their singly purified phenolic constituents inhibit cell proliferation, modulate cell cycle arrest, and induce apoptosis (programmed cell death) in cancer cells with little or null cytotoxic effects in normal cells, including human oral, breast, colon, and prostate cancer cell lines in a dose-dependent manner (Seeram, 2008).

However, resveratrol is a stilbene produced in plants as a response to fungal infection and thus acts as phytoalexin, the primary dietary source of resveratrol in the human diet being table grapes, wine, and peanuts. Resveratrol naturally occurs in two isomeric forms, *cis* and *trans*, with the *trans* form being the most common and exhibiting greater biological activity (Figure 2.7). Resveratrol was first identified in 1976 from grapevines whose production was induced by UV light, although climactic conditions, grape cultivar, and the amount of fungal infection by *Botrytis cinerea* influenced the concentration of resveratrol in the grape skin. Since red grapes produce higher amounts of resveratrol than white grapes, red wines contain important content of resveratrol. The increased consumption of resveratrol-containing food has been associated with improved health, which is related to a diverse range of biological activity such as antioxidant, cardioprotector, anticancer, and anti-inflammatory activity, and modulation of cellular signal transduction (King et al., 2006).

As stated in Section 2.3, there is much information about the evolution of the organoleptic and nutritive parameters during fruit growth and ripening, while very few efforts have been made to study the evolution of bioactive compounds and antioxidant activity during the phases of fruit development. Figure 2.8 shows the changes in total phenolics and the corresponding antioxidant activity at the latest phases of growth and ripening of some fruits, and that the total phenolics increase as maturity advances in pepper, sweet cherry, and plums (both yellow and red cultivars) but decline in tomato. This behavior in total phenolics is reflected in the total antioxidant activity (TAA) from the hydrophilic extracts (H-TAA), which evolves in a similar way and at the same time as the loss of green tonality and occurrence of their typical color, red or yellow. In addition, Figure 2.8 shows variations in both total phenolic content and H-TAA depending on the fruit type, with pepper having the highest values and tomato the lowest ones. Moreover, a direct relationship (R^2 = 0.76–0.99) has been found between the total phenolic

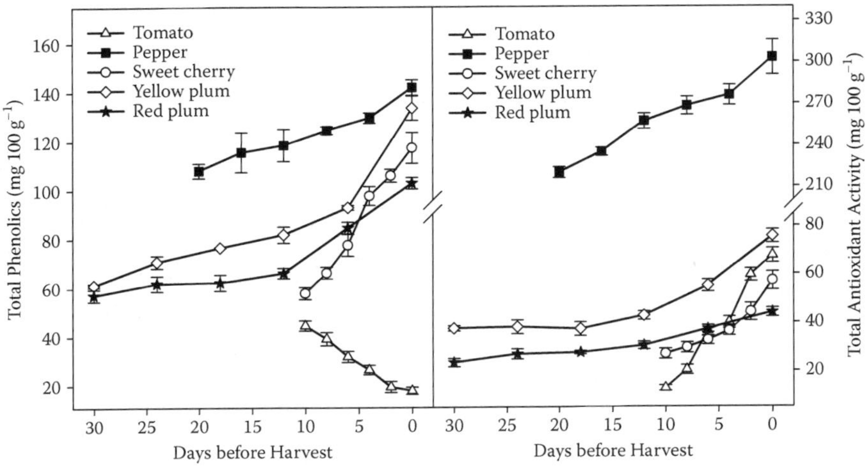

Figure 2.8 Evolution of total phenolic concentration and total antioxidant activity (TAA) of hydrophilic extracts (H-TAA) during the ripening process on-plant of different fruits.

compounds and the H-TAA during the ripening of plums, peaches, peppers, nectarines, and sweet cherries (Gil et al., 2002; Cevallos-Casals et al., 2006; Deepa et al., 2007; Díaz-Mula et al., 2008; 2009a). Table 2.7 summarizes the content of total phenolics and H-TTA and lipophilic total antioxidant activity (L-TTA) in a wide range of fruits at commercial harvest and indicates that pepper and strawberry show the highest H-TTA, watermelon shows the highest L-TTA, and pomegranate shows the highest polyphenol content.

Anthocyanins (Greek *anthos* = flower and *kianos* = blue) are responsible for the red, blue, and purple color of some flower and fruits, and have been described as potent antioxidants. The distribution of the six common anthocyanidins in fruits (Figure 2.3) is Cy (50%), Dp (12%), Pg (12%), Pn (12%), Pt (7%), and Mv (7%), while the 3-glucoside derivative is the most common found in nature (Castañeda-Ovando et al., 2009). Anthocyanins have shown higher antioxidant activity than vitamin C or E or other phenolic compounds, with cyanindin being the most common anthocyanidin and 3-glucoside the most active anthocyanin with antioxidant activity. It seems that this higher antioxidant capacity is due to their ability to capture free radicals by donation of phenolic hydrogen atoms. As shown in Figure 2.9 for two sweet cherry (Cristalina and Santina) and two plum (Larry Ann and Black Diamond) cultivars, the anthocyanin concentration increases at the latest stages of ripening on tree, showing variations between plant species and even cultivars, although for all of them, the anthocyanin accumulation in sweet cherry and in the plum skin is highly correlated with H-TAA (Figure 2.9, insert) indicating that anthocyanin

Table 2.7 Total Phenolic Content (mg 100 g^{-1}) and Antioxidant Activity (mg 100 g^{-1}) in a Collection of Fruits Typical of the Mediterranean Diet at Commercial Ripening Stage

Fruit	Total phenolics	Hydrophilic total antioxidant activity	Lipophilic total antioxidant activity
Kiwifruit	39.65 ± 1.41	45.52 ± 2.60	12.72 ± 0.55
Lemon	45.55 ± 2.51	13.39 ± 1.44	9.78 ± 2.49
Apple	23.62 ± 1.21	29.72 ± 2.05	14.67 ± 2.1
Melon	26.36 ± 2.64	14.51 ± 0.62	6.5 ± 0.63
Orange	43.54 ± 3.92	97.76 ± 5.79	11.14 ± 1.01
Nectarine	26.01 ± 1.32	31.14 ± 3.42	13.83 ± 1.55
Pear	11.13 ± 0.15	12.64 ± 2.14	9.30 ± 0.51
Banana	15.91 ± 0.35	17.46 ± 1.16	6.41 ± 1.34
Green pepper	99.05 ± 3.98	145.06 ± 3.98	14.77 ± 1.35
Red pepper	142.16 ± 3.41	235.98 ± 9.41	26.29 ± 2.09
Grapefruit	83.28 ± 2.58	22.37 ± 1.84	12.06 ± 0.39
Watermelon	12.06 ± 0.66	8.84 ± 1.05	56.05 ± 3.01
Pomegranate	499.44 ± 17.80	85.08 ± 4.96	16.70 ± 0.53
Red tomato	17.86 ± 1.47	9.44 ± 0.41	29.70 ± 3.90
Grape	61.43 ± 1.36	146.06 ± 3.37	24.10 ± 2.61
Strawberry	75.22 ± 1.45	246.76 ± 5.86	43.02 ± 4.72

could be the main phenolic compounds with antioxidant activity. This seems to be a general behavior of red-purple fruits, since correlations were also found between the values of the antioxidant capacity and the anthocyanin content in blackberries, red raspberries, black raspberries, and strawberries (Wang and Lin, 2000). These authors also found differences attributable to the ripening stage, species, and cultivars. Very recently, various transgenic approaches have been taken to increase the flavonoid levels in tomato fruit by overexpressing either the structural or regulatory genes involved in the biosynthetic pathway, and then transgenic fruit started to synthesize anthocyanins at the end of the green stage and continued to accumulate these pigments during subsequent ripening, ultimately reaching an intense, uniform purple coloration both in the peel and in the flesh with concentration ≈300 mg 100 g^{-1} of total anthocyanins (Gonzali et al., 2009). These purple tomatoes had increased H-TAA compared with the red tomatoes, which is attributable to the high production of anthocyanins.

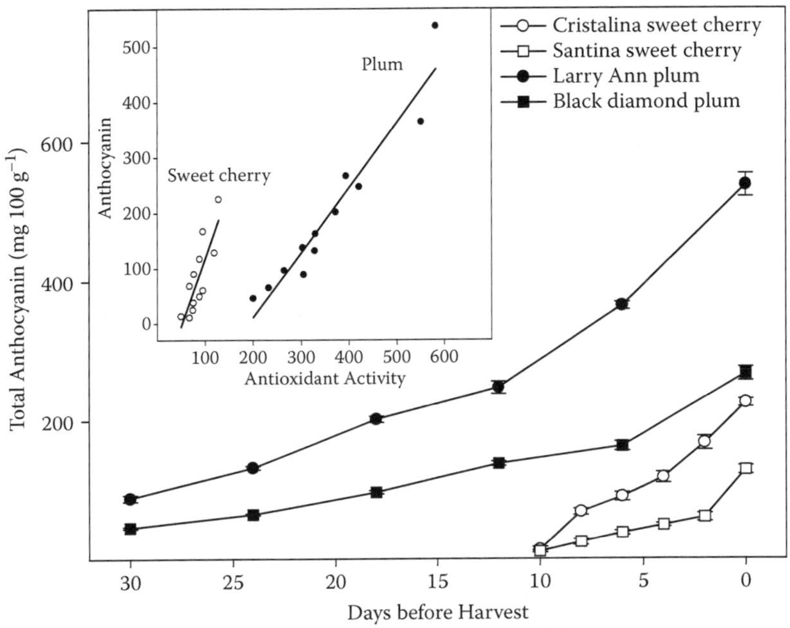

Figure 2.9 Evolution of total anthocyanin concentration during sweet cherry and plum ripening on tree, and correlation between anthocyanin concentration and antioxidant activity in hydrophilic extracts (insert graph).

2.3.5.2 Carotenoids

Carotenoids are a group of lipid-soluble natural pigments present in fruits and vegetables that impart colors from yellow to red and are originated from the condensation of isoprenyl units (see Section 2.3.1). The main physiological effect of carotenoids in humans has been classically attributed to their role as pro-vitamin A, since those carotenes with a ß-ring end group are converted to vitamin A (retinol) by the action of an intestinal mono-oxygenase. Thus, vitamin A (Figure 2.10) is a C_{20} carotenoid cleavage product essential for animal survival as both a chromophore in vision (retinaldehyde) and a hormone (retinoic acid). The primary source of vitamin A in the diet comes from fruits and vegetables in the form of ß-carotene. However, in the last decade several epidemiological studies suggest that carotenoids also have important roles in a range of diseases, including age-related macular degradation, cataract, cardiovascular diseases, blue light filter protectors, and some types of cancer due to their function in cell differentiation and proliferation regulators or cell-to-cell communication stimulators (Krinsky and

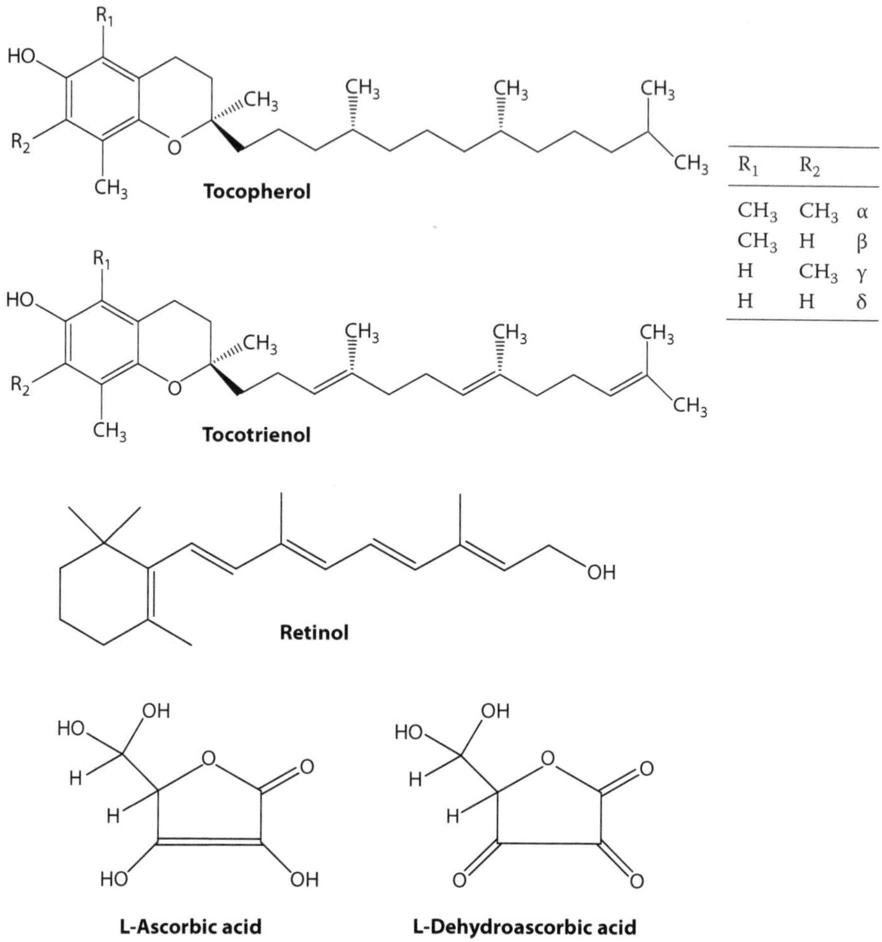

R_1	R_2	
CH_3	CH_3	α
CH_3	H	β
H	CH_3	γ
H	H	δ

Figure 2.10 Chemical structures of the main vitamins present in fruits.

Johnson, 2005; Taylor and Ramsay, 2005; Voutilainen et al., 2006), and improve bone and joint health by increasing alkaline phosphatase activity and osteopontin in osteoblastic cells (Lister et al., 2007) due to their antioxidant properties.

Of the over 600 carotenoids found in nature, about 40 are present in the human diet but only 14 of them have been identified in blood or tissues (Krinsky and Johnson, 2005). In this regard, the most studied carotenoids have been ß-carotene, lycopene, lutein, and zeaxanthin. Lycopene, a carotenoid with non–pro-vitamin A activity, has been found to have both greater antioxidant capacity and stronger inhibition of cancer cell proliferation than other carotenoids (Nguyen and Schwartz, 1999; Omoni and Aluko, 2005). The biological mechanism for these protective effects is still unclear, and several hypotheses have been proposed: (1) Carotenoids can be converted to retinoids having pro-vitamin A activity, (2) they can modulate the enzymatic activities of lipooxygenases and then act as immunomodulatory and anti-inflammatory molecules, and (3) they can behave as antioxidant compounds. Accordingly, there is considerable evidence about the interaction of carotenes *in vitro* with free radicals through their capacity for scavenging singlet oxygen, peroxyl radicals formed from lipid peroxidation, and other radicals such as nitrogen dioxide ($NO^{\bullet}_2$), thiyl ($RS^{\bullet}$), and sulphonyl ($RSO^{\bullet}_2$), which thus suggests activity as an antioxidant. These mechanisms and others support the *in vivo* evidences, especially in the clinical trials using ß-carotene and lycopene as a source of carotenoids. Miller et al. (1996) studied the antioxidant ability of several carotenoids (carotenes and xanthophylls) against the $ABTS^{\bullet +}$ radical and established the following sequence from high to low: lycopene > ß-cryptoxanthin ≈ ß-carotene > lutein ≈ zeaxanthin > α-carotene > canthaxanthin. They concluded that lycopene exhibited threefold more antioxidant activity than vitamin E and that carotenes are more efficient quenchers than xantophylls, with the exception of ß-cryptoxanthin, probably due to the influence of the increasing polarities of the functional groups in the terminal rings as well as the lower double bonds of the xanthophylls (Figure 2.5).

As provided in Section 2.3.1, carotenogenesis occurs parallel to the loss of chlorophyll during fruit ripening and renders the yellow, orange, and red color of several fruits such as tomato, pepper, yellow plums, peaches, nectarines, and apricots. When antioxidant capacity of fruit and vegetables is carried out separately on hydrophilic and lipophilic extracts the antioxidant activity derived from water-soluble (H-TAA) or lipo-soluble molecules (L-TAA) can be separately evaluated. L-TAA has also been correlated with total carotenoids (R^2 = 0.73–0.99) in both flesh and peel of plum cultivars (Díaz-Mula et al., 2008) as well as in tomato fruits (Lenucci et al., 2006), vegetables, and legumes (Wu et al., 2004; Cho et al., 2007).

2.3.5.3 Vitamins

Vitamins are a class of nutrients that are essentially required by the human body for its biochemical and physiological functions. Since humans do not synthesize vitamins they must be supplied by the diet in the appropriate concentration. Vitamins are subdivided into fat-soluble and water-soluble, the vitamins A, D, E, and K being lipophilic and vitamins C and B complex are hydrophilic. Tocopherols (vitamin E), together with carotenoids are the two most abundant groups of lipid-soluble antioxidant vitamins in fruits and vegetables, while vitamin C is a hydrophilic compound with contrasted antioxidant capacity and proceeds also from the diet. This is one of the main reasons for a rapidly growing market of vitamin-enriched foods (mainly beverages).

Natural vitamin E comprises eight different forms, namely α-, ß-, γ-, and δ-tocopherols and α-, ß-, γ-, and δ-tocotrienols. The tocotrienols have an unsaturated isoprenoid side chain, while the tocopherols contain a trimethyltridecyl tail (Figure 2.10). These compounds are exclusively synthesized in photosynthetic tissues but are predominantly accumulated in the seeds. Thus, plant oils represent the major sources of vitamin E in the human diet, α-tocopherol being predominant in olive and sunflower oils, γ-tocopherol in corn oil, and δ-tocopherol in soybean oil, whereas the tocotrienols are the major vitamin E components of palm oil. Several functions of vitamin E in plants have been described, including its ability to prevent nonenzymatic lipid oxidation and photo-oxidative stress to adapt to low temperatures and to modulate signal transduction. In animals, vitamin E was discovered as an essential factor for reproduction in rats, although its main function is the prevention of lipid oxidation and other oxidative processes associated with many diseases (DellaPena and Pogson, 2006; Sen et al., 2007; Zingg, 2007). In fact, vitamin E has been recognized as one of the most important antioxidants due to its capacity to scavenge directly ROS and nitrogen species and to up-regulate the activities of antioxidant enzymes. In this sense, vitamin E inhibits ROS-induced generation of lipid peroxyl radicals, thereby protecting cells from (1) peroxidation of polyunsaturated fatty acids in membrane phospholipids, (2) oxidative damage of plasma in very low-density lipoprotein, cellular proteins, and DNA, and (3) membrane degeneration. Accordingly, a dietary deficiency of vitamin E reduces the activities of hepatic catalase and glutathione peroxidases and reductases; induces liver lipid peroxidation; and causes neurologic and cardiovascular disorders, which can be reversed by dietary vitamin E supplementation (Fang et al., 2002; Zingg, 2007).

Vitamin C was first isolated in 1928 by the Hungarian biochemist and Nobel Prize winner Szent-GyorGyi. Ascorbic acid (vitamin C) is a familiar molecule due to its dietary significance since a diet devoid of it causes scurvy. Humans and other animals are dependent on vitamin C in their diet due to loss of a functional form of the last enzyme (L-gulono-1,4-lactone oxidase) of the biosynthesis pathway of ascorbic acid (Valpuesta and Botella, 2004). Ascorbic acid has four isomers but only the L-ascorbic and L-dehydroascorbic acids have physiological activity as vitamin C (Figure 2.10). Since dehydroascorbic acid can be easily converted into ascorbic acid in the human body, it is very important to measure both isomers to determine the vitamin C capacity, for which dehydroascorbic supposes ~10% of total vitamin C. Apart from the vitamin role of ascorbic acid, vitamin C has great importance as an antioxidant, being highly effective in inhibiting lipid peroxidation initiated by peroxyl radical and acting as radical scavenger of ROS. Ascorbic acid acts as antioxidant at two levels: (1) in the cytosol, in which ascorbate acts as a primary antioxidant to scavenge free radical species that are generated as by-products of cellular metabolism, and (2) in cellular membranes, in which ascorbic acid may play an indirect antioxidant role to reduce the α-tocopherooxyl radical to α-tocopherol, thus recycling the latter (May, 1999). Thus, these two vitamins (C and E) can be effective partners in reducing the destructive processes of lipid peroxidation. The strong antioxidant activity of ascorbic acid is considered responsible for its effect in lowering the risk of some degenerative and cardiovascular diseases. Ascorbic acid is widely distributed in nature, the main food sources of vitamin C being fruits, with large variations among the different species. Thus, citrus species, kiwifruit, pepper, and other leafy vegetables are considered to have the highest content of vitamin C (100–200 mg 100 g^{-1}), compared with the 1–10 mg 100 g^{-1} found in pomegranate, pear, stone fruits, and apple (Gebhardt and Thomas, 2004). Many preharvest factors influence the vitamin C of horticultural crops, as well as the genotype of each cultivar. Thus, during fruit ripening discrepancies about the ascorbic acid behavior have been reported based on differences in ascorbic acid metabolism, the discordances being attributed to the fact that different species follow different maturation models, which are genetically determined, as well as to the strong influence of the climatic conditions and cultural practices. The biosynthesis and accumulation of ascorbic acid in fruits are of great importance, not only because of the nutritional value of ascorbic acid but also because it modulates fruit growth and ripening. The ascorbic acid pool is affected by synthesis, transport, catabolism, and recycling processes, contributing specifically in the different plant tissues (Ishikawa et al., 2006). However, the biosynthesis pathway and control of ascorbic acid are not well elucidated, and catabolism is still unknown, especially in fruits. Therefore a deeper understanding of ascorbate metabolism is needed to achieve larger increases in vitamin C in plants. It is generally accepted that immature green fruits contain higher concentrations of ascorbic acid than mature ones, in which the diminution of ascorbic acid coincides with the beginning of the color changes, as has been observed in tomato (Serrano et al., 2008b) and pepper (Yahia et al., 2001), although in the latter ascorbic acid concentration increased as did the developmental process and color changes from green to red (Serrano et al., 2010). Nagy (1980) also reported that immature citrus fruits contained the highest concentration of vitamin C, whereas ripe fruits contained the least. Although vitamin C concentration decreases on a fresh weight basis during maturation of citrus fruits, the total vitamin C content per fruit tended to increase because the total volume of juice and fruit size increased with advancing maturity. However, ascorbic acid content increases with ripening on plant in apricot, peaches, and papayas but decreases in mangoes and apples (Lee and Kader, 2000). Generally, during ripening of climacteric fruits the availability of ascorbic acid seems to be a regulatory factor for ethylene production, with the decrease in ascorbic acid being related to the down-regulation of ACO, the key enzyme in ethylene biosynthesis (Davey et al., 2000; De Gara, 2004). In addition, the ripening process is accompanied by some oxidative events that are required to confer organoleptic characteristics to mature fruits, such as hydrogen peroxide production coinciding with the onset of ripening, and thus ascorbic acid would oversee this radical turnover during fruit ripening.

2.3.5.4 Thiol-SH compounds

Other micronutrients with contrasted antioxidant activity are those compounds with sulphur-containing radicals, from which glucosinolates are the most recognized moieties. The glucosinolates are the main health-promoting phytochemicals of cruciferous species, the most important being *Brassica* vegetables such as broccoli. A hundred of different glucosinolates have been identified although all of them share a common structure comprising a sulphonated moiety, a ß-D-thioglucose, and a variable side chain with amino-acid nature. Glucosinolates are derived from amino acids and can be classified according to the amino acid precursor from which they originate. The three major classes of glucosinolates are aliphatic (derived from L-methionine homologues), aromatic (derived from L-phenylalanine homologues and L-tyrosine) and indolic (derived from L-tryptophan). The most important glucosinolates found in *Brassica* vegetables are those derived from methionine.

The glucosinolates are chemically stable and biologically inactive while they remain sequestered within subcellular compartments throughout the plant. However, tissue damage caused by pests, harvesting, food processing, and chewing initiates contact with the endogenous enzyme myrosinase (thioglucoside glycohydrolase; EC 3.2.3.1). This leads to rapid hydrolysis of the glucosidic bond, releasing glucose and an unstable intermediate, which undergoes a spontaneous rearrangement to form a complex variety of breakdown products, the most important being isothiocyanates followed by indoles, nitriles, and thiocyanates (Johnson, 2002). Figure 2.11 shows an example of the most studied glucosinolates and their hydrolysis product involved in human nutrition for each chemical class. These autolytic breakdown products have exhibited protective effects against many types of cancer, in both *in vivo* and *in vitro* studies, by modulating the induction of detoxification enzymes and the inhibition of activation enzymes (Cartea and Velasco, 2008; Traka and Mithen, 2009).

The main factors that influence the levels of glucosinolates in vegetables are cultivation, storage, and processing conditions. Understanding the mechanism by which environmental, postharvest, and processing conditions affect the production of bioactive components can lead to

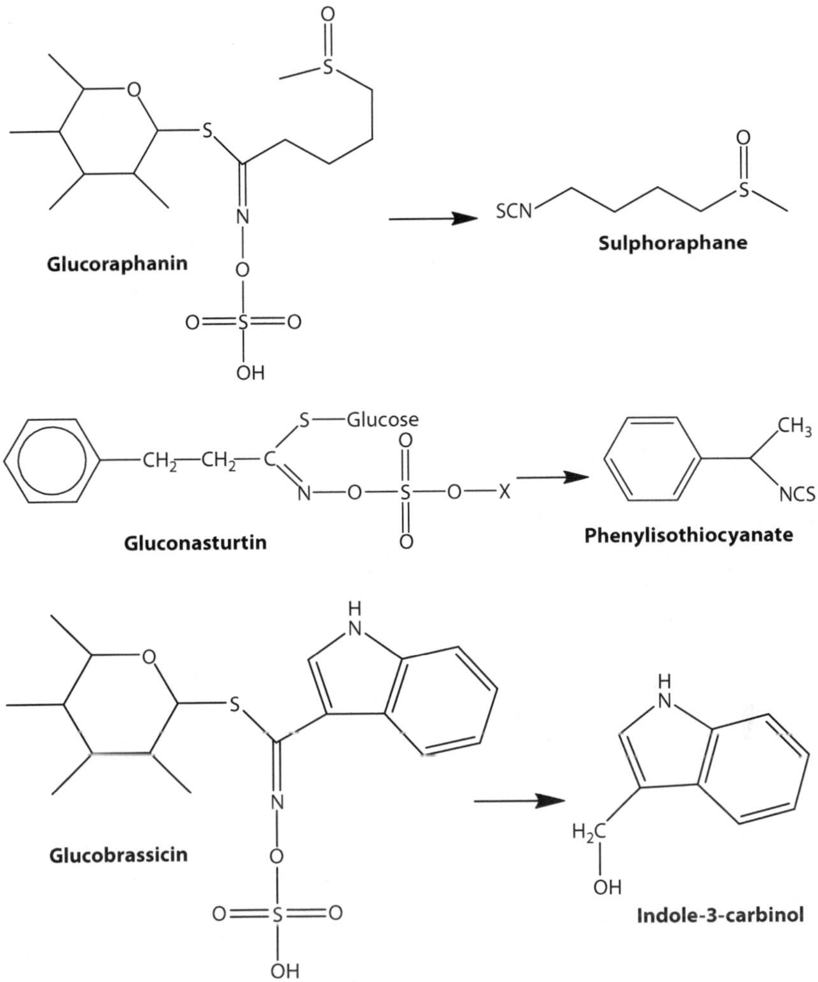

Figure 2.11 Some examples of glucosinolates and their hydrolysis products involved in human nutrition.

genetic control of these factors and the development of a product with high health-promoting activity (Moreno et al., 2007). In addition to the genetic influence, ecophysiological factors such as the climate parameters of irradiation, temperature, and water and nutrition supply have a strong influence on the glucosinolate composition of vegetables. All factors are responsible for the wide variation in the formation and content level of phytochemicals at preharvest and varying phytochemical contents at harvest.

2.3.6 Health-related interactions of fruit phytochemicals

From the previous sections, it can be concluded that there are a wide range of phytochemical compounds with antioxidant properties and health-beneficial effects. However, the question is whether a purified phytochemical has the same health benefit as does the whole fruit or vegetable, in which the phytochemical is present. Recent reviews have shown that there are additive and synergic effects of bioactive compounds in fruits and vegetables that confer altogether more antioxidant and anticancer activity, among other diseases, than the sum of the individual components. The additive effects occur when two or more compounds in a mixture interact to provide a global effect, which is equal to the sum of the individual component effects, while the synergic effects appear when the mixture has greater activity than the sum of the individuals. These synergic interactions could be explained by the fact that some of the mixture component would improve solubility, absorption, safety, stability, and bioavailability of the active principle(s).

Currently, it is believed that dietary supplements do not have the same health benefits as a diet rich in fruits and vegetables, because the individual antioxidants studied in clinical trials do not appear to have consistent preventive effects when taken alone. One of the most documented examples is the relationship between lycopene and prostate cancer; tomato fruit ingestion confers cancer chemoprotective effects but it is not clear if lycopene alone is able to have a similar effect (Liu, 2003; Lila and Raskin, 2005; Seifried et al., 2007). Thus, consumers should have a diverse diet based on fruits and vegetables rather than on dietary supplements, which are expensive and do not contain the balanced combination of bioactive compounds, in order to improve their nutrition and health-beneficial effects.

2.3.7 Physiological changes

Fruit ripening physiology has been classically defined as either climacteric or nonclimacteric, which differ in their pattern in both ethylene production and respiration rates. In this sense, climacteric fruits, such as tomato, avocado, banana, peach, and plum (Table 2.1), show a sharp increase in respiration rate and ethylene production at the onset of ripening. For these fruits, ethylene is considered to be the plant hormone responsible for the ripening process. On the contrary, nonclimacteric fruits, such as sweet cherry, pomegranate, pepper, grape, and citrus fruits (Table 2.1), show comparatively low profile and a gradual decline in their respiration pattern and ethylene production through the ripening process (Lelièvre et al., 1997; Giovannoni, 2001; 2004; 2007; Adams-Phillips et al., 2004; Barry and Giovannoni, 2007).

Ethylene is a very simple molecule with two carbon atoms linked with a double bond and naturally occurs as gaseous form. The first indications of a gaseous compound affecting plant tissues were reported in the nineteenth century, with the observation that illuminating gas streetlights caused senescence and defoliation in neighboring trees. In the early twentieth century (1901), Neljubov identified ethylene as the causative agent of this effect, and he is recognized as the discoverer of this plant hormone. Later, Gane (1934) proved that plants produce ethylene, although this compound could be quantified only after the establishment of gas chromatography (1959). Ever since the discovery of ethylene, continuous efforts have been made to clarify its biosynthesis pathway. Ethylene biosynthesis, perception, signal transduction, and regulation at biochemical, genetic, and biotechnological levels are well documented and covered by a number of excellent reviews (Sisler and Serek, 1997; Bleecker and Kende, 2000; Ecker, 2002; Wang et al., 2002; Stearns and Glick, 2003; De Paepe and Van der Straeten, 2005; Yoo et al., 2009). In higher vascular plants, ethylene is synthesized from the amino acid methionine, which is converted to SAM by the addition of adenine and consumption of ATP. SAM is then transformed to ACC by the enzyme ACS with the generation of the byproduct 5′-methylthioadenosine, which is recycled to methonine (Yang's cycle). Thus, ethylene can be produced at high rates even with a small pool of free methionine. Finally, ACC is oxidized to ethylene by ACO (formerly named *ethylene-forming enzyme, EFE*). The main step controlling ethylene biosynthesis is ACS and the subsequent pool of ACC. Early studies reported the up-regulation of this pathway (Figure 2.12) by observations of ACC accumulation and increases in the activities of both ACS and ACO enzymes (Yang and Hoffman, 1984; Abeles et al., 1992; Kende, 1993). More recently, it has been reported that ACS and ACO are encoded by multigene families. The expression of ACS genes is differentially regulated by several environmental, developmental, and hormonal signals, while for ACO activity the presence of CO_2 is necessary, although the exact mechanism for this is still unclear (Bleecker and Kende, 2000; Wang et al., 2002; Chang and Bleecker, 2004). In climacteric fruit, once the ethylene is being synthesized at low amounts, the internal production of ethylene rapidly increases. This is very important, since the onset of the ripening process of these fruits is considered to begin at this stage, and there is a positive feedback regulation in which ethylene promotes its own synthesis. This phenomenon is the so-called autocatalytic ethylene production (Yang and Hoffman, 1984).

As a hormone, ethylene binds to a receptor and the signal is transduced through a complex mechanism to trigger specific biological responses. Over the past decade, continuous efforts have been made to identify and isolate the ethylene receptor, using *Arabidopsis* as a model, although the complete set of signaling components is still unknown. Ethylene binds to

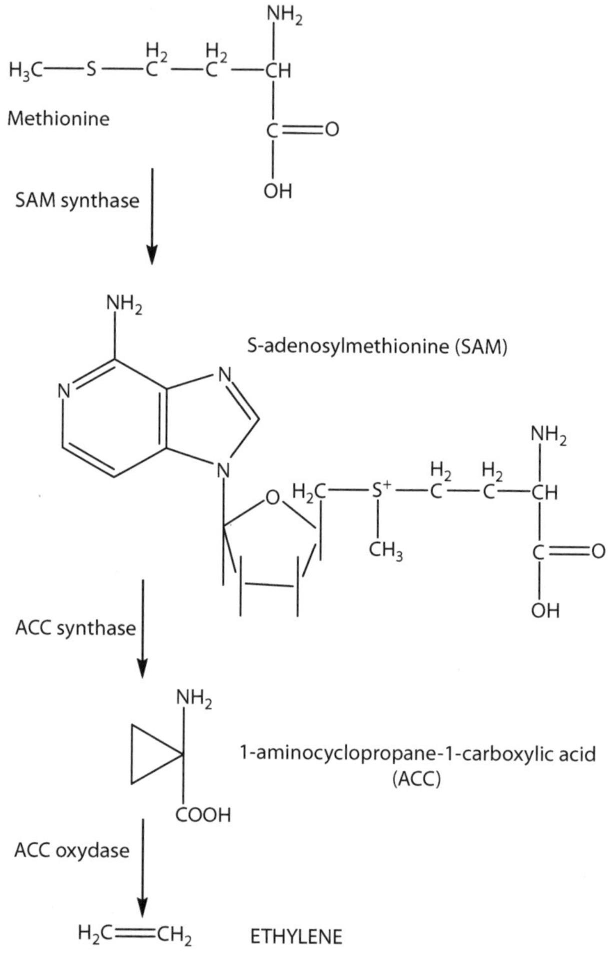

Figure 2.12 Ethylene biosynthesis pathway.

its receptors using copper as co-factor (Guo and Ecker, 2004). Tomato fruit is a good model system for the study of ethylene response, offering a number of advantages due to the well-characterized roles of ethylene in the control of its ripening. In tomato, a gene family composed of six members with major domains has been reported for the ethylene receptor (Klee and Tieman, 2002; Adams-Philips et al., 2004). Although the ethylene receptor is being well characterized, and the use of an increasing number of transgenic plants is providing new information of ethylene control (Stearns and Glick, 2003), there are still gaps in our knowledge on the differential responsiveness of a specific tissue to ethylene. More details about ethylene receptors will be given in Chapter 8 (Section 8.2).

Currently, ethylene biosynthesis and action can be blocked by chemical compounds that differ in their structure and act at different levels, such as modifying ACS and ACO activities, blocking receptor sites, diverting SAM through polyamine biosynthesis, and removing ethylene (Martínez-Romero et al., 2007a).

Climacteric fruits synthesize small amounts of ethylene during the growing period (0.1–0.2 μL kg^{-1} h^{-1}) but can increase markedly (up to 1000-fold) with the ripening process. In general, climacteric fruits have high rates of ethylene production and are also highly sensitive to this plant hormone (at concentrations of 0.03–0.1 μL L^{-1}). Conversely, nonclimacteric fruits produce very low amounts of ethylene and exhibit low sensitivity to this plant hormone (over 0.2 μL L^{-1}). However, some nonclimacteric fruits such as *Citrus* show a good response to exogenous ethylene, the phenomenon being used for the degreening agricultural practice (Goldschmidt et al., 1993). The distinction between climacteric and nonclimacteric fruits is not absolute, since there are also a number of species in which different varieties and cultivars exhibit both climacteric and nonclimacteric behavior. Thus, plum cultivars have generally been categorized as climacteric fruit, although Shiro, Golden Japan, and TC Sun behave as suppressed-climacteric fruits (Abdi et al., 1997; Zuzunaga et al., 2001; Díaz-Mula et al., 2008). Accordingly, melon fruits comprise both climacteric and nonclimacteric genotypes. Thus, *Cucumis melo* var. *cantalupensis* has a fast ripening rate and a short shelf life with high ethylene production rate, while *C. melo* var. *inodorous* is unable to produce autocatalytic ethylene and has a slow ripening rate associated with a long shelf life. In addition, the inheritance of the climacteric character seems to be dominant, since crossing climacteric with nonclimacteric melons generates climacteric melons, although the genetic control involved is still unknown (Pech et al., 2008).

As commented previously, ripening of climacteric fruits is widely accepted to be regulated by ethylene, although there are ethylene-dependent and -independent ripening pathways (Barry and Giovannoni, 2007; Pech et al., 2008). Thus, in many fruits such as tomato, apple, banana, and melon pulp coloration, sugar accumulation, and loss of acidity are ethylene-independent processes, whereas degreening and yellowing of the rind, softening of the flesh, development of peduncle abscission zone, aroma formation, and climacteric respiration are totally or partially ethylene-dependent. Thus, antisense ACO melons and apples from plants silenced for ACS or ACO exhibited strong reduction of softening, but significant residual softening still persisted, indicating the presence of an ethylene-independent component of softening. Moreover, in antisense ACO tomatoes ethylene production was inhibited at 97%, but not softening, which could also show that the 3% of residual ethylene was sufficient for active cell wall degradation events. The inhibition of the ethylene-dependent component of softening can also be achieved with 1-MCP, which caused total inhibition of softening in pear and only a moderate reduction in kiwifruits and plums. These examples point out that the relevance of ethylene-dependent or -independent component of softening is different among fruit species and probably among cultivars. In this sense, it has been shown that depolymerization of pectins and xyloglucans are strongly ethylene-dependent, although specific genes of each family of the cell wall degrading enzymes have been categorized as ethylene-dependent, totally ethylene-independent, and partially ethylene-dependent.

However, chilling injury (CI) caused by storage of many tropical and subtropical fruits at low but nonchilling temperatures has been shown to be ethylene-dependent in melon, avocado, pineapples, and Shamouti oranges, while in Fortuna mandarins ethylene treatments enhanced resistance to CI, showing that the role of ethylene in CI may vary from one fruit to another (Pech et al., 2008). However, chlorophyll degradation and synthesis of pigments such as anthocyanins and carotenoids are also ethylene-dependent processes, even in nonclimacteric fruits as grape berries, pepper, and citrus fruits. These results support the hypothesis that although ethylene synthesis does not increase during the ripening of these fruits, alteration in ethylene responsiveness might be able to mediate physiological changes associated with ripening in them (Adams-Phillips et al., 2004; Barry and Giovannoni, 2007).

Clearly, ethylene is required for the normal ripening of many fruits and in its absence the ripening process fails to occur, rendering the product unacceptable. However, once initiated, ripening is a one-way process and ethylene stimulates over-ripening and decay, leading to rapid loss of fruit quality. Then, in postharvest storage conditions it is important to control ethylene effects, not only in fruits but also in vegetables and ornamental crops in order to maintain their quality and enlarge storage possibilities.

Respiration is the oxidative breakdown of complex substrate molecules normally present in plant cells, such as starch, sugars, and organic acids, to simpler molecules such as CO_2 and H_2O. When glucose is used as substrate, the reaction can be written as follows:

$$C_6H_{12}O_6 + 6\ O_2 + 38\ ADP + 38\ Pi \rightarrow 6\ CO_2 + 6\ H_2O + 38\ ATP + 686\ kcal$$

Then, the primary purpose of the respiration is to maintain an adequate supply of ATP to obtain energy and intermediate molecules that are required to sustain the myriad of anabolic reactions essential for the maintenance of cellular organization and membrane integrity of living cells.

The components of this reaction have various sources and destinations. Glucose proceeds from stored simple sugars or polysaccharides, such as starch. The O_2 diffuses into the tissue from the surrounding atmosphere and is used to oxidize glucose, while CO_2 diffuses out of the tissue and the water produced is simply incorporated into the aqueous solution of the cell.

The internal factors affecting respiration are type and maturity stage of the fruit commodity. Even different varieties of the same product can exhibit different respiration rates. In general, both climacteric and non-climacteric commodities have higher respiration rates in the early stages of development that steadily decline during maturation, but in climacteric fruits a rise occurs that coincides with ripening or senescence (Yang and Hoffman, 1984). The respiration rate is usually very high during the early stages of fruit development and decreases as plant organs mature on tree, as can be observed in plums (Zuzunaga et al., 2001) and tomato (Serrano et al., 2008b), for which respiration rate peaked at pink stage of ripening and deceased in pink, light red, and red fruits. The respiration rate of citrus fruits continuously declines during fruit ontogenity and remains nearly constant during natural maturation or in detached mature fruits (Rodrigo and Zacarías, 2006). In addition, the respiratory intensity of sweet cherry depended on the cultivar and agroclimatic conditions during the development of the fruit, in which a relationship has been established between respiratory intensity and the date of harvesting, with late-harvested cultivars having reduced respiration rate compared to early fruits (Jaime et al., 2001).

It is well known that respiration rate of fruits strongly determines their transit and postharvest life, since at the senescent stage of climacteric fruit development there is a rise in respiration, presumably in order to obtain more energy for metabolic processes. Therefore, this situation must be avoided when the produce is being submitted to prolonged storage.

chapter three

Changes in fruit quality attributes during handling, processing, and storage

3.1 Introduction

The agricultural products can be classified as (1) durables, comprising cereal grains, oilseeds, and grain legumes; and (2) perishables, comprising succulent storage organs such as fleshy fruits, vegetables, rhizomes, and tubers. The harvested commodities are essentially plant organs with physiological functions quite different from tissues of the mother plant. As the ripening-senescence process sets in, the produce quality deterioration and the susceptibility of the stored products to decay caused by microbial spoilage and pathogens increase progressively. In this sense, the required fruit quality will depend on the final use and it is well accepted that the postharvest quality is determined by preharvest factors and appropriate handling, processing, packaging, and retailing. In today's modern society, fruits are exposed to a wide range of events commencing with the separation from the mother plant and finishing up on plates, all of them affecting the produce freshness and quality. For the fresh produce market, specific minimum quality standards exist in many countries; however, owing to the international nature of the fresh produce market, there is a trend toward international standardization of quality grades. The European Commission was one of the first organizations to develop international standards for fresh fruits (MAFF, 1996). Many of these standards have been adopted by the Organization for Economic Cooperation and Development (OECD). Usually, standards required for multiple retail outlets are considerably more stringent than these minimum standards, and will be defined for the supplier by the retailer. From the point of view of fruit quality, the factors that limit storage and shelf life fall into the following categories: weight loss, appearance, texture, flavor/aroma, and decay. In addition, occurrence of mechanical damage along the handling process will accelerate the changes in the above factors with a faster reduction in fruit quality.

3.2 What is quality?

There is an increasing consciousness of quality, particularly in the fruit and health sector, which strongly demands research activities regarding the production of defined quality, the preservation of quality during marketing, and the possibilities to evaluate quality parameters and to integrate this into production processes. During the postharvest chain (from harvesting to retailing) the concept of fruit quality is frequently used, but its significance is different depending on the level at which is used: growers, producers, handlers, packers, distributors, retailers, markets, and finally and the most important consumers. However, for all of them the term *quality* is related to the degree of excellence and absence of defects of a fresh produce, which implies sensory attributes (appearance, color, texture, flavor, and aroma), and nutritive (chemical components used to obtain energy) and functional (vitamins and other non-nutrients phytochemicals) properties. Shewfelt (1999) suggested that the produce characteristics determine the quality, but the consumer's acceptability is determined by its perception and satisfaction. Thus, quality can be oriented to the product or to the consumer's point of view. Product-oriented quality is generally measured with the aid of analytical determinations, while consumer-oriented quality is based on acceptability or willingness to purchase the fresh produce. Products offered to consumers in the market should fulfill certain external requirements that are perceived by the senses of sight and touch because they are important for the purchase decision. In this sense, dietary guidelines recommending the consumption of fresh fruits (5-a-Day Campaign) will not be successful if consumers show certain dissatisfaction with the product quality, which limits the fruit consumption due to the development of undesirable characteristics.

With regard to overall quality, it is much clearer that quality of fresh fruit or vegetable changes from harvest to consumption. These changes are due to physiological or technological processes related to fruit ripening and ending with senescence, and thus determine the shelf life of a particular fruit. The increase in the storage life of fruits is carried out through the development of new postharvest technologies aimed at reducing the rate of deterioration and maintaining the desirable characteristics of the fruits, leading to a great expansion of the opportunities for the industry to supply high-quality fruits to local and export markets. However, the development of most effective handling procedures and innovative postharvest technologies to ensure the quality without compromising the safety and nutritional value of fruits depends on a better understanding of fruit biology and physiology. In this sense, it is necessary to get better knowledge about the main changes occurring during the normal postharvest life of fruits that lead to quality deterioration: weight loss, visual appearance, softening, loss of flavor and aroma, and decay. All these quality traits will be enhanced if mechanical damage occurs along the commercialization process (from harvest to consumers).

3.3 Weight loss

Preharvest conditions largely affect fruit quality, chemical composition, texture, and postharvest moisture loss (Gómez-Galindo et al., 2004). At time of harvest, the water status of the produce is usually high but after harvesting there are two factors that lead to fruit weight loss: (1) water can no longer be taken up from soil due to the interruption of the plant's natural life cycle, and (2) water transpiration, which is a physical process by which water vapor can permeate the stomas and epidermis. Water is also lost through lenticels, which are gaps in the periderm formed to enable gas exchange for respiration. If the epidermis or periderm is damaged, water loss can be massively exacerbated. The rate of postharvest water loss is dependent primarily on the external vapor pressure deficit, although other factors will influence the situation. Products with a large surface to volume ratio, such as leaf crops, will lose greater percentages of their water far quicker than large spherical fruits. The specific structure of the cuticle and the extent of suberization in the periderm appear to be more important than thickness in improving resistance to the movement of water vapor. Produce varies in the percentage of water that can be lost before quality is markedly reduced (Acked, 2002). Fruits with thick peels, for example, citrus species and bananas, can lose a considerable amount of moisture from the skin without compromising edible quality. Figure 3.1 shows some examples of weight loss of a wide range of fruits after 1 week of storage at 20°C: Lemon, pepino, and tomato had significantly lower percentages of weight loss (below 5%) than stone fruits (apricot, peach, nectarine, and plum). Thus, fruit species is another key factor that determines the rate of weight loss; the cultivar is also significant, since between the Black Diamond (BD) and Golden Japan (GJ) plums, the latter experienced much lower loss of weight. The appearance of the fruit will, however, deteriorate steadily with increasing water loss. Other thin-skinned fruits are more susceptible to water loss, for example, table grapes (Ben-Yehoshua, 1987). When fruits exhibit considerable weight loss, the quality of the product is then regarded as poor due to loss of turgidity, and consumers do not accept a fruit that is soft, dull, and wrinkled. During postharvest, turgidity is a necessary condition for the fresh appearance of the fruit since texture properties and color attributes can affect consumer purchase negatively. Thus, storage conditions will be of crucial importance to maintain the tissue turgidity, for which temperature and relative humidity are among the main factors. In this sense, the optimal storage conditions for each particular fruit need to be set up, which will be addressed in Chapter 4.

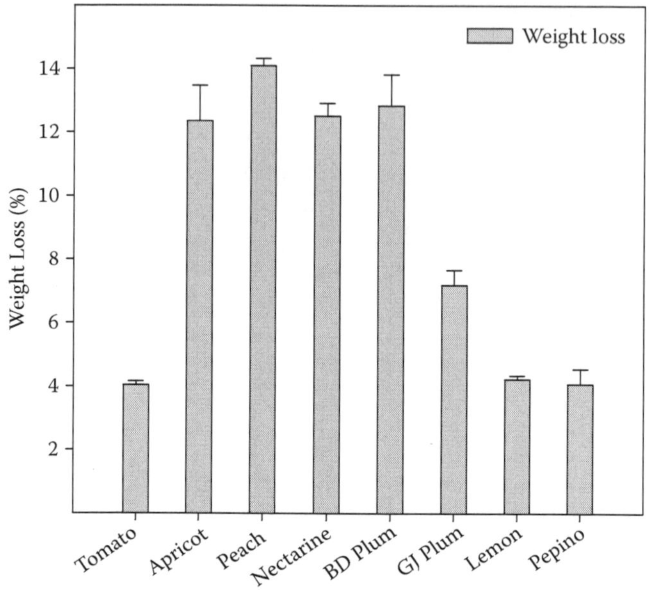

Figure 3.1 Percentage of weight loss in some fruit types after a storage period of 7 days at 20°C. BD and GJ mean Black Diamond and Golden Japan plum cultivars, respectively.

3.4 Appearance

Appearance is the vital factor for consumers in deciding the purchase of fresh produce. In developing countries, consumers expect that fresh fruits have near perfect visual appearance. The display of fruits is characterized by uniformity of size, shape, and color. Essential components of visual quality include color and color uniformity, glossiness, absence of defects in shape or peel, and freedom from diseases. From these components, color contributes more to the assessment of quality than any other single appearance factor.

Natural colors from fruits and vegetables have always been part of human's everyday diet. They have been consumed for generations and help humans to identify food and evaluate its palatability. Color mainly defines the aesthetic value of food, predetermines consumers' expectation of flavor and taste, and modulates appetite. Therefore, color is a major issue for the food industry and the manufacturer will try best to retain the natural appearance of the raw material. However, during storage of fruits color may be altered through the action of light, temperature, oxygen, metal ions, and endogenous enzymes (Stintzing and Carle, 2004). In addition, the color of fruits and vegetables will vary during seasons depending on their intra- and infraspecific variabilities, the edaphic factors at the site of cultivation, and postharvest treatments.

To investigate color quality in a systematic way it is necessary to objectively measure color, as well as pigment concentration. In this context, color denotes the visual appearance of the product whereas pigments or colorants are the chemical compounds that impart the observed color. The CIEL*a*b* system (International Commission on Illumination, Vienna) has been adopted by the food industry for measuring color of food products. While this system does not necessarily give an accurate definition of color, it is very effective for measuring color differences and tracking color changes during storage (Wrolstad et al., 2005).

Most fruits experience color changes as part of the ripening process. Unripe fruit is usually green (the so-called ground color) and in many types of fruit, the green color becomes lighter during ripening and maturation owing to breakdown of chlorophyll, for example, in apples, pears, grapes, and papaya. These color changes affect both peel and pulp tissues, and in many cases the color of the fruit is a strong indicator of the eating quality and shelf life, for example, tomatoes, plums, sweet cherries, and bananas. Figure 3.2 shows the color changes in the peel of several fruits from values at harvest and after 7 days of storage at 20°C. The increase in a* parameter reflects the change from greenish to orange-red while the decrease in Chroma is related to peel darkening. Accordingly, four sweet cherry cultivars picked at two ripening stages (partially ripe and ripe)

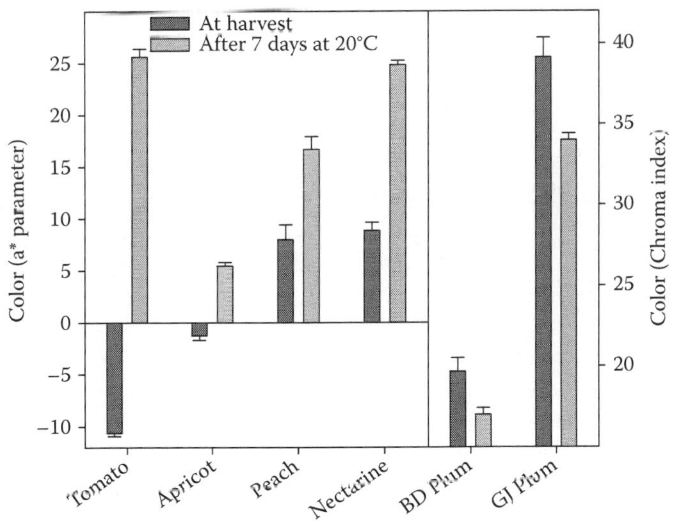

Figure 3.2 Color expressed as a* parameter or Chroma index at harvest and after a period of 7 days at 20°C in some fruit types. BD and GJ mean Black Diamond and Golden Japan plum cultivars, respectively.

showed reductions in color parameters after 6 days of storage at room temperature (Hue angle from ≈40 to 16, on average), which were correlated with an increase in anthocyanin levels (Gonçalves et al., 2007).

3.5 Texture

Fruit *texture* is not an easy term to define since it is composed of a wide range of attributes including type of tissue, water content, and cell wall composition, among others. Bourne (1980) wrote, "The textural properties of a food are that group of physical characteristics that are sensed by the feeling of touch, are related to the deformation, disintegration and flow of the food under the application of a force, and are measured objectively by the functions of force, time and distance." According to this definition, the role of the consumers for produce acceptance is crucial, since they desire the same product but with differences in textural properties.

It is generally accepted that changes in texture occur normally during growth and development on tree (Chapter 2, Section 2.3.3) but go on during postharvest storage of fruits, with changes in texture being due to changes in the chemistry of the middle lamella and primary cell wall components—pectins, cellulose, and hemicelluloses—that accelerate fruit softening. The primary cell wall of fruits undergoes structural and compositional changes as the fruits soften during ripening (Brady, 1987). During softening, pectins are solubilized and sequentially disassembled by increasing the rate of depolymerization of several pectin classes and are accompanied by a net loss of some neutral sugars, particularly galactose and/or arabinose. Hemicelluloses, and especially xyloglucans, can also suffer some degradation that will affect the cellulose microfibrils, since xyloglucans are tightly bonded to the cellulose complex.

As explained in Chapter 2, the breakdown of the cell wall and dissolution of the middle lamella that accompanies fruit ripening are at least partially caused by the degradation of pectic polysaccharides by enzymes capable of altering cell wall texture such as PME, endo- and exo-PG, α- and β-GAL, cellulase, α-L-arabinosidase, β-glucosidase, β-xylosidase, α-L-fucosidase, α-L-rhamnosidase, arabinoxylanase, feruloyl esterase, and XET (Brownleader et al., 1999; Brummell, 2006; Goulao and Oliveira, 2008). However, differences exist in the type and extent of the modification of the polysaccharides of the cell wall and in the expression and regulation of cell wall–modifying enzymes depending on the fruit type and even among cultivars of the same fruit species. Figure 3.3 shows some examples of the values in fruit firmness of a wide range of fruits at harvest and after 7 days of storage at 20°C: Lemon and pepino showed significantly lower percentages of firmness loss (26–40%) than tomato (55%) or stone fruits (apricot, peach, nectarine, and plum), with 70–90%. In this sense, fruit species is an important factor determining the rate of softening. It

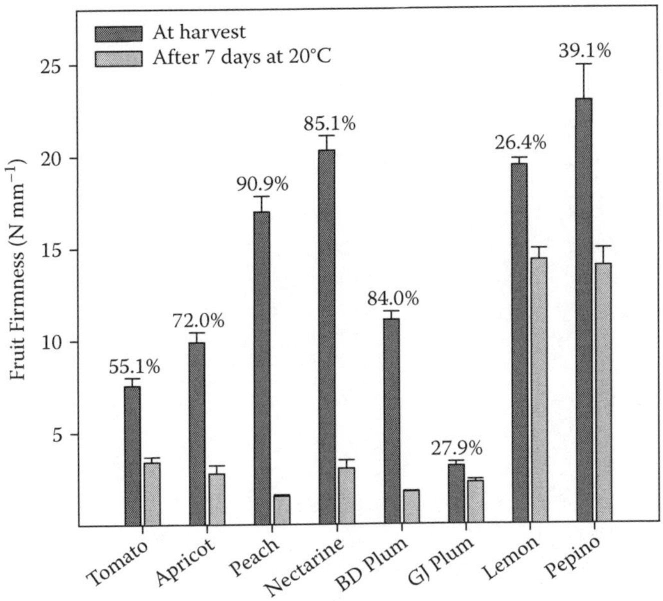

Figure 3.3 Fruit firmness at harvest and after a period of 7 days at 20°C in a wide range of fruits. Percentage number above bars indicates the firmness loss with respect to value at harvest for each fruit. BD and GJ mean Black Diamond and Golden Japan plum cultivars, respectively.

is interesting to point out that different cultivars from the same species could also show a different behavior, since Black Diamond plum exhibited much higher firmness loss (85%) than Golden Japan plums (28%).

During the last decades, research efforts have been focused on the role of PG and PME as the main responsible enzymes for the ripening-associated pectin modifications that lead to softening during postharvest storage, mainly due to their significance in tomato as the climacteric model fruit. The development of tomato transgenic plants with modified ethylene biosynthesis and perception and with modified expression PG and PME has supported the idea that ethylene regulation of fruit cell wall metabolism is a central feature of climacteric fruit ripening and plays an important role in fruit softening. In addition, the PME action for the de-esterification of pectin in the cell wall softening could be a prerequisite to the action of PG, while the expression of both enzymes is regulated by ethylene (Bennett and Labavitch, 2008).

Excessive fruit softening is one of the main factors responsible for the limitations of shelf life, storage, and marketability, and thus a poor relationship between firmness at harvest and after storage occurs in those fruits with accelerated softening pattern (stone fruits), while in those commodities with moderate softening rate there is a positive correlation (Goulao and Oliveira, 2008).

The accelerated softening also contributes to the increased occurrence of physical damages during handling and to higher susceptibility to pests and diseases. In fact, it was reported very recently that the cell wall disassembly during tomato ripening was mediated cooperatively by PGs and expansins (EXPs), and then the tomato susceptibility to the necrotropic pathogen *Botrytis cinerea* increased, while the simultaneous suppression of these degrading enzymes in transgenic fruits led to a dramatic reduction in the susceptibility to this fungus (Cantu et al., 2009). Interestingly, the suppression of just one enzyme (either PG or EXP) did not reduce the decay occurrence.

3.6 Flavor, taste, and aroma

In addition to their external appearance and texture changes in fruits, aroma and flavor are becoming key factors that determine the choice to purchase a fruit. Apart from sugars and organic acids, aroma volatiles contribute also to fruit flavor. When a fruit is consumed, the interaction of taste, odor, and textural feeling provides an overall sensation that is best defined by *flavor*. Flavor results from compounds that are divided into categories: those responsible for taste and those contributing to odors, the latter often designated as aroma substances. However, there are compounds that provide both sensations. When it is generally accepted that "flavor life" of the product either has not been reached or has been exceeded before consumption, the main consequence is a dissatisfaction and lower demand for a particular fruit by consumers but there are also commercial consequences.

The compounds responsible for taste are generally nonvolatile at room temperature. Therefore, they interact only with taste receptors located in the taste buds of the tongue. The four important basic taste perceptions are sour, sweet, bitter, and salty. Taste is a fruit attribute considered as a quality indicator too and cannot be separated from other characteristics of the produce. In most cases, the taste of fresh fruits is usually disregarded by consumers, probably due to an internal attribute that cannot be determined by nondestructive taste measurement, as well as the large variation among the fruits harvested at the same time. It is important to point out that taste is being used currently to differentiate one cultivar from another, with economic repercussions. Most growers and marketers use the Brix determination to measure the total soluble solids (TSS), which primarily estimates the sugars content in a particular fruit and thus provides the degree of sweetness. In this sense, consumers are quite familiar with sweetness as a preferable attribute. However, in recent years the perception of taste by consumers is not only related to the content of sugars, and total acidity (TA) is becoming an important factor. For that reason, the ratio between TSS and TA (TSS/TA) is being used as a criterion for ripening index and the degree of a fruit acceptance. A clear example was the reports by Crisosto et al. (2002; 2003) about testing the consumer acceptance of sweet cherries and data counteracted with trained panelists. The main conclusion was that consumer acceptance was related to cherry skin color, with fruits harvested at full bright red and full dark colors being the most scored, but these maturity stages were correlated to the content of soluble solids (16–20%) and values of TA <0.80%. Nevertheless, although TA plays a role in consumer acceptance, within a given TSS range, the importance of TA measurement is less relevant than TSS because TA changes are small in comparison to TSS changes during the cherry maturation/ripening period within a given orchard.

During postharvest there is a general increase in the content of soluble solids, as has been reported for nectarines, apricots, kiwifruits, and strawberries (Aubert et al., 2003, Aubert and Chanforan, 2007; Park et al., 2006; Hernández-Muñoz et al., 2006). This increase in soluble solids is much higher in those fruits that accumulate larger amounts of starch during development on plant, such as mango or bananas. Starch is the principal polysaccharide of green bananas, undergoing important changes during ripening. The average starch content drops from 70 to 80% in the preclimacteric (prior to starch breakdown) period to less than 1% by the end of the climacteric period, while sugars, mainly sucrose, accumulate to more than 10% of the fresh weight of the fruit (Arvanitoyanni and Mavromastis, 2009). In mango, about 7% of starch is accumulated during development, which suffers metabolism to sugars only after harvest for most cultivars (Simão et al., 2008). As shown in Figure 3.4, apricots and nectarines showed these increases in TSS after 7 days of storage at 20°C, while two plum cultivars remained without significant changes. However, different behavior has been reported for tomato cultivars with either maintenance or increases (Kaur et al., 2006) and even decreases, as observed in Figure 3.4 for Rambo cultivar.

The behavior of fruit acidity during postharvest ripening is clearer, since a net decrease in TA has been reported for all the assayed fruits, as can be observed in Figure 3.4 for a range of climacteric fruits, although the magnitude of the diminution is greatly dependent on the fruit species. Other fruits that show reductions in TA during postharvest storage are kiwifruit, strawberry, nectarine, and several apricot cultivars (Aubert et al., 2003, Aubert and Chanforan, 2007, Park et al., 2006; Hernández-Muñoz et al., 2006). The reduction of the acidity associated with postharvest ripening has been attributed to the fact that organic acids are substrates for the respiratory metabolism in detached products.

As addressed in Chapter 2 (Section 2.3.4) aroma substances are volatile compounds that are perceived by the odor receptor sites of the olfactory

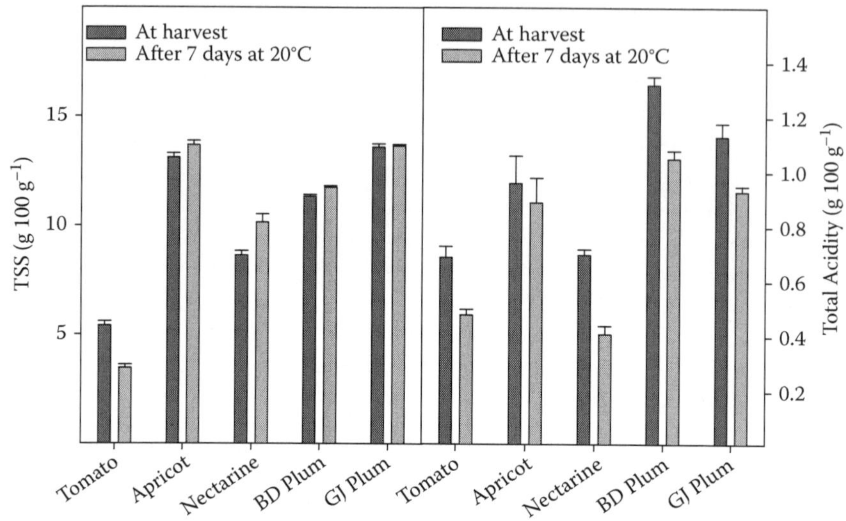

Figure 3.4 Total soluble solids (TSS) and total acidity (TA) at harvest and after a period of 7 days at 20°C in some fruit types. BD and GJ mean Black Diamond and Golden Japan plum cultivars, respectively.

system at the nasal cavity. The concept of aroma substances, like the concept of taste substances, should be used loosely, since a compound might contribute to the typical odor or taste of one food, while in another food it might cause a faulty odor or taste, or both, resulting in an off-flavor. In this sense, one of the major problems in postharvest storage and handling of fruits is the development of off-flavors and loss of authenticity. The appearance and sensation of off-flavors are highly associated with over-maturation and the accumulation of the ethanol fermentation products acetaldehyde and ethanol, which are also volatiles. In general, the higher the storage temperature, the greater is the production of acetaldehyde and ethanol.

In the case of tomato, although 400 compounds have been identified as volatile constituents, only a limited number are essential to flavor: hexanal, (E)-2-heptenal, (E,E)-2,4-decadienal, 6-methyl-5-hepten-2-one, geranylacetone, 2-isobutylthiazole, 1-nitro-2-phenylethane, geranial, and methyl salicylate. From these volatiles, the first eight increased and only methyl salicylate decreased during postharvest storage at 20°C of three tomato cultivars (Krumbein et al., 2004). These authors proved that the intensity of the attribute "tomato-like" aroma increased during storage but so did the undesirable attribute "moldy," and suggested that 2-isobutylthiazole could be responsible for the "off-flavor" occurrence detected in stored tomatoes, which would affect to the sensory quality, and on the contrary, the increase in gernaylacetone would contribute to the "tomato-like" flavor.

Similarly, the storage at 20°C of 28 apricot cultivars induced a general increase in volatile compounds (1.4–8 fold), the most discriminating compounds being lactones (γ-decalactone, γ-nonalactone, γ-octalactone, γ-hexalactone, and γ-jasmolactone), which increased 1–45 fold and were responsible for the fruity aroma of apricot (Aubert and Chanforan, 2007). For this fruit, esters of butyl and hexyl acetates were also found as contributors to apricot aroma. In the case of nectarines, the level of volatiles in the postharvest ripened nectarines could be equal to or higher than the level of volatiles in the tree-ripening fruits. Nevertheless, although the volatile level, in particular lactones and C13-norisoprenoids, were notably higher in samples ripened at 20°C than in those attached to the tree, no differences by sensory evaluation were detected among them with respect to the intensities of "peach odor" or "peach aroma" (Aubert et al., 2003).

3.7 Bioactive compounds

There is little information about the changes in the bioactive molecules with antioxidant activity during the postharvest ripening at ambient temperatures, and in some cases contradictory results have been reported. In kiwifruit, no significant changes in total phenolic concentration and antioxidant activity were found during postharvest storage at 20°C (Park et al., 2006), while in mangoes the content of total phenolic increased although the antioxidant activity remained unchanged (Kim et al., 2009).

In a study of four sweet cherry cultivars during two consecutive years, total phenolics increased after 6 days of storage at ambient temperature in "Van" and "Saco" cultivars but decreased in "Burlat" and did not change in "Summit," suggesting that genotype can have a important influence on the phenolic behavior, apart from ripening stage or harvest year (Gonçalves et al., 2004). The diminution in total phenolics was reflected in neochlorogenic acid (the main polyphenol in sweet cherries belonging to the hydroxycinamate group), which decreased in "Burlat" and increased in the remaining cultivars.

With respect to ascorbic acid, on general, freshly harvested fruits and vegetables contain more vitamin C than those held in storage (Lee and Kader, 2000). However, ascorbic acid concentration and total antioxidant activity (TAA) increased during postharvest ripening at 20°C in the Japanese plum Tegan Blue (Khan et al., 2009).

3.8 Decay

Fruit and vegetables contain a wide range of organic acids (Chapter 2, Section 2.3.2) and high water activity, and thus are good substrates for microbial spoilage. However, the low pH of fruits leads to their spoilage being predominantly by fungi, while vegetables, in contrast, have pH values closer to neutrality and thus both fungi and bacteria cause spoilage (Moss, 2008). In general, mold spoilage of fruits does not lead to health hazard, since the commodities are usually rejected, but the economic losses are considerably important due to decay occurrence.

Fungal pathogens exploit through main routes to penetrate the host tissue: (1) through wounds caused by biotic and/or abiotic agents during growth or storage, (2) through natural openings such as lenticels, stem-ends, and the pedicel-fruit interfaces, and (3) by directly breaching the host cuticle. The incidence of fruit decay during postharvest is the result of preharvest latent infection or contamination at harvest, which is manifested during storage, transport, or marketing of the fleshy fruits leading to a net reduction of the postharvest shelf life. An active pathogen can start its attack process immediately after spores land on the host tissue or can remain inactive for months until the harvested fruits ripen, this period being designated as *quiescent stage* (Prusky and Lichter, 2008). Thus, the agricultural industries aim to offer fresh produce that has high-quality standards and is less prone to postharvest decay. There are a wide range of factors that influence the occurrence of decay and its severity that can be grouped at three levels: at preharvest (type and amount of inoculums, cultivar, climatic and environmental conditions, and ripening stage at harvest), at harvest (manual or mechanical methods), and at postharvest (handling procedures, storage conditions, and postharvest treatments).

3.8.1 Preharvest factors

It is clear that preharvest factors influence postharvest decay, and thus the initial step in reducing postharvest decay is to gain an effective control of fungi in the field and at the time of harvest. Accordingly, most growers, producers, and packers have developed a series of guidelines called Good Agricultural Practices (GAP), which start at bloom and finish with the harvest of each commodity. More recently, Good Postharvest Practices have been suggested to be established during the postharvest life of agricultural products (Michailides and Manganaris, 2009).

Because they are rich in moisture and nutrients, mature fruits are good hosts for several microorganisms, especially some typical fungi and bacteria of the harvested and stored fruits and vegetables, although in most cases the microorganisms come from the field. In fact, the primary source of inoculums is the seed and the obtained plants are accompanied by the pathogens along the growth cycle, which are quiescent but express the symptoms later during storage. The examination of the scientific literature reveals that many of the airborne fungi are among the most important decay agents that affect harvested fruits developing and causing decay. The main fungal species in fruits belong to the genera

Table 3.1 The Main Fungal Pathogens of the Fruits and the Corresponding Diseases

Fungal species	Fruit target	Diseases
Alternaria citri	Citrus fruits	Stem-end rot
Alternaria alternata	Tomato, apple, grapes, pepper, melon, plum, peach, nectarine, apricot, pear, sweet cherry	Fruit rot, dark spot Sooty mold
	Avocado, mango, papaya, persimmon	Stem-end rot, black rot
Penicillium expansum	Apple, pear	Blue mold
Penicillium digitatum	Citrus fruits	Green mold
Penicillium italicum	Citrus fruits	Green mold
Penicillium spp.	Tomato, melon	Green mold
Aspergillus niger	Tomato, grape, date, melon	Black rot, brown rot
Fusariumm verticilloides	Banana, pineapple	Black heart
Botrytis cinerea	Strawberry, raspberry, grape, persimmon, tomato, pepper, melon, stone fruits, pome fruits	Gray mold
Cladosporium herbarum	Date, grape, pome and stone fruits, papaya, fig, tomato, pepper, melon	Olive-green mold Sooty mold
Colletotrichum gloesporoides	Avocado, mango, papaya, guava, Citrus fruits	Anthracnose
	Pome and stone fruits	Bitter rot
Monilinia fructicola	Stone fruits	Brown rot
Monilinia fructigena	Pome fruits	Brown rot
Mucor piriformis	Tomato, strawberry, raspberry, melon	Watery soft rot
Rhizopus stolonifer	Strawberry, raspberry, sweet cherry, grape, avocado, papaya, tomato, pepper, melon	Watery soft rot

Alternaria, Botrytis, Cladosporium, Colletotrichum, Aspergillus, Penicillium, Monilinia, Rhizopus, Mucor, and *Fusarium.* Table 3.1 summarizes the main fungi responsible for diseases in specific fruits and it can be observed that stone fruits (peach, nectarine, plum, sweet cherry, and apricot), pome fruits (pear and apple) and the *Solanaceae* tomato and pepper are the main hosts for fungal development and incidence of decay. It is well accepted that the severity of the infection is directly correlated with the level of the inoculums, and therefore increased spore concentrations usually lead to higher rates of infection and lesion formation, as could be observed in tomato for *Botrytis cinerea* (Eden et al., 1996). Thus, two ways to minimize postharvest decay are the reduction of inoculums in the field and minimization of injury and damage to tissues postharvest. In this case a close relationship exists between the spore load on the fruit surface and the availability of wounds for penetration. In this sense, proper sanitation in the field, packinghouses, and storage facilities will help to reduce the occurrence and spread of the disease (Barkai-Golan, 2001).

One of the preharvest factors that may affect postharvest quality is the cultivar, since the cultivars among each plant species can vary greatly in their susceptibility to diseases. In fact, one of the aims of plant breeding and genetic engineering is to incorporate resistance genes in new varieties of crops. Differences in cultivar characteristics can markedly affect the keeping quality of the fresh produce. Thus, large variations in postharvest decay among apple cultivars has been related to differences in the wounding resistance of their skins, a feature that may be of major importance for decay pathogens that depend on a wound to initiate infection (Spotts et al., 1999).

Environmental conditions during growth, such as extremely high or low temperature, wind, rain, and hail, can affect the crop and determine not only the yield but also the quality of the stored commodity. High temperature was found to increase *Botrytis cinerea* infection of tomatoes via the flowers because it increased the rate of flower development and senescence (Eden et al., 1996). Environmental conditions may also affect the pathogens directly. Many pathogens persist in the soil or survive on plant debris in the field, from which winds and rain may be directly responsible for dispersing to potential hosts. Some cultural practices, such as pruning of fruit trees and destruction of crop debris, can markedly affect the survival of pathogenic fungi, as can the application of preharvest fungicides, which reduce the level of infestation by directly killing the microorganism. However, preharvest chemical sprays with the same chemical that is designated for postharvest application can enhance the production of new fungal strains resistant to that fungicide (Barkai-Golan, 2001).

The ripening stage at harvest is a key factor determining the susceptibility of the fruit to develop decay. On a general basis, as ripening advances the fruits become more susceptible to pathogen attack, which could be also related to the increased susceptibility to be injured. During the ripening process, the typical changes in acidity, sugars, softening, and water availability (Chapter 2) could induce enhancements in the susceptibility to disease, especially near the onset of senescence. In addition, a special role of ethylene (the ripening plant hormone) is attributed to decay occurrence in fruits, both climacteric and nonclimacteric ones. One example is the use of ethylene as a degreening agent in the *Citrus* industry. Degreening is a common commercial practice in many parts of the world that is used to enhance the appeal of the fruits for consumers by the removal of the green color from the peel of orange and lemon fruits by exposure to ethylene after harvest. Usually, ethylene is applied at 5–10 μL L^{-1} during a period of 1–5 days at temperature 20–22°C and relative humidity of 90–95% (Smilanick et al., 2006), and rapid chlorophyll degradation with concomitant carotenoid synthesis occurs during the treatment, although this environment is optimum for developing green mold by *P. digitatum* with losses between 4–30% of total fruits. To solve this problem, either preharvest fungicide application or thermal curing methods during postharvest are currently employed. The mechanism by which the exogenous ethylene induces decay in citrus is not well elucidated, although it has been hypothesized that ethylene might stimulate fungal growth as well as the activation of several hydrolytic enzymes, such as PG and cellulase, at the cell wall and that the inhibition of the natural antifungal activity of the peel by ethylene should not be discharged (Barkai-Golan, 2001).

3.8.2 Harvesting factors

Mature fruits are more sensible to injuries induced during the harvesting process and therefore more susceptible to the attack of those pathogens that require a damaged tissue to facilitate the penetration. Manual harvesting is the predominant method for highly perishable fruits destined for the fresh produce market, and therefore appropriate trained personnel can keep damage to a minimum, with the disadvantages of the high economic and time costs. The other alternative is mechanical harvesting, which even when used correctly can cause substantial damage to the commodity, which may serve as suitable areas of penetration for the pathogens. Mechanical harvest is used to handle large quantities of commodities rapidly and the systems include trunk shake-and-catch and many times are aided by the use of abscission agents, as for oranges (Burns et al., 2006), although mechanized harvest of apples can predispose the stem cavity to blue mold decay by *P. expansum*, which could be reduced by the use of biocontrol (Peterson, 2005).

3.8.3 Postharvest factors

The postharvest diseases causing spoilage of fruits are widespread due to improper transportation and handling procedures (enhanced levels of injuries or wounds). The harvested produce might be infected by pathogens prior to harvest under field conditions or they may get infected during transit and storage. It is estimated that in the developed countries, about 25% of all perishable fruits harvested are lost between harvest and consumption, while this percentage increases up to 50–70% in underdeveloped countries. Thus, appropriate postharvest management is of special importance to provide commodities with high quality standards and reduced incidence of decay.

The presence of a pathogen on the surface and its penetration will not ensure that the disease will be developed. The development of the fungi will appear when the conditions are optimal, the main factors being appropriate temperature and relative humidity (RH), the presence of available nutrients, suitable pH value, and other environmental conditions. The germination of the spores and mycelium growth is strictly dependent on the temperature, which is considered the limiting factor for the development of the disease. On a general basis, the optimal temperature for growth of most storage fungi is 20–25°C, although some species prefer higher or, more rarely, lower temperatures. However, the optimum temperature for growth is not necessarily identical to the optimum for germination. The deviations of the optimal temperature will prolong the required time for initiation of the germination, the mycelium growth, and the duration of the incubation period of the disease, that is, the time until the appearance of decay symptoms (Barkai-Golan, 2001).

The high RH required for the protection of fruits from dehydration and weight loss can stimulate pathogen development during storage. The severity of decay is enhanced by the condensation of mist over the fresh fruit or vegetable surface. In this sense, the susceptibility of many fruits to fungal decay is enhanced when the pathogens encounter tissues with elevated levels of turgidity, as occurs under high RH. In many cases, the increased decay rate should be attributed to moisture held within the wounds, lenticels, or stomata under these conditions. Fungal spores use this moisture for germination previously to their penetration into the tissues. This is the main reason that some fruit commodities, such as grapes and strawberries, cannot be washed during the handling process, since the excess of humidity will favor the decay occurrence.

With respect to pH, most of the fruits are characterized by low pH (pH<5), this factor being the most important for the general resistance to bacterial decay, but it favors the postharvest development of various fungi. In fact, fungi cause most of the decays in harvested fruits, whereas bacteria are important mainly in vegetables. However, the ripening stage at harvest influences the fruit susceptibility to fungal decay, and for most of the cases this susceptibility increases as ripening process advances, which could be related to the enhanced occurrence to be injured. It is clear that TA, nutrient availability, and tissue turgidity change during the ripening process and especially when senescence is initiated, these changes being related to the enhancement of fungal decay more in mature fruits than in immature ones.

Finally, the plant hormone ethylene plays a key role in the fungal decay of fruits. Generally, an increase in ethylene production is observed during the interaction between a host and a pathogen. It has been suggested that ethylene released during infection represents an early response of plants to the perception of a pathogen attack and can be associated with induction of a defense reaction. However, ethylene is considered to be very important in the development of disease symptoms, although the specific role is still unknown. One of the most studied interactions between fungi and ethylene has been *B. cinerea*, which causes grey mold. Fungal hyphae can penetrate through wounds or natural openings of the plant tissue and spread from previously colonized dead tissues into healthy tissues. Usually, grey mold development is associated with an increase in ethylene production from the infected tissues, which is most often attributed to the host plant (Elad and Eversen, 1995), although the release of ethylene by *B. cinerea* has been also reported (Cristescu et al., 2002). These authors postulated that *B. cinerea* produced greater amounts of ethylene as conidia inoculated *in vitro* or in the climacteric tomato fruit exhibited an increased ethylene concentration. More recently, infected table grapes with *B. cinerea* exhibited higher productions in both ethylene and respiration rate, which were attributed to the fungal growth, since grapes are nonclimacteric fruits (Martínez-Romero et al., 2007b).

Thus, both respiration and ethylene evolution are important indicators of the physiological state of the fruit, and their enhancement following infection highlights its effects on the postharvest ripening and senescence processes.

3.9 Mechanical damage versus fruit quality

Injury is the heaviest stress, at least at the cellular level, and happens not only in the natural environment but also is frequently involved in harvesting and postharvest handling of agricultural products. Physical injury is possibly the most important cause of loss in quality in fresh produce by the indirect effect of creating a wound in the surface of the produce.

This wound is an ideal entry point for many postharvest pathogens as described previously. Injury also allows water loss, which compromises the quality of the produce. Furthermore, physical injury stimulates ethylene production in plant tissues, which can lead to premature yellowing or ripening of commodities.

Mechanical damage is considered as a type of stress that occurs during the postharvest manipulation of fruits. This stress is accompanied by physiological and morphological changes that affect the fruit commodity. Mechanical damage of fruits and vegetables, as a consequence of inappropriate harvest, manipulation, and transport techniques, is one of the most common and severe defects; it has great economic repercussions, mainly due to negative changes in organoleptic attributes (skin and flesh browning and off-flavors) and internal breakdown reactions. Fresh fruits need to be manipulated at different stages from the orchard to the industry before reaching consumers. At each of these stages, injuries can be induced resulting in quality reduction. These injuries could be either externally visible and easily detectable or nonexternally visible because internal bruising is masked by external color.

The definition of mechanical damage is not completely clear and authors give different definitions; however, there is a general coincidence: mechanical damage is caused by one or more loading types. In this sense, Bollen et al. (1995) described two different types of mechanical damage during fruit postharvest handling: (1) impacts during fruit harvest, selection, manipulation, and transport and (2) compression loads during packing lines or storage. Other researchers have considered more types of mechanical damage sources: abrasions between fruit and accompanied materials (stones, stems, and insects); impacts with other fruit or with containers or machinery (conveyor belt); and puncture and prolonged vibrations during transportation.

The development of mechanical damage depends on whether the displacement exceeds the elastic limit, resulting in cell-wall rupture and a reduced tissue integrity, such as has been observed to occur in peaches, tomatoes, pears, apples, papayas, mandarins, lemons, and cucumbers (Martínez-Romero et al., 2004). Consequently, citosolic contents leak from the internal cells and release to the intercellular spaces, resulting in a net increase of weight loss (Miller, 1992). The next events are related to the activation of the enzymes present in the extruded cellular content that are responsible for browning (peroxidase [POX]; and polyphenoloxidase [PPO]) or to tissue degradation by the action of hydrolytic enzymes such as PG and PME. Finally, mechanically damaged tissues are the key factor determining pathogen invasion that results in decay.

Mechanical damage causes physiological changes at hormonal, genetic, and biochemical levels besides at the physical level. Some of the modifications that occur naturally during fruit ripening are accelerated after the mechanical damage has been induced, especially at the senescence stage. However, different signals can be used as indicators or markers of the mechanical stress, such as ethylene, polyamines (PAs), and abscisic acid (Martínez-Romero et al., 1999). Ethylene plays a key role in the fruit response against mechanical stress, with stress increasing ethylene levels in climacteric and nonclimacteric fruits. The response of this hormone immediately follows the mechanical damage (between 2–3 hours) and lasts 2–10 hours. This ethylene is the so-called wound ethylene, as it has been observed, for example, in damaged peaches with compression forces of 30, 40, and 50 N, in which the ethylene emission was proportional to the impact intensity 3–5 h after the mechanical damage was induced. Also, apricots artificially damaged with compression forces of 25 N showed higher ethylene production along storage than nondamage controls and an advancement of the climacteric peak of ethylene production was found compared with nondamaged apricots (Martínez-Romero et al., 2004). This higher ethylene emission rate is attributed to the increase of ACC synthesis by activation of the enzyme ACS and its posterior conversion to ethylene (Miller, 1992). Accordingly, studies over the last decade showed that production of wound ethylene in fruits is controlled by a coordinated expression of both ACS and ACO genes; the latter was revealed often to have a positive feedback control by ethylene. There are indications that the wound-stimulated activity of the enzymes of the ethylene biosynthesis pathway is mediated by post-transcriptional/translational control and/or enzyme turnover (Druege, 2006).

Another physiological parameter that could be affected by mechanical damage is the increased respiration rate. It is well known that respiration rate is a sensitive physiological indicator of mechanical stress or wounding in both vegetative tissues and fruits, with production being linearly correlated with the number of impacts and the increasing loads in blueberries and sweet cherries (Burton and Schulte-Paso, 1987). The high CO_2 production was also correlated with the percentage of fruit decay. Another indirect indicator of damage is weight loss, as has been studied in several fruits, including lemons, oranges, peaches, apricots, and blueberries (Martínez-Romero et al., 2004). The increased weight loss in damaged fruits is perhaps due to changes in their biophysical properties: modification of cellular arrangements and tissue permeability, occurrence of small fissures connecting the fruit internal and external atmospheres (which would accelerate gas transfer, particularly water vapor), and increased respiration rate (Woods, 1990).

There are other quality parameters that could be affected by mechanical damage, such as TSS, which was found to increase in kiwifruits (Mencarelli et al., 1996) and was more evident at high temperatures. Thus, the increase in TSS could be explained simply by lower moisture contents existing at high temperatures due to weight loss. Another experimental observation made in mechanically damaged fruits (postulated as an indicator of the mechanical damage) is the increase in PPO and POX activities, which are responsible for significant decrease in the content of total phenolic compounds observed in mango (Ketsa and Atantee, 1998). In nondamaged fruits, the phenolic compounds are localized mainly in vacuoles while POX is localized mainly in the cell walls and PPO in the chloroplast. If fruits are mechanically damaged, the cell wall structures are deteriorated and the phenolic compounds may leak and get in direct contact with highly active POX and/or PPO. These enzymes oxidize the phenolic compounds to brown melaninic compounds that will brown the damaged tissue (Friedman, 1996). The final result of these enzymatic reactions may be the synthesis of lignin, which may form complexes with other compounds such as carbohydrates, proteins, and pectins, resulting in strong lignin complexes (Ketsa and Atantee, 1998).

In summary, to avoid the occurrence of mechanical damage and its physiological and technological implications, it is necessary to detect the critical points where the impact, compression, and vibration energies originating the mechanical damage are produced in order to reduce the quality loss occurring during fruit handling.

chapter four

Cold storage and fruit quality

4.1 Introduction

Fruits and vegetables are well known to be highly perishable, the rate of deterioration being dependent on the respiration rate, which varies primarily with the type of produce, the temperature, and the level of physiological stress caused by harvesting or postharvest processing. Thus, it is necessary not only to chill the product but to cool it as quickly as possible after harvest in order to arrest the deteriorative and senescence processes and to maintain a high level of quality that ensures customer satisfaction. In fact, temperature control is the single most important factor to maintain quality and reduce the deterioration rate of harvested commodities, since it is widely accepted that the rate of deterioration after harvest is closely related to the respiration rate of the harvested product and this is dependent on temperature (Kader, 2002).

4.2 Effect of low temperature storage on fruit metabolism

The main effect of the low temperature application during postharvest storage is a reduction of the fruit metabolism and consequently a delay of the evolution of the parameters related to fruit ripening and quality loss (Chapter 3). One of the main parameters determining the metabolic activity of a fruit is its respiration rate, which is usually associated with the commodity deterioration. Respiration rate of a produce is dependent on a wide range of variables, of which temperature is considered the most important in modulating this physiological parameter. As can be seen in Figure 4.1, the respiration rate of apple, orange, lemon, and banana increased as the assay temperature was enhanced, although differences exist among fruit types. Thus, at 30°C oranges showed a respiration rate of ~40 mg kg^{-1} h^{-1} while banana showed ~170 mg kg^{-1} h^{-1}. Moreover, differences were also found in the temperature at which the maximum respiration rate was achieved, this temperature being 50°C for apple and orange, 45°C for lemon, and 40°C for banana. The diminution of the temperature led to a reduction in the respiration rate for all fruits, and calculated Q_{10}, that is, the reduction of the reactions between two

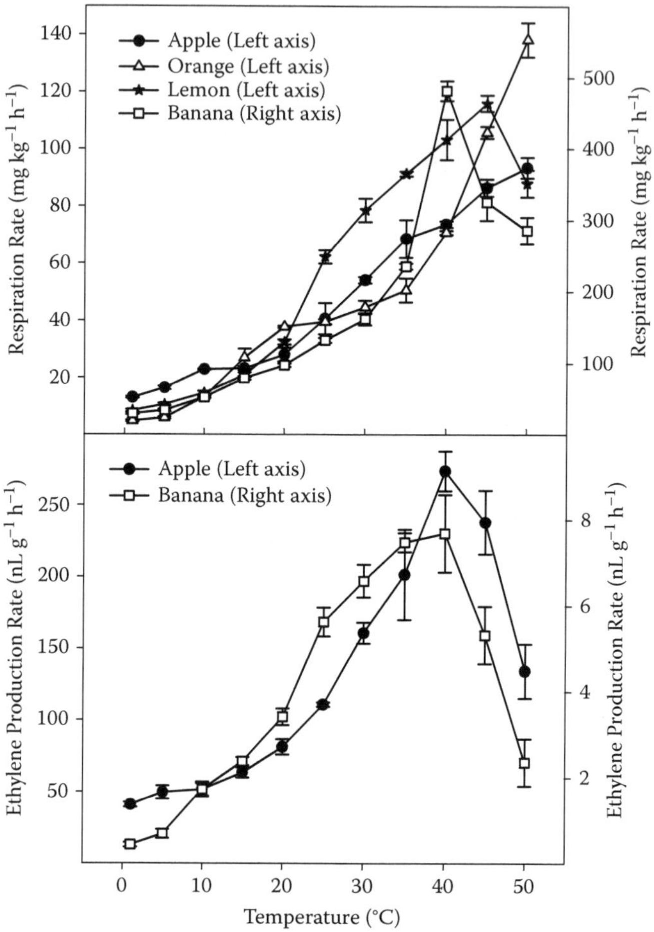

Figure 4.1 Respiration and ethylene production rates in some fruits as affected by temperature. Data are the mean ± SE of determinations made in five fruits.

temperatures that differ in 10°C, was 1.63 for apple and 1.9 for the other fruits. Interestingly, at the lowest temperature (1°C) there were still differences among fruits and respiration rates followed the same sequence, with banana having the highest and orange the lowest (≈40 and 5 mg kg^{-1} h^{-1}, respectively).

The reduction in storage temperature has the added advantage of reducing the production and sensitivity of ethylene, with special interest in the climacteric fruits since this hormone accelerates the ripening process and senescence in them. In fact, the maximum ethylene production in the assayed climacteric fruits (banana and apple) was obtained at 40°C, and the reduction of the temperature significantly decreased the ethylene production (Figure 4.1), although differences existed between two fruits for whichever temperature. Thus, at 40°C banana produced the highest rate (≈230 nL g^{-1} h^{-1}) compared with the apple (≈9 nL g^{-1} h^{-1}).

These effects in slowing down the rates of respiration and ethylene production by lowering temperature lead to a delay in the evolution of the parameters related to fruit ripening and quality, such as color, acidity, and texture. Thus, apricots and tomatoes stored at 20°C showed a threefold higher increase in color a* parameter than those fruits stored at 2 and 8°C, respectively, over 7 days (Figure 4.2). Accordingly, the decrease in acidity was fourfold higher at 20°C than at 2 or 8°C in apricot and tomatoes, respectively (Figure 4.3). The softening process is also affected by temperature, as can be seen in Figure 4.4 for a wide range of stone fruits, in which the firmness loss was ~80–90% after 7 days at 20°C, while these losses oscillated between 6 and 30% when these fruits were stored at 2°C for the same period.

According to this evidence it is clear that fruit and vegetable products need to be stored at low temperatures as soon as possible after harvesting in order to reduce the metabolic activity of plant tissues. Some postharvest cooling techniques with some advantages and disadvantages depending on the fruit commodity characteristics will be addressed in the next section.

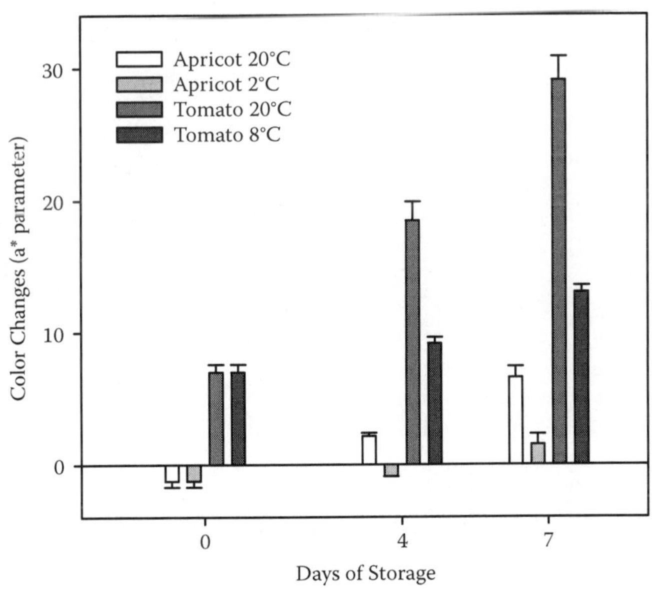

Figure 4.2 Color (a* parameter) evolution in apricot fruits during postharvest storage at 2 or 20°C and in tomato fruits at 8 or 20°C.

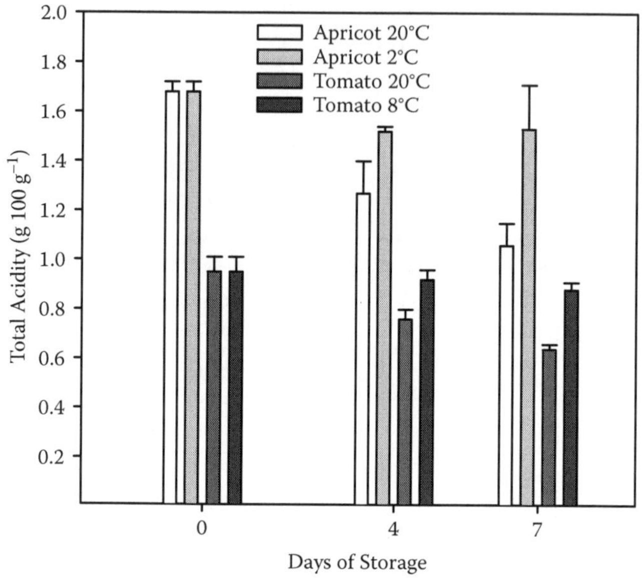

Figure 4.3 Total acidity evolution in apricot fruits during postharvest storage at 2 or 20°C and in tomato fruits at 8 or 20°C.

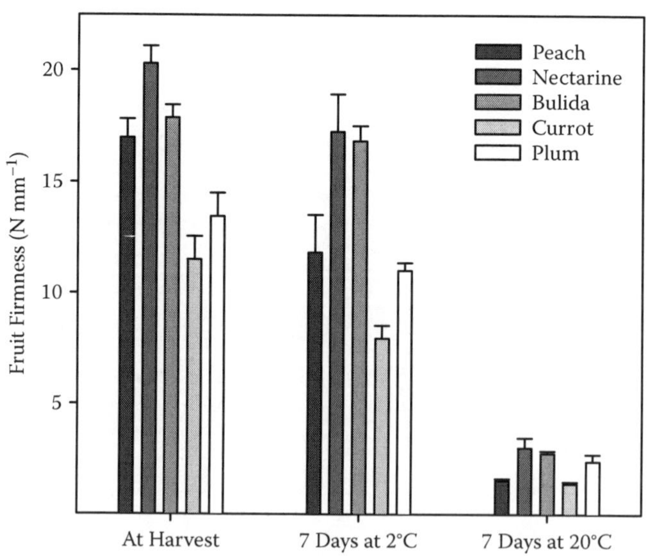

Figure 4.4 Fruit firmness at harvest and after 7 days of storage at 2 or 20°C in some stone fruits. Bulida and Currot are apricot cultivars.

4.3 Cooling rates

The rate of cooling produce depends primarily on many factors including rate of heat transfer, difference in temperature between the produce and the cooling medium, thermal properties of the produce, size and shape of the produce, nature of the cooling medium, type of packaging (if any), and stacking arrangement. The rate of cooling of a particular product is not constant but diminishes exponentially as the temperature difference reduces; that is, product cooling follows a logarithmic function, with rapid cooling initially followed by a slower and slower rate. All cooling rate graphs follow a similar basic curve. However, because the rate of cooling varies over time, two single parameters have been adopted to describe the cooling process: cooling coefficient (C) and half-cooling time (Z). The temperature ratio (*Y*) is the unaccomplished temperature change at any time in relation to the total temperature change possible for a particular cooling condition. It is calculated according to the formula: $Y = (T - T_{\mathrm{m}})/(T_{\mathrm{i}} - T_{\mathrm{m}})$, where the subscripts *i* and *m* represent initial and cooling medium temperatures, respectively, and *T* indicates the temperature at any point in the product. The cooling coefficient represents the change in product temperature per unit change of cooling time for each degree temperature difference between the product and its surroundings, and can be calculated by the following formula, with the cooling time θ expressed in hours: $C = (\ln Y_1 - \ln Y_2)/(\theta_1 - \theta_2)$.

The half-cooling time is the time required to reduce the temperature difference between the product and its surroundings (cooling medium) by one-half (Z). Theoretically, the half-cooling time is independent of the initial product temperature and remains constant throughout the cooling period. Therefore, if it takes 2 hours to reduce a crop temperature to 50% of its original value, it will take a further 2 hours to reduce it to 25%, a further 2 hours to reduce it to 12.5%, and so on. Another useful parameter is the seven-eighths (7/8) cooling time (S), which is the time required to reduce the temperature difference between the product and its surroundings by seven-eighths. This is also independent of the initial product temperature and is of more practical use in commercial cooling operations because the temperature of the produce at the seven-eighths cooling time is acceptably close to the required storage or transport temperature and is equal to three half-cooling times. Figure 4.5 shows an example for plum cooled in a forced-air cold chamber at 0.5°C. The initial fruit temperature was 24°C and the half-cooling time (Z) was 15 min, while the required time for the 7/8 was 66 min.

However, in systems where the cooling rate is rapid, the temperature change in the interior of the produce lags considerably behind the change in surface temperature, especially for bulky products such as melons. In

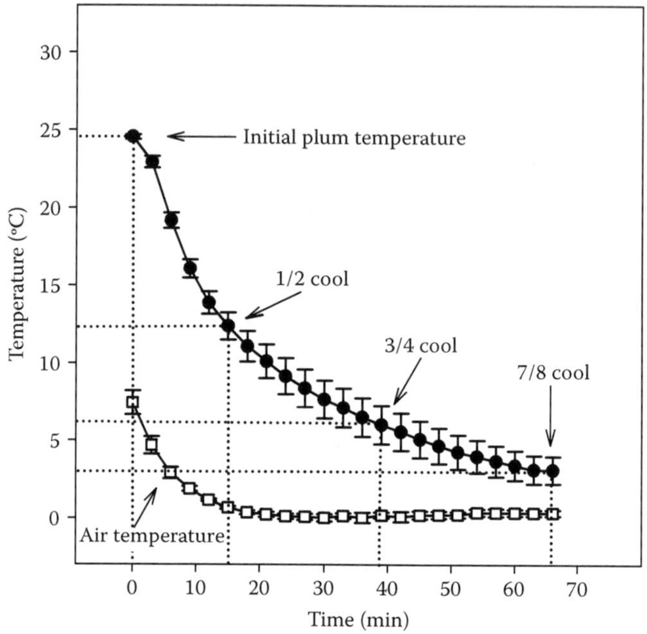

Figure 4.5 Temperature change in plums cooled in a forced-air cold chamber over time showing the half (1/2), three-fourth (3/4), and seven-eighth (7/8) cooling times.

these cases the limiting factor is the rate of heat conduction from the core to the surface of the product. This positional lag effect can alter the relative difference in time between *S* and *Z* such that *S* may range from 2*Z* (3/4) to 3*Z* (7/8).

Mathematically, the half-cooling time is expressed as $Z = \ln(0.5)/C$, or it can also be calculated by $Z = [-0.693 \times \text{target cooling time (h)}]/\ln[(T_2 - T_m)/(T_1 - T_m)]$. Similarly, the 7/8 cooling time is expressed as $S = \ln(8j)/C$, where *j* is the lag factor and *C* is the cooling factor, and thus is core temperature divided by the surface temperature, and may vary from 1 to 2 (Brosnan and Sun, 2001).

4.4 *Precooling techniques*

The precooling process is the removal of field heat by a cooling treatment to reduce the temperature of horticultural commodities promptly and rapidly after harvest, which rapidly reduces respiration rate and thus the deterioration rate. The distinction between cooling and precooling is that the latter one involves technologies separate from normal cooling in a refrigerated environment, which is not considered a precooling process because the time required to cool the product is too long. In addition, it is necessary to take into account that some products may be cooled by any of these methods without suffering any loss in quality, while others can be affected adversely depending on the type of cooling technique applied. Moreover, the choice of cooling method is also greatly influenced by the type of packaging used (if any). The produce may be in a box, bin, or bag, which will alter and affect its cooling requirement to achieve rapid temperature reduction. In this sense, the material and packaging design, such as the presence of particular vent holes, have a great effect on the cooling rates. The proper cooling equipment must also be considered depending on product volume to be cooled per season, per day, or per hour, since invariably some cooling techniques are much faster than others and therefore have different throughput of produce. Finally, the construction and operating cost vary greatly among cooling methods and thus the expense of the chosen cooling technique must be justified by higher selling prices or other economic benefits.

Figure 4.6 shows several precooling systems applied to lemon fruits. It can be observed that efficacy in reducing the fruit temperature is highly dependent on the precooling system used. Thus, the fastest method was hydro-cooling with a 7/8 cooling time of 50 min, followed by forced air. Moreover, the air rate influences the cooling time, since the 7/8 was 77 minutes with air at 6.5 L/s and increased up to 132 minutes at a flow rate of 1.5 L/s. It is interesting to point out that the slowest method for cooling lemon fruits was the cold room, with a required time of 500 minutes to

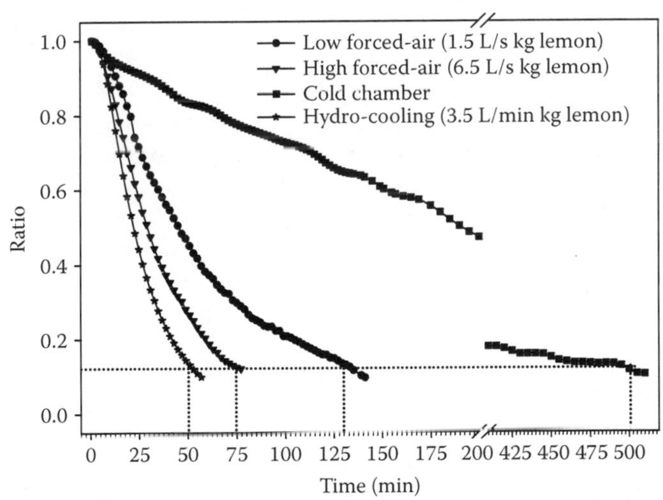

Figure 4.6 Cooling ratio over time of lemon fruits using several precooling systems: forced-air (at low or high air rates), hydro-cooling, and cold chamber. Dotted lines show the 7/8 cooling times.

reach the 7/8 cooling temperature. In this sense, any precooling system will reduce the produce temperature at higher rates than cold rooms. Therefore, cooling rates and appropriate storage temperatures are commodity dependent and different technologies of precooling fruit and vegetables are available, as discussed in the following sections (Brosnan and Sun, 2001; Vigneault et al., 2008).

4.4.1 Room cooling

Room cooling is one of the most widely used forms of cooling horticultural produce, but it should not be considered a precooling method, since room cooling is a natural heat transfer between a mass of produce and the surrounding cool environment, while precooling processes use methods to enhance the heat transfer from the produce. During room cooling, produce in boxes (wooden, fiberboard, or plastic), bulk containers, or various other packages are placed in a refrigerated room where they are exposed to cold air. Typically the cool air is discharged from evaporators near the ceiling and travels across the top and between containers before returning to the evaporator. An air velocity of at least 1–2 m/s is needed to provide the necessary turbulence to efficiently remove field heat and therefore attain adequate cooling. Air velocity should be reduced to 0.05–0.1 m/s for subsequent storage to prevent excessive moisture loss. Better air distribution can be achieved with several small evaporators evenly spaced along one wall than with one large evaporator.

Room cooling has the advantage of using the same room for cooling and for long-term storage of the produce, thus reducing overall handling requirements and costs. However, for the best cooling rates to be achieved more space is required among containers than is good for storage management and thus some rearranging of the produce after cooling may be necessary to utilize the storage space fully. The time to cool the produce to the recommended storage temperature may range from a few hours to several days, depending on produce characteristic and the presence of packages, this cooling time being shorter if the produce is unpacked, since the produce is directly exposed to the cold air. In general, crops that are harvested in the cool season or have low respiration rates are suitable for this method, which has a potential economy, since the refrigeration load is distributed over a longer period and air-flow requirements are often less than for the fast cooling. Nevertheless, room cooling is not recommended for crops that have a high respiration rate or are harvested in the warmer months, since significant quality deterioration may take place during the cooling period.

Standard room cooling can be modified to improve performance by installing a false ceiling in the room and forcing cold air to go into the space between the false ceiling and the roof. Cones in the ceiling conduct the air downwards and pallets are arranged in a manner so that the air from the cones is forced down the corners of the pallets and the air then spreads into the channels between the stacked units. The floor should be marked to ensure the pallets can be properly placed. Another useful modification is the addition of cooling bays. The cooling room is sectioned off into bays by installing partitions and leaving a central aisle for easy access during forklift operations. The flow rate may be controlled for each bay, so warm produce can receive large air flows for cooling and subsequently the flow rate for cooled produce can then be adjusted for optimum storage conditions. In this way, cooled produce in one bay is not warmed by the addition of warm produce in another bay due to the partitions.

4.4.2 Forced-air cooling

Forced-air cooling is a method of precooling applicable to a wide range of produce requiring relatively rapid removal of field heat, since it may be 4 to 10 times faster than room cooling, as can be observed in Figure 4.6, and it results in a more uniform temperature distribution in the pallet. This method works well for small-scale operations due to its cost effectiveness, compared with hydro-cooling or vacuum cooling, and its high cooling rate. Forced-air cooling or pressure cooling is a modification of room cooling in which packages of produce are exposed to higher air pressure on one side than on the other, leading cold air to be forced through the produce rather than just surrounding the produce containers as is done in room cooling. An air circulation system is used to create a static pressure difference across the containers, with a typical value of 12 mm, which produces a more uniform air distribution. Air circulation systems should be selected to operate with these criteria for static pressure and air flow by placing the containers with vent holes in the direction of the moving air and using packaging materials that do not interfere with the free movement of air through the containers (Vigneault et al., 2006).

Forced-air tunnel systems are the most used form of forced-air cooling, in which two rows of palletized containers are placed parallel to each other across an aisle, which is covered on the top and along one end to create a tunnel. A fan is placed at the free end to pull the air out of the tunnel, creating a static pressure difference across the containers. The cool air around the outside of the pallets is pulled through the void in between the produce and into the plenum. The fan may be a portable unit that returns the air to the room or a permanent fan that directs the air back directly to the cooling coils. In the case of the portable fan, the warm air is allowed to return to the room before it is cooled, which may cause condensation on previously cooled produce. To avoid condensation problems, the position of the portable unit must be chosen to direct the warm air to the intake of the cooling system. In the case of permanent fans, the containers must be rearranged after cooling to prevent possible dehydration.

The cooling rate is affected by numerous variables including product size, shape and thermal properties, product configuration (bulk or packages), carton vent area, initial and final desired temperature and air flow rate, and temperature and RH of the storage area. With respect to produce size, Figure 4.7 shows the differences between plum and sweet cherry fruits with respect to the cooling rates in a forced-air cooling system, with values of 7/8 cooling time being 58 and 21 min, respectively. Thus, the fruits with lower size (sweet cherry, 28 mm) experienced a faster cooling rate than plum (50 mm). However, in a given system the velocity of the cool air is the main controlling factor to achieve the desired cooling rate, since no change can be made in certain fixed factors, such as produce properties. In fact, as can be seen in Figure 4.6, the cooling rate of lemon fruit was twofold faster when flow rate was increased from 1.5 to 6.5 L/s. A net disadvantage of the forced-air precooling method is the commodity moisture loss during the process, which is related to the air flow. Nevertheless, new forced-air systems are available now that have a moisture content to avoid excessive produce water loss.

Many other configurations of forced-air systems exist and the main objective of each configuration is to reduce the distance separating the

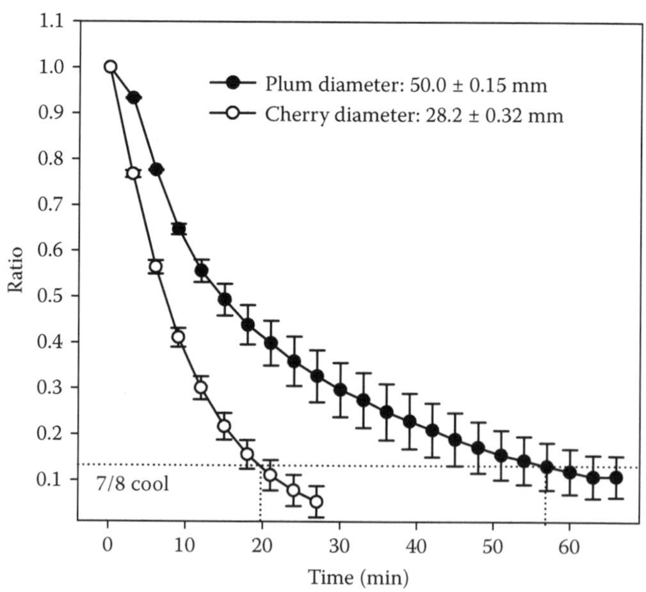

Figure 4.7 Effect of fruit size on cooling ratio over time of plum and cherry fruits using a cold chamber with air forced as precooling system. Dotted lines show the 7/8 cooling times.

circulating air and each individual piece of warm produce by increasing the air flow rate, air turbulence, or air distribution uniformity, or decreasing the energy and the time required. Finally, another aspect of forced-air cooling is that converting the existing facilities is often simple and inexpensive and, in turn, the cost associated with this precooling technology is minimal (Brosnan and Sun, 2001; De Castro et al., 2005; Vigneault et al., 2008).

4.4.3 *Hydro-cooling*

Hydro-cooling involves cooling produce, in bulk or in a small container, with cold water, which is generally kept at 0–0.5°C using mechanical refrigeration to increase the cooling efficiency. This method is very effective for a wide range of produce as water has a much higher heat capacity than air and comes into closer contact with the produce (Silva et al., 2006). In general, cooling times range from 10 minutes to 1 hour, which is from 2 to 20 times faster than forced-air cooling (Figure 4.6). Furthermore, as water can be used efficiently as a temporary heat sink storage system, some hydro-cooling facilities can handle up to 300,000 kg/day during the peak season. In addition, this precooling system has the net advantage of eliminating the commodity moisture loss occurring in the forced-air cooling process. Thereafter, water could be an advantage for some ready-to-eat produce that require washing and need to be gently dried. There are two methods of hydro-cooling: immersion in a cold water bath and shower cooling.

Immersion systems are continuous flow and useful for produce that have a higher density than water and therefore remain submerged. In immersion systems the produce, in bulk or in containers, is conveyed through a tank of cold water and lifted out at the end of the tank by an inclined conveyor. As the conveyor speed is usually too slow to provide adequate water movement around the produce, circulating pumps or propellers are used to promote heat removal from the produce. This is the most rapid hydro-cooling system, due to the fact that moving chilled water completely surrounds the exterior surface of the produce and hence facilitates quicker temperature reduction. However, cooling time varies proportionally to produce volume. In fact, the relationship between volume and time needed to cool fruits and vegetables has been proposed as an index that could be used to estimate cooling time (Teruel et al., 2004).

Flotation of lower density produce in cool circulating water is also used for produce such as cucumbers, squashes, and tomatoes. However, when the produce is immersed in cool water, the air contained inside some commodities decreases sufficiently in volume to create a suction capacity. This factor can be seen in Figure 4.8, in which two different products, lemon and pepper, were hydro-cooled by immersion in cold water at 1°C and the cooling rate was much faster in pepper than in lemon, with

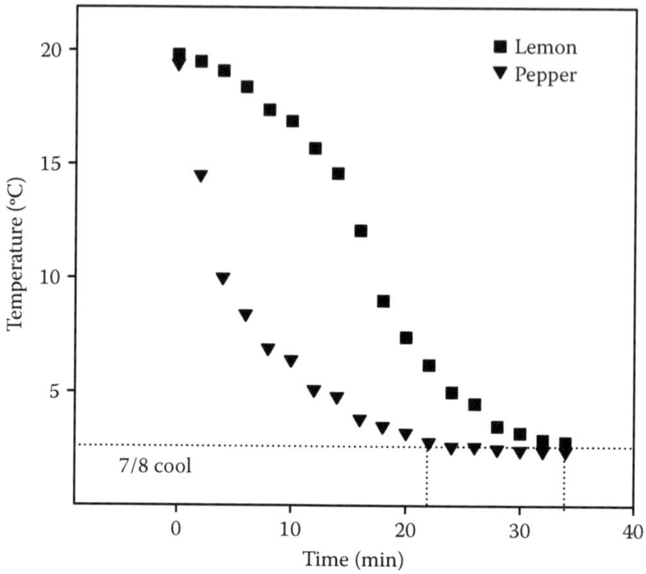

Figure 4.8 Effect of air internal spaces on cooling over time of lemon and pepper fruits using a hydro-cooling dipping as precooling system. Dotted lines show the 7/8 cooling times.

the 7/8 cooling time being 22 and 34 minutes, respectively. Thus, the air inside the pepper facilitates the heat transfer and the cooling efficiency could be increased.

Shower coolers involve overhead spraying of the produce with cold water, and may be batch or continuous systems. The water is either pumped onto an overhead perforated pan and then allowed to drip onto the produce or showered through spray nozzles. The pumping requirements for spray nozzles are much higher than they are for a perforated pan. When water is applied from overhead, the distance of the water falls before hitting the produce should not exceed 150–200 mm depending on the fragility of the produce, since drop heights exceeding this range can damage some products. Produce that are in pallet bins or field bins should be covered with a perforated cover for protection as necessary. In a batch operation, palletized containers are placed in the hydro-cooling system and water is sprayed from the top. The design of hydro-cooling system requires accurate estimation of the hydro-cooling times for each fruit or vegetable, as well as the corresponding refrigeration loads (Becker and Fricke, 2002).

Water quality is a very important consideration in hydro-cooling systems, since pathogens contained in the water may then be pulled into the commodity resulting in disease (Vigneault et al., 2000). Therefore, water should be taken from a clean source and disinfected by adding chlorine

(100–150 ppm), and the system should be sanitized regularly. In addition, screens and filters should be used to remove debris and dirt from the water before it is recycled. In fact, a net reduction in the mold inoculums on the produce surface can be achieved by proper water chlorination and system cleanliness.

Taking into account these considerations, hydro-cooling methods work well on both bulk and packaged produce, although both must be water tolerant. However, to achieve high energy efficiency, the hydro-cooler system must operate at maximum capacity and inside a cold room, due to the great amount of refrigeration required within a short time to reach the desired cooling effect. Thus, since hydro-coolers have a relatively high cost, they must be operating for considerable periods each year to be economically justified (Brosnan and Sun, 2001; Vigneault et al., 2004; 2008).

4.4.4 *Contact-icing*

Contact-icing involves filling packed containers or pallet-boxes or covering these containers with ice, and is one of the oldest and simplest cooling methods. The contact between ice and produce causes cooling of the produce with the cooling time being proportional to the contact efficiency between the ice particles and the produce. There are several different methods of filling the containers with ice, the simplest being to keep the ice on the top of individual packages, although with this method cooling is rather slow as the ice is only in contact with the top layer. In addition, it is not efficient for large operations due to the amount of labor involved in opening the containers, adding the ice and then closing the containers. Moreover, the coating of ice may block vent spaces; thereby restricting air movement and leaving the center of the load warm. Thus, top icing of individual packages should be used only after precooling and prior to shipping to assist in cooling and maintaining a high relative humidity.

An improvement to top icing is pallet box icing by layer, by crushing ice and produce in alternate layers in the pallet box. This method of icing is more labor intensive than top icing but the cooling is faster and more uniform, since the produce is better surrounded by ice and cools faster. Finally, the use of liquid-icing, consisting of a slurry of cold water and ice drenched over the pallet of produce or pumped into the containers through the hand holds, also provides much faster cooling than top icing of individual packages. As the water drains out, ice is distributed throughout the container filling the spaces between the produce, and very good contact between the ice and the produce results in good heat removal. In addition, the cold water of the slurry has a substantial effect on the cooling of the produce.

The main advantage of icing is that produce does not dry as it is cooled. In addition, package icing can maintain low product temperature during transit and therefore refrigerated transportation may not be necessary for short transport duration. However, produce undergoing contact-icing should be tolerant to wet conditions at 0°C for long periods of time and the containers must be water resistant and large enough to accommodate the amount of ice required to cool the produce (Goyette et al., 2000; Brosnan and Sun, 2001; Vigneault and Goyette, 2001; Vigneault et al., 2008).

4.4.5 Vacuum cooling

Vacuum cooling is one of the most rapid cooling methods and it is suitable for produce that have large surface area to mass ratios and easily release water, such as lettuce and other leafy vegetables, sweet corn, celery, green beans, and mushrooms, as well as for cut flowers, which can be cooled in 20–30 minutes (McDonald and Sun, 2000; Rennie et al., 2001). Produce is placed in an air-tight chamber and the pressure in the chamber is decreased to the point that water boils at low temperature. For example, a pressure of 0.610 kPa (4.6 mm Hg) permits water to boil at 0°C. As the energy needed for the phase change of water from liquid to vapor comes from the sensible heat of the produce, the produce cools down close to the boiling temperature in a very short time.

The vacuum cooling itself occurs in two fairly distinct phases. In phase one, the pressure in the vacuum chamber is reduced from an atmospheric one to about 2 kPa and during this time the evaporation is low and relatively little cooling takes place. Phase two starts at approximately the pressure at which the flash point occurs, and as the pressure continues to be reduced the water in the produce begins to vaporize and the produce starts to cool rapidly. This vapor must be removed quickly by using a condenser in the chamber in order to prevent saturation of the air and keep the overall cooling cycle to a reasonable length. However, the evaporation of water results in weight loss of the produce. Thermodynamically, each temperature decrease of 6°C results in a 1% reduction in the weight of the produce due to moisture loss. As this can have detrimental effects on produce quality, the produce can be wetted before vacuum cooling or sprayed with a fine mist during cooling.

The rapid cooling achievable by the use of vacuum cooling makes it more attractive and gives it a distinct advantage over other precooling systems. In addition, vacuum cooling can achieve uniform cooling throughout a package or lot of produce and gives the best results in terms of energy efficiency as heat is removed only from the product that is being cooled. Nevertheless, the main drawback of vacuum cooling is its limited capacity due to the air-tight room and vacuum requirements, which eliminates the possibility of developing any continuous flow vacuum processing system. Moreover, the expensive equipment required makes vacuum cooling more expensive than other precooling techniques, being feasible only for large growers or organizations. However, portable vacuum coolers are also available, which are not as expensive and therefore may be justified (McDonald and Sun, 2000; Brosnan and Sun, 2001; Vigneault et al., 2008).

4.4.6 Cryogenic cooling

In cryogenic cooling the produce is cooled by conveying it through a tunnel in which liquid nitrogen or solid CO_2 evaporates, producing boiling temperatures of –196 and –78°C, respectively. However, at the above temperatures the produce will freeze and thus be ruined as a fresh market product. This problem is prevented by careful control of the evaporation rate and conveyor speed. Cryogenic cooling is relatively cheap to install but expensive to run due to the high cost of liquid nitrogen, dry ice, and other suitable nontoxic substances. Its main application is in cooling crops such as soft fruits with a seasonal production period. Hence, by using cryogenic cooling the grower would not incur the high capital costs associated with alternative cooling techniques over such period of use (Brosnan and Sun, 2001).

4.5 Chilling injury

Rapid produce cooling after harvest is essential in the preservation of most fresh commodities, since temperature has the single greatest effect on the respiration rate and thus in the deterioration rate of produce. As explained previously, there are a number of precooling methods, each one having different advantages for each particular produce and/or practical applications. Thus, factors that must be taken into account when selecting a precooling method include produce deterioration rate, sensitivity to water contact, temperature of freezing, temperature of chilling, sensitivity to water loss, economics, and the expected storage duration. Due to the combination of these factors, some precooling methods are not suited for certain produce. In addition, it must be also to taken account that some produce are sensitive to low temperatures, suffering damage know as *chilling injury* (CI).

CI is primarily a physiological disorder occurring in crops of tropical and subtropical origin, when they are stored at low temperatures. CI is not the same as freezing injury, which is a result of damage from ice crystals formed in tissues stored below their freezing point. However, CI occurs when sensitive commodities are stored at temperatures below 10–13°C, although the critical temperature for CI varies with the commodity. Therefore, crops that are susceptible to CI often have a short storage life as low temperatures cannot be used to slow deterioration and pathogen growth, which has serious economic consequences on the agro-industry. CI may occur in the field, in transit and distribution, and in retail and home refrigerators. Moreover, the effects of short periods of exposition to chilling temperatures may be cumulative in some commodities. However, this physiological disorder develops faster and more intensely when sensitive fruits are stored at temperatures between 2 and 10°C (killing temperature zone) than when they are stored at 0°C or below, but above their freezing point. Therefore, fruit maximum storage life can be achieved near or below 0°C depending on the soluble solids content of the fruit (Serrano et al., 1996; Crisosto et al., 1999; Lurie and Crisosto, 2005).

The primary cause of CI is thought to be damage to plant cell membranes, including disorganization of mitochondria and chloroplast, which sets off a cascade of secondary reactions, including ethylene production, increased respiration, reduced photosynthesis and interference with energy production, accumulation of toxic compounds, such as ethanol and acetaldehyde, and altered cellular structure (Kratsch and Wise, 2000). Thus, for example, pomegranate fruits developed CI during cold storage and subsequent shelf life at 20°C, which was evident after 15 days of storage and became more severe as storage time advanced, with increasing visual skin browning and electrolyte leakage (Mirdehghan et al., 2007b). It has been reported that low temperature induces changes in cell membrane lipids from a liquid-crystalline to a solid-gel state, which lead to an increase in membrane permeability and leakage of ions (Gómez-Galindo et al., 2004). In fact, in pomegranate skin, membrane lipid composition changed during cold storage, with significant losses in saturated, mono-unsaturated, and especially in poly-unsaturated fatty acids after 45 days of cold storage plus 3 days at 20°C (Figure 4.9). In addition, the ratio unsaturated/saturated fatty acids decreased from an initial value of 1.27 to 0.72 after 90 days of storage and was highly correlated with the increase in electrolyte leakage (Mirdehghan et al., 2007b).

As plant structures differ in both susceptibility to damage and ability to repair their membranes, these CI symptoms vary greatly among commodities. In general, if the produce is stored below the critical temperature for short periods, the organ can repair the damage, but if exposure is prolonged irreversible damage occurs and visible symptoms often result. In addition, injury occurs sooner and is more severe the lower the temperature below the threshold temperature and the higher the time of exposure.

Potential symptoms of CI are surface lesions, pitting, sunken areas and discoloration (which occurs most frequently in produce with a firm and thick peel such as citrus or cucumbers), water-soaking of tissues (occurring most frequently in fruit and vegetables with thin or soft peels such as peppers, asparagus, and grapes), water loss, desiccation, shriveling, internal discoloration, mealiness and browning in the flesh (especially in peaches and nectarines), and tissue breakdown. Other reported symptoms are failure of fruit to ripen or uneven or slow ripening, accelerated senescence and ethylene production, shortened storage or shelf

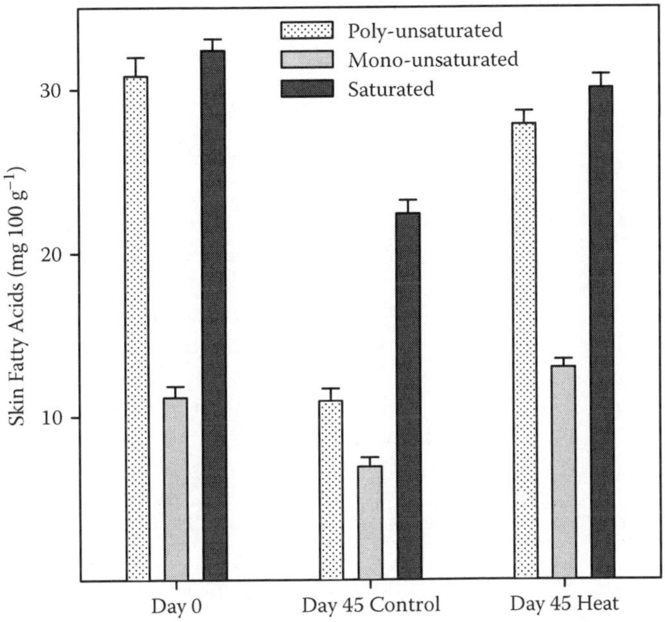

Figure 4.9 Total fatty acid concentration (mg 100 g^{-1}): saturated, mono-unsaturated, and poly-unsaturated in pomegranate skin at harvest and after 45 days of cold storage plus 3 days at 20°C in control and heat-treated (water dipping at 45°C for 4 min) fruits before cold storage.

life, compositional changes affecting flavor and texture, loss of growth or sprouting capability, wilting, and increased decay due to leakage of plant metabolites, which encourage growth of microorganisms, especially fungi. Some examples of fruits susceptible to CI when stored below a critical temperature as well as the recommended storage temperature (which varies with cultivar, storage duration, maturity, and prestorage conditions) and the CI symptoms are displayed In Table 4.1.

However, detection and diagnosis of CI is often difficult, as products often look sound when removed from the chilling temperature, but symptoms may occur when the produce is placed at higher temperatures or may take several days to develop, and even may not be visible externally. In addition, CI symptoms vary depending on a wide range of factors, such as fruit species and cultivar, ripening stage at harvest, and duration of storage and prestorage conditions (Saltveit and Morris, 1990; Lurie and Crisosto, 2005; Sevillano et al., 2009).

Table 4.1 Examples of Fruits and Vegetables Susceptible to Chilling Injury (CI), Showing Recommended Minimum Storage Temperature and Potential CI Symptoms

Commodity	Recommended minimum storage temperature (°C)	Potential chilling injury symptoms
Apple	0–7	Core or flesh browning, fermented flavor, spongy texture.
Avocado	7–13	Darkening of vascular tissues, discoloration of flesh and skin, off-flavors and odors, abnormal ripening.
Banana	> 13	Brown to black peel discoloration, off-flavors, abnormal ripening.
Cantaloupe	2–5	Pitting, surface decay.
Cucumber	7–10	Pitting of surface, lenticel area affected first, followed by *Fusarium* and other rots.
Grapefruit	10–15	Brown pitting of rind, watery breakdown of internal and external tissues, fermented odor.
Honeydew melon	7–13	Water-soaking of the rind, softening, graying or browning; surface becomes soft and sticky resulting in increased decay.
Lemon	10–14	Same as for grapefruit, plus red blotch.
Lime	9–12	Same as for grapefruit.
Mango	> 13	Grayish skin discoloration, pitting, uneven ripening, poor flavor, increased susceptibility to *Alternaria* rot.
Orange	2–5	Same as for grapefruit.
Papaya	7–13	Pitting, olive or brown discoloration, abnormal ripening.
Peach/nectarine	–0.5–1	(Critical temperature 2–8) Internal breakdown, mealiness, abnormal ripening, flesh browning or reddening.

Table 4.1 Examples of Fruits and Vegetables Susceptible to Chilling Injury (CI), Showing Recommended Minimum Storage Temperature and Potential CI Symptoms

Commodity	Recommended minimum storage temperature (°C)	Potential chilling injury symptoms
Pepper	7–13	Water-soaked appearance, sheet pitting, darkening, predisposition to *Alternaria* and *Botrytis*.
Pineapple	7–13	Flesh watery, followed by browning or blackening.
Tomato—ripe —green	7–13 > 13	Rubbery texture, watery flesh, irregular ripening, seed browning.
Watermelon	10–15	Pitting, loss of flavor, fading of red color.
Zucchini	5–10	Surface pitting, rapid decay.

Sources: *Produce Handler's Guide*, Agriculture and Agri-Food Canada; Kader, 2002, *Postharvest Technology of Horticultural Crops*, University of California; Hardfenburg et.al., 1986, *The Commercial Storage of Fruits, Vegetables and Nursery Stocks*, U.S.D.A. Saltveit and Morris, 1990; Serrano et al., 1996; Lurie and Crisosto, 2005; Artés et al., 2007; Sevillano et al., 2009.

4.5.1 *Role of ethylene in stimulating chilling injury*

The role of ethylene in the development of CI has been proposed due to the similarity among symptoms of ripening and those of CI, such as alterations in the structure and composition of cell membranes and the associated oxidative stress. In addition, in many cold-sensitive fruits and vegetables chilling temperatures stimulate ethylene biosynthesis, the precursors of ethylene and the activities of the enzymes implicated in the biosynthetic pathway, especially when fruits are reconditioned at room temperature after cold storage (Lederman et al., 1997; Serrano et al., 1997; Rodriguez et al., 2001; Lafuente and Sala, 2002). This increased ethylene production can be interpreted in two different ways, either as a simple response to low temperatures or as an inducer of CI in sensitive species. The observation that ethylene treatments of different climacteric and nonclimacteric fruits induce the manifestation of CI and the fact that CI is reduced by treatments with the ethylene antagonist 1-MCP or in genetically modified cantaloupe Charentais melon having inhibited autocatalytic ethylene production seem to support the latest hypothesis and to confirm the induction of CI by ethylene (Pesis et al., 2002; Candan et al., 2008; Sevillano et al., 2009). However, this theory cannot be generalized for every plant species sensitive to CI, since in some horticultural products a protective effect of ethylene against CI has been observed (Wang et al., 2006a).

4.5.2 Minimizing chilling injury

Although CI is most easily prevented by storing susceptible crops above their critical temperatures, this is not always possible when only one storage facility is available for several crops. In addition, as longer storage time could be achieved by reducing storage temperature, many researchers have been focused to find methods to reduce and or delay the severity of CI in sensitive commodities, and some strategies and/or treatments have shown promising results, although not all of them will be appropriate for all crops. For instance, by minimizing the length of time the crop is exposed to the chilling temperature the damage can be reversed and no visual symptoms will occur. Preconditioning, that is, stepwise cooling of the commodity, can allow the fruit to adapt to the cooler temperatures and also minimize CI development. Another strategy is intermittent warming (IW), consisting of warming the commodity to room temperature at intervals during storage and before permanent injury has occurred, which will allow the product to recover and prevent CI symptoms. This treatment may, however, cause undesirable softening and increased decay since it may cause condensation on the product. Heat treatment also prevents CI. Thus, heating pomegranate fruits (by immersion in hot water at 45°C for 4 min) reduced CI symptoms and electrolyte leakage, as well as the loss of saturated, mono-unsaturated, and poly-unsaturated fatty acids in the skin that occurred in control fruits (Figure 4.9). Thus, skin of heat-treated pomegranates exhibited a higher ratio of unsaturated/saturated fatty acids than control husks over all storage time. This increase in the degree of unsaturation of membrane lipids has been described as a mechanism of acclimatization to low temperatures, which would lead to maintenance of membrane fluidity at low temperature and could be responsible for lower electrolyte leakage and skin browning (Mirdehghan et al., 2007b).

The effect of these and other postharvest treatments, such as polyamines (PAs), 1-MCP, and storage under modified atmosphere, on reducing fruit susceptibility to CI will be commented on in Chapters 7, 8, and 9, respectively. However, cultivar selection is also important, since certain cultivars are more resistant to chilling than others. In this sense, a great variation in susceptibility to CI among peach, nectarine, and mango cultivars has been reported (Phakawatmongkol et al., 2004; Lurie and Crisosto, 2005) and thus a selection of cultivars with low sensitivity to CI might be a factor to be taken into account in breeding programs.

Likewise, proper preharvest nutrition can minimize chilling susceptibility, for instance, by using calcium treatment, which may stabilize cellular membranes leading to reduction of CI in certain commodities. In fact, lower incidence of CI was negatively correlated with total calcium concentration in fruits of pineapple varieties and even in different parts of a single fruit (Hewajulige et al., 2003). However, calcium foliar sprays on peach and nectarines showed no effect on CI symptoms (Crisosto et al., 2000). With respect to nitrogen fertilization during fruit growth, no relation with CI has been found in peach or nectarine cultivars (Lurie and Crisosto, 2005), while in avocado excessive nitrogen concentration increased CI symptom severity (Van Rooyen and Bower 2005).

Fruit exposure to sun light also has a great influence on decreasing the incidence of CI on sensitive fruits, such as nectarines and peaches (Lurie and Crisosto, 2005). Thus, the use of more efficient training systems that allow for more sun-light penetration into the center and lower canopy areas as well as leaf removing around the fruits could reduce the number of shaded fruits and in turn lead to an increase in postharvest life. Related to this issue, preharvest high temperatures have also been found to reduce CI in some fruits, such as avocado and muskmelon, although in grapefruit and kiwifruit CI has been found to be greater in fruit taken from the exterior canopy, with direct sun exposure and higher temperature (Woolf and Ferguson, 2000).

Maturity/ripeness selection is also an important factor to be taken into account, since in general riper fruit are less susceptible to CI than unripe ones. Thus, it has been shown that ripe tomatoes, bananas, and avocados tolerate lower temperatures than unripe fruit, and that peaches and nectarines that are ripened for 1–2 days after harvest prior to storage are less susceptible to low temperatures. In addition, special storage conditions can also reduce CI. Thus, high humidity can minimize desiccation due to CI. Controlled or modified atmospheres (generally $O_2 < 5\%$, $CO_2 > 2\%$) can slow plant metabolism and slow CI development in certain crops (e.g., peaches, nectarines, okra, avocado). CA can also allow longer storage of chilling sensitive crops, although they may in some cases cause further stress and increase CI susceptibility (e.g., apple cultivars, cucumber, tomato, asparagus, and citrus). Finally, other methods that are still in experimental stages include treatment with hormones or other chemicals to stabilize plant membranes and induction of chilling resistance by exposure to other stresses such as high temperature or low O_2 concentration. The next chapters will address specific effects of several postharvest treatments and storage technologies on increasing cold storage possibilities, as well as their effects on reducing CI occurrence.

chapter five

Heat treatments

5.1 Introduction

Heat treatment as postharvest tool was used in the first decades of the 20th century after the First World War in the citrus industry in the United States. Hot water (44–48°C) was used in the washing tank and not only cleaned the fruit but was also observed to partially control green and blue molds (*Penicillium digitatum* and *P. italicum*) (Fawcett, 1936). From this time, postharvest heat treatments have been used commercially on a limited scale to control fungal diseases and pest infestation of horticultural crops. In the 1990s, Ben-Yehoshua and his colleagues in Israel initiated the studies of the application of heat following a casual unexpected observation that a large number of grapefruit that were stored in a room whose temperature fluctuated during the day, at times exceeding 37°C and with mean temperature above 30°C for several days, had much less decay than fruit stored at the optimal temperature of 11°C. They introduced the concept of *curing* as the establishment of a short period of heat treatment (36°C for 3 days) during the first 48 hours after harvest that would reduce decay in storage (Ben-Yehoshua and Porat, 2005). With the development of selective synthetic and systemic fungicides, heat treatment was abandoned because fungicides were more effective, easier to apply, and cost less. However, nowadays there is an increasing concern about the use of synthetic fungicides due to the public perception that pesticides are harmful to human health and environment. This negative perception has promoted governmental policies restricting the use of fungicides (Tripathi and Dubey, 2004) and have contributed, together with the increase of pathogen resistance, to the development and implementation of strategies for reducing dependence on agrochemicals. In this sense, the use of heat treatments is actually considered an environmentally friendly method of decay control, either alone or in combination with other methods. In addition, this treatment has also been shown to have beneficial effects on delaying the evolution of parameters related to postharvest fruit ripening and preserving fruit quality and increasing storage time, with interesting possibilities of commercial application in the horticultural industry.

5.2 Means of heat application

There are three main methods for applying heat treatments: hot water, hot air, and vapor heat. Hot water has been used classically for fungal control and vapor heat was developed specifically for insect control, while hot air is used for both fungal and insect management (Lurie, 1998). However, in the last two decades research has been continuous on these methods, on new techniques, and on the responses to high temperature treatments of fruit and vegetables (Ferguson et al., 2000). On a general basis, heat is applied as a prestorage treatment prior to short- or long-cold storage period by using hot water, hot air, or vapor heat.

5.2.1 Hot water

Hot water baths and dips are the simplest way of heat treatment with a fast energy transfer, and fungal spores and latent infections present in the surface or in the first cell layers under the fruit skin can be controlled. Postharvest dip to control decay is usually achieved with temperature over 40°C and variable exposure time. It is interesting to point out that tolerance temperature for most fruits is 50–60°C for up to 10 minutes, since higher temperatures and time would induce heat damage. The beneficial effect of prestorage hot water immersion treatment to prevent rot development has been shown in numerous temperate, subtropical, and tropical fruit, vegetables, and flowers. This method has a number of advantages that include relative ease of use, short treatment time, reliable monitoring of fruit and water temperatures, and the killing of skin-borne decay-causing agents (Fallik, 2004).

The two main commercial hot water treatments are hot water immersion and hot water rinsing and brushing. In general, the main components of a hot water immersion unit are the treatment tank, a heat exchanger unit, water circulation system, and temperature controller. In contrast to hot water immersion, a new technology based on a brief hot water rinsing and brushing to clean and disinfect fresh harvested produce was first introduced commercially in 1996 (Fallik et al., 1996). Fresh produce is rinsed by nozzles from above with pressurized recycled hot water, while rolling on brushes made from medium-soft synthetic bristles. An improved version of this machine (to improve the cleaning and disinfecting process and to increase treatment capacity) contains 18–20 parallel brushes.

5.2.2 Hot air

Hot air treatment is similar to vapor heat treatment but does not have the moisture component and is a more recent development. Improvements in temperature and moisture monitoring and air delivery have advanced forced hot-air treatments (Tang et al., 2007). Hot air can be applied by placing fruit or vegetables in a heated chamber with a ventilating fan, or by applying forced hot air where the speed of air circulation is precisely controlled. Hot air, forced or not, heats more slowly than hot water immersion or forced vapor heat, although forced hot air will heat produce faster than a regular heating chamber. The hot air chamber has been utilized to study physiological changes in fruits and vegetables in response to heat. Forced hot-air treatments are being devised for commodities normally subjected to vapor heat treatment, and have also been applied to new commodities. Their disadvantages are the long treatment durations and sophisticated equipment needed for operation and the fact that not all horticultural commodities are suitable for this treatment (Lurie, 1998).

5.2.3 *Vapor heat*

Vapor heat is a method of heating commodities with air saturated with water vapor at temperatures of 40–50°C to kill insect eggs and larvae as a quarantine treatment before fresh market shipments (Lurie, 1998). Heat transfer is by condensation of water vapor on the cooler fruit surface. This method is disputed because the vapor condensing heat-transfer coefficient is far higher than the coefficients of air and water (Lu et al., 2007). This explains why high humidity in vapor heating can sometimes damage the fruit undergoing treatment, whereas the slower heating and lower humidity of forced hot air may cause less damage.

5.3 *Heat treatments and fruit quality storability*

The application of heat treatments to fruit commodities and its effect on physiological, biochemical, nutritive, and quality parameters has been widely studied in recent years. Heat treatments can also be used to inhibit ripening processes or to induce resistance to CI and external skin damage during storage, thus extending storability and marketing (Lurie, 1998; Paull and Chen, 2000).

There is no general rule for the combination of heat treatment/exposure time to gain a specific effect on a particular fruit type. As can be seen in Table 5.1, temperature in the range of 39–53°C and duration 10 minutes to 12 hours is needed to achieve an effective decay control in tomato, orange, mango, and pear and to reduce mechanical damage before handling in plum, while higher temperatures act as quarantine insect method (46–58°C). In addition, it is interesting to point out that in very recent years, hot treatments have shown a positive effect on increasing nutritive and functional properties of some fruits such as pomegranate, tomato, mango, and kumquat.

Table 5.1 Some Heat Applications and Their Effects in Several Fruit Commodities

Effect	Fruit	Heat treatment	Reference
Alleviate CI	Peach	Hot air 38°C, 12 h	Jin et al., 2009.
	Pomegranate	Hot water 45°C, 4 min	Mirdehghan et al., 2006.
		Hot air 33°C, 3 days	Artés et al., 2000.
	Plum	Hot water 40–50°C, 25–40 min	Abu-Kpawoh et al., 2002.
	Tomato	Hot water 39–45°C, 60 min	McDonald et al., 1999.
	Orange	Hot water 53°C, 6 h or 48°C, 12 h	Erkan et al., 2005.
	Banana	Hot water 42°C, 15 min	Promyou et al., 2008.
Quarantine insects and	Sweet cherry	Hot water 46–58°C, 0.25–18 min	Feng et al., 2004.
De-infest	Pitaya	Hot air 46.5°C, 20 min	Hoa et al., 2006.
Reduce decay	Tomato	Hot water 39–45°C, 60 min	McDonald et al., 1999.
	Orange	Hot water 53°C, 6 h or 48°C, 12 h	Erkan et al., 2005.
	Mango	Hot water 52°C, 10 min	Dang et al., 2008.
	Pear	Hot water 46°C, 10–20 min	Zhang et al., 2008.
Reduce mechanical damage	Plum	Hot water 45°C, 10 min	Serrano et al., 2004a.
Increase nutritive and bioactive compounds	Pomegranate	Hot water 45°C, 4 min	Mirdehghan et al., 2007b.
	Tomato	Hot air 34°C, 24 h	Soto-Zamora et al., 2005.
	Mango	Hot water 46°C, 70 min	Kim et al., 2009.
	Kumquat	Hot water 50°C, 2 min	Schirra et al., 2008.

5.3.1 *Fruit ripening*

On a general basis, the effect of heat treatments on fruit ripening is a delay of some parameters related to fruit physiology (ethylene production and respiration rate) and quality deterioration (softening, color evolution, increase in soluble sugars, and reduction in acidity), the overall quality of fresh produce exposed to an appropriate temperature and time being significantly better than in nonheated commodities. However, sometimes there is a more advanced evolution in some ripening characteristics, since heat acts as a stress-environmental condition inducing tissue injury, with negative effects on quality (Paull and Chen, 2000). Table 5.2 shows that mild heat treatments (38–55°C) are preferred to reduce the ripening process and/or maintain fruit organoleptic quality, although the duration is widely variable, from seconds (for apple) to several minutes (4–60 minutes, for pomegranate, tomato, sweet cherry, pitaya, and mango) and even to several hours (12 hours for peach).

In climacteric fruits, the inhibition of ripening by heat may be mediated by its effect on the ripening hormone ethylene and the enzymes responsible for its biosynthesis, ACS and ACO (Lurie, 1998; Serrano et al., 2004a). This can be seen in Figure 4.1 (Chapter 4), which shows that temperature over 40°C led to maximum ethylene production in both apple and banana, while from this temperature, any increase (45 or 50°C) conducted a significant reduction in ethylene emission. The mechanism by which heat delays and/or inhibits ethylene production is variable. Thus, temperatures in the range of 35–38°C tend to accumulate ACC and to decrease ethylene production due to inhibition of ACO activity. However, higher temperatures induce lower concentration of ACC through inhibition of ACS activity. This means that ACS is less sensitive to heat treatments

Table 5.2 Response of Several Fruits to Heat Treatments with Respect to Organoleptic Parameters Related to Ripening

Fruit	HM	Tª (°C)	Time	Firmness	Color	Sugars	Acidity
Tomato[1]	Water	42	60 min	=	↑	=	↓
Peach[2]	Air	38	12 h	=	ND	↑	=
Apple[3]	Water	55	15 s	↑	↓	=	=
Sweet cherry[4]	Water	48	10 min	=	↓	=	↓
Pomegranate[5]	Water	45	4 min	↑	↓	↑	↑
Pitaya[6]	Air	46.5	20 min	↑	=	ND	ND
Mango[7]	Water	50	30 min	↑	↓	↑	↓

Note: HM (Hot method), ↑, ↓ and = mean higher, lower, or unaffected with respect to controls. ND = not determined.

[1]McDonald et al., 1999, [2]Jin et al., 2009, [3]Fallik et al., 2001, [4]Drake et al., 2005, [5]Mirdehghan et al., 2006; 2007b, [6]Hoa et al., 2006, [7]Djioua et al., 2009.

than ACO. In addition, the differences in response to heat between ACS and ACO may be related to difference in their turnover rates (Paull and Chen, 2000). In fact, it is clear that the effect of heat temperature on ethylene biosynthesis is reversible, since fruits exposed to high temperature over a long period can recover their ability to synthesize ethylene when they are removed from heat, and even the rates of ethylene are higher in heated than in nonheated produce (Lurie, 1998). Thus, in a wide range of fruits (papaya, apple, melon, and mango) a full recovery of ACO activity occurred within 3 days after removal from heat, for which new protein synthesis was required as well as reactivation of previously synthesized mRNA, which were attenuated during the heating process.

Table 5.2 shows the response of several heat treatments on some parameters related to organoleptic quality, such as firmness, color, sugars, and acidity. Most of the assayed fruits gave a similar response during postharvest storage, with decreased fruit softening, color evolution, and acidity losses, but little effect on sugar concentration. However, there are some exceptions to these general effects of heat treatments, such as the enhancement of color found in tomato (McDonald et al., 1999), the increase in total acidity in pomegranate (Mirdehghan et al., 2006; 2007b), and the absence of effect on fruit firmness recorded in tomato, sweet cherry, and peach (McDonald et al., 1999; Drake et al., 2005; Jin et al., 2009).

As stated in Chapter 3, the postharvest storage of fruit is accompanied by loss of cell wall integrity due to breakdown of pectic substances leading to an increase in soluble pectin and decrease in fruit firmness. The softening process was significantly reduced in heat-treated fruit (either by immersion or hot air), although effectiveness was highly dependent on maturity stage before practicing the heat treatment. In addition, the beneficial effect of heat treatments on maintaining firmness has been observed not only in whole fruits but rather in fresh-cut produce, such as kiwifruit (Beirão-da-Costa et al., 2006), melon (Lamikanra and Watson, 2007; Aguayo et al., 2008), peach (Koukounaras et al., 2008), and mango (Djioua et al., 2009). In Figure 5.1 the effect of hot water treatment at 45°C for 10 minutes in lemon and plum is displayed, showing that after 14 days of storage at 15°C control plums and lemons had lost ≈30% and 50% of their initial firmness, respectively, while the firmness loss in heat-treated fruits was only 10%. The mechanism by which prestorage heating may affect the cell wall structure and thus maintain fruit firmness is not clear yet, although some hypotheses have been postulated. Possibly, the heat treatment would activate the use of endogenous Ca^{2+} to form calcium-pectate with low methoxyl pectins generated by the activation of pectinesterase by heat, thus delaying the action of cell-wall degrading enzymes, mainly PG and PME, as was reported for apples (Conway et al., 1994). In addition, a direct effect of heat treatment on these enzymes has been also proposed (Lurie, 1998; Paul and Chen, 2000; Serrano et al., 2004a).

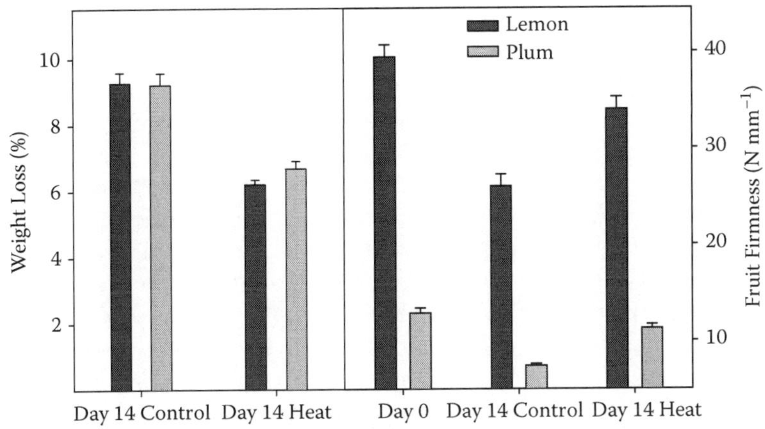

Figure 5.1 Weight loss (%) and fruit firmness (N mm^{-1}) in lemon or plum after 14 days of cold storage at 2°C in control and heat-treated (water dips at 45°C for 10 min) fruits.

More recently, heat-treated strawberries (45°C for 3 hours) showed delay in softening by reduction of EGase, β-xylosidase, PG, and β-GAL activities, while PME activity was enhanced (Vicente et al., 2005). This broad effect of heat treatments on cell-wall degrading enzymes could slow down pectin solubilization by reducing pectin cleavage and by increasing the amount of putative sites for calcium bridge formation at the cell wall. In this sense, inhibition in solubilization of the carbonate-soluble pectin fractions is considered one of the main factors contributing to firmness retention due to heat treatment. The hot method used for application seems to affect fruit firmness, since strawberries air heated at 45°C for 15 minutes retained the fruit firmness but similar dip treatment failed (Lara et al., 2006). These authors postulated that cell wall yields increased during storage but these increases were the same in control and heated fruits, and higher yields for cell wall material were not related to fruit firmness. In fact, the decrease in solubilization of pectic polymers as a consequence of heat treatment could be responsible for the firmness retention through inhibition of cell-wall degrading enzymes. In an attempt to go further about the effect of heat treatment on the activity and gene expression of a set of enzymes associated with cell-wall degradation in strawberry, Martínez and Civello (2008) concluded that the application of heat treatment (45°C, 3 hours in air) delayed postharvest softening in strawberry fruit through a reduction in the expression of a set of genes and enzymes that are involved in cell wall metabolism—β-xylosidase, EGase, and β-GAL—their expression being reduced during the first hours of treatment but recovered after 24 h, while the activity of PG remained unaffected. Thus, heat treatment modified the gene expression patterns in heated fruits, which in turn provoked a reduction in cell wall catabolism and delayed the normal fruit softening.

Another effect that accompanies and influences negatively the fruit quality during storage is weight loss, which can be reduced by the use of heat treatments. As an example, Figure 5.1 shows that weight loss of lemons and plums after 14 days of cold storage was 50% lower in heat treated fruits than in nonheated ones, which could be considered an additional positive effect of heat application. Other fruit commodities in which reduced weight loss was obtained after heat treatments were fresh-cut melon (Lamikanra et al., 2005) and blueberries (Fan et al., 2008), among others. However, this is not a general effect for heat treatments, since in other fruits either the weight loss was unaffected, as in the case of strawberry and pitaya (Hoa et al., 2006; Lara et al., 2006), or enhanced with respect to control, as reported for mandarins, pomegranates, and mangoes (Schirra and D'hallewin, 1997; Artés et al., 2000; Dang et al., 2008). Interestingly, the hot method also affected the fruit mass loss, since air-heated oranges significantly increased the weight loss compared with hot water-treated for the same combination of temperature-time (Erkan et al., 2005). However, occurrence of mechanical damage greatly induces increases in weight loss (Chapter 3), but the application of hot water at 45°C for 10 minutes significantly reduced the weight loss of mechanically damaged plums (Serrano et al., 2004a) by reducing the ripening-related membrane changes, such as microviscosity and the increase in fatty acid saturation. It has been postulated that the reduced weight loss by using water as a heat treatment might be the result of water uptake during the treatment.

The color and nutritive constituents (sugars and organic acids) changes that occur during postharvest storage of fruits are also affected by heat treatments (Table 5.2) with delays in color evolution and little or no effect on the content of sugars and acids. Figure 5.2 summarizes some effects on quality parameters in breba fig fruit heated 10 minutes in water at 45°C, the heat treatment being effective in inhibiting the softening compared with control (a 30% firmness loss), and in reducing the ripening index increase (a 20% less increase with respect to control), although heat treatment accelerated the color changes, which were associated with a net increase in anthocyanin concentration. In the case of climacteric fruits, the delay in these quality parameters has been attributed to the reduced ethylene production. However, the exact mechanism of action by which heat application affects these quality parameters is still unknown, although partial evidence has been obtained. The effect on color has been attributed to the activation of several enzymes, such as chlorophyllase, or the synthesis of new enzymes (Lurie, 1998), although this issue deserves further in-depth research. The increase of sugars following heat treatments was probably due to the solubilization of neutral sugars from pectic polymer residues but was dependent on the maturity stage at harvest, as reported

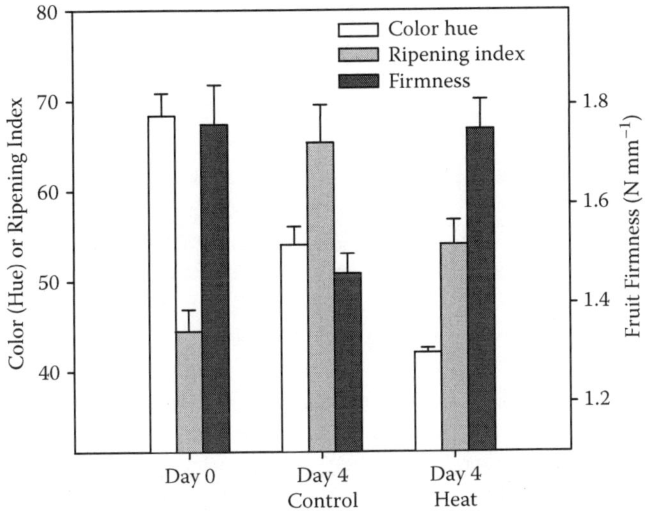

Figure 5.2 Color (Hue parameter), ripening index (TSS/TA), and fruit firmness of breba fruits at day 0 (harvest) and after 4 days of cold storage at 2°C in control and heat-treated (water dips at 45°C for 10 min) fruits.

for kiwifruit slices (Beirão-da-Costa et al., 2006). In ripe kiwifruit cell walls, the main neutral sugars are galactose, glucose, and xylose, some arabinose and rhamnose, and traces of manose and fucose. At a partially mature stage, when fruits are firm, the pectic polysaccharides remain unbroken, with many neutral sugar residues. The application of a mild heat treatment probably activated enzymes such as α-galactosidase (α-GAL), glucosidase, and arabinase (ABN) that will promote the release of these neutral sugars, thus making fruits sweeter. When kiwifruit is fully ripe most of these sugars are already solubilized as result of the maturation process, and so heat treatment has only a marginal effect. On the contrary, in mandarins, heat treatment lead to a decline in sugars, which was attributed to the increase in the respiratory rate in heat-treated fruits (Holland et al., 2002). Accordingly, some authors have postulated that accelerated acidity loss might be connected to the acceleration of the metabolism induced by the treatment, especially increased respiration rate by heat treatment, as observed for tomato (Polenta et al., 2006). Nevertheless, during storage of fruits the changes in nutritive compounds (sugars and organic acids) seem to be variable and dependent on the fruit species, treatment time, and storage conditions. Thus, in sweet cherry the levels of glucose and malic acid decreased during cold storage plus 2 or 4 days shelf life at 20°C, and the hot water treatment (50°C, 2 minutes) did not modify this pattern of these constituents (Alique et al., 2005). Accordingly, glucose, fructose, and sucrose did not change during storage of kumquat at 17°C for 21 days and were not significantly affected by hot water dip at 50°C for 2 minutes (Schirra et al., 2008).

Flavor and aroma are also other fruit quality components determining the produce acceptability by consumers, but there is little evidence about the relationship between flavor/aroma constituents and heat treatments. The earliest report (McDonald et al., 1999) on tomato revealed that heat treatments decreased the levels of hexanal, *cis*-3-hexenal and *trans*-2-hexenal, while increases were found in *trans*-2-heptenal and *cis*-3-hexenol, leading to a general reduction in flavor volatiles. Accordingly, in the case of oranges, heat treatment (48.5°C for 5 h, the usual for disinfecting) significantly reduced the concentrations of α-pinene, β-myrcene, and limonene (Obenland et al., 1999), all three of these compounds contributing positively to orange flavor, and thus the reduction in the amount of these volatiles by heat could potentially have a negative effect on flavor, with limonene being especially important due to its abundance in orange. Moreover, storage conditions and length resulted in volatile compound loss in apple mainly due to loss of substrates or enzymes essential for the formation of esters as well as to some kind of evaporation of aroma compounds. A 4-day heat treatment at 38°C of apple fruits markedly reduced total volatile and volatile ester emission, although the diminution was temporal since volatiles were again increased 24 hours after treatment or removal from cold storage (Fallik et al., 1997). Thus, heat treatment temporarily inhibited but did not destroy (or destroyed but allowed resynthesis of) the enzyme systems catalyzing volatile compound synthesis. In mango, the hot method also influenced greatly the concentrations of the main flavor and aroma compounds after 3 weeks of cold storage at 13°C, since hot air (40°C, 8h) induced reductions in sesquiterpenes, lactones, and alcohols, but did not modify monoterpenes, aldehydes, or esters. On the contrary, hot water (52°C, 10 minutes) led to increases in monoterpenes and aldehydes but did not change the remaining volatile groups (Dang et al., 2008). Thus, the loss of volatiles in heat-conditioned fruits might be due to the combined degrading effects of high air temperature and prolonged exposure compared with the hot water application.

Contrarily, in blueberries hot water treatments (45, 50, or 60°C) for 15 or 30 s led to significant increases in the headspace concentrations of a wide range of volatiles, the most important being ethanol, ethyl acetate, and ethyl 2-methylbutanoate, which are considered stress-induced volatiles (Fan et al., 2008). In summary, the impact on flavor and aroma compound varies with species, temperature, duration, and method of the heat treatment, and thus volatiles are changed with some being enhanced more than others but significant losses are also reported, which can be temporal or definitive.

5.3.2 *Bioactive compounds with antioxidant activity*

With the new millennium, the role of fruit consumption in human health and well-being has progressively increased (Chapter 2). However, the use of noncontaminant and environmentally friendly technologies is more accepted by consumers in contrast to chemical preservation. Accordingly, heat treatments and their effect on enhancing the bioactive phytochemical content with antioxidant activity have been subjects of much attention in recent years with research efforts on postharvest heat treatment increasing steadily, although the information on the influence of heat treatments on nutritional and bioactive compounds is scarce. In this sense, heat treatments have been postulated as physical elicitors that affect the biosynthesis of phytochemicals and antioxidant properties of horticultural crops (Schreiner and Huyskens-Keil, 2006). Figure 5.3 shows the effect of hot water treatment in pomegranate (45°C for 4 minutes) and the results obtained at harvest and after 45 days of cold storage in bioactive compounds (total phenolics, total anthocyanins, and ascorbic acid) and the antioxidant activity. Arils from heat-treated pomegranates exhibited higher H-TAA than controls, which was correlated primarily to the high

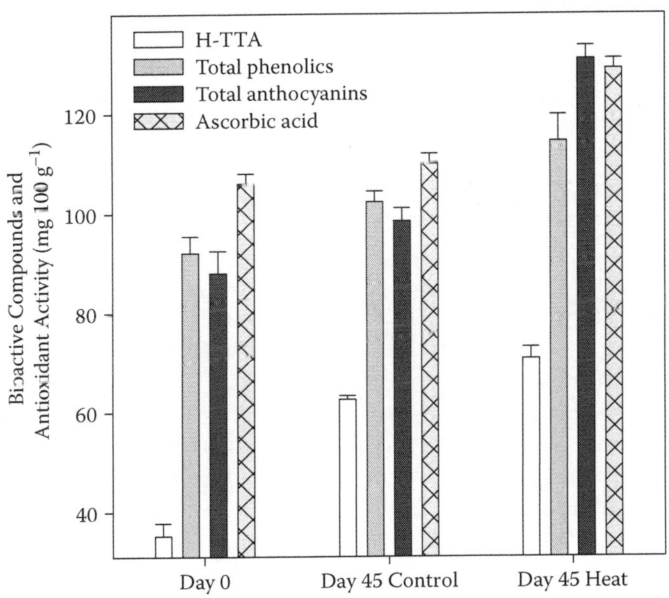

Figure 5.3 Bioactive compounds (total phenolics, total anthocyanins, and ascorbic acid) and total hydrophilic antioxidant activity (H-TAA) of pomegranates at day 0 (harvest) and after 45 days of cold storage at 2°C in control and heat-treated (water dips at 45°C for 4 min) fruits.

levels of total phenolics and to lesser extent to ascorbic acid and anthocyanin contents. Additionally, the levels of sugars (glucose and fructose) and organic acids (malic, citric, and oxalic acids) also remained at higher concentrations in arils from treated fruits. Thus, with this simple and noncontaminant technology, the functional and nutritive properties, after long periods of storage, could then be even greater than in recently harvested fruits, thus providing a high content in health-beneficial compounds to consumers after the intake of these fruits (Mirdehghan et al., 2006). However, large variations in this behavior have been reported for other fruit commodities, heat treatment procedures, and storage conditions.

With respect to heat treatments and total phenolics, air-heat treatment in peaches (38°C, 12 h) significantly increased the content of total phenolics after 3 and 4 weeks of storage and also prevented the increase in PPO activity and accelerated the decrease in POX activity that usually occur in nonheated fruits (Jin et al., 2009), although in fresh-cut peaches hot water dips were ineffective in preventing the loss of total phenols and their corresponding antioxidant activity (Kuokuonaras et al., 2008). However, hot water treatment in tomato (35°C, 12 h), melon (55°C, 5 minutes), and mango (42°C, 24 h) inhibited PPO and POX activities leading to delayed anthocyanin degradation and protection of color pigment changes by maintaining the anthocyanins in their red-pigmented form with high antioxidant activity during postharvest storage. This antioxidative system could also be activated by the induction of superoxide dismutase (SOD) activity (Schreiner and Huyskens-Keil, 2006). Total phenolic compounds were increased also in citrus peel after heat treatments at different temperature-time combinations, with the highest increase being found after 30 minutes at 150°C, which was attributable to the heat capacity to liberate the phenolic compounds covalently bound (Jeong et al., 2004), and for that reason 50°C did not exert any beneficial effect in liberating the polyphenols. These authors also found good correlations with radical scavenging activity either in ethanol or water extracts, which was enhanced at the higher temperature and null at 50°C. The gas chromatography-mass spectrometry (GC-MS) analysis revealed that heat treatment favored the occurrence of 2,3-diacetyl-1-phenylnaphthalene, ferulic acid, and p-hydroxybenzaldoxime in the ethanol extracts, while 5-hydroxyvaleric acid, 2,3-diacetyl-1-phenylnaphthalene, vanillic acid, and ferulic acid were newly detected when Citrus peel was heated at 150°C for 30 minutes. None of these phenolics were present in raw material.

The relationship between carotenoids and heat treatments has revealed different behavior, with increases in total carotenoids and the content of β-carotene and lycopene during storage of tomato heated with air at 34°C for 12 h, which might indicate that heat treatment induced faster fruit ripening once the heat stress was removed and a promotion of the tomato antioxidant system (Soto-Zamora et al., 2005; Yahia et al., 2007).

On the contrary, total carotenoids decreased during storage of kumquat, although heat treatment increased the concentrations of β-cryptoxanthin and decreased lutein with respect to control fruit but did not significantly affect β-carotene and zeaxanthin. After storage, as a result of some changes in the individual carotenoids, lower levels of total carotenoids were recorded in heat-treated fruits in comparison to their initial values (Schirra et al., 2008).

There is also some evidence about heat application and the content of vitamins during storage of fruits, with increases, decreases, or no changes. Thus, tomato heat-treated with air (34°C, 24 h) exhibited lower ascorbic acid and α-tocopherol than control fruits, the diminution being enhanced when 38°C and 12 hours were used, which was related to acceleration of the ripening process (Yahia et al., 2007). However, the method used for heat treatments seems to affect the content of vitamin C in stored oranges, since air-heated oranges improved the ascorbic acid compared with hot water-treated fruits for the same combination of temperature-time up to 2 months, although prolonged storage did not show quantitative differences between control and heated fruits (Erkan et al., 2005). In kumquat, the levels of ascorbic acid remained unchanged during storage at 17°C while vitamin E (α-tocopherol and γ-tocopherol) increased, but hot water treatment (50°C, 2 minutes) did not modify this vitamin behavior (Schirra et al., 2008). The application of hot air (45°C, 3 h) in strawberry showed higher antioxidant capacity than the control immediately after harvest and lasted until day 7 of storage, which was correlated to the increase in ascorbic acid in response to heat treatments. However, after 14 days there were no differences between control and heated fruits (Vicente et al., 2006). In fresh-cut peaches, the hot water treatment was ineffective in avoiding the diminution of ascorbic acid as well as the antioxidant activity (Koukounaras et al., 2008).

5.3.3 Minimizing chilling injury

As stated in Chapter 4 (Section 4.5), CI symptoms occur when sensitive commodities are stored at low temperatures that induce several physiological disorders affecting fruit quality negatively. Postharvest researchers have focused their attention for many years on the availability of appropriate tools to minimize or to inhibit these adverse effects. Among these technologies, prestorage heat treatments are considered one of the most effective means to counteract the undesirable effects of low temperature in chilling-sensitive produce and thus extend the shelf life.

Plant cells sensitive to low temperatures show as a common response the disruption of membrane integrity, with the lipids in the bilayer having a high percentage of saturated fatty acid chains, and membranes with this composition tend to solidify into a semi-crystalline state at a temperature well above 0°C. In addition, prolonged low temperature storage also affects membrane proteins and enzymes, for which protein–protein and protein–lipid interactions may be weakened by a decrease in the relative strength of hydrophobic bonding, leading to subunit dissociation and/or polypeptide unfolding (Gómez-Galindo et al., 2007). The net consequence of CI is the production of reactive oxygen species (ROS) causing lipid peroxidation and DNA damage primarily together with a decrease in the defense enzymatic system, especially the SOD and catalase (CAT) activities, which are in charge of keeping ROS at low levels. Thus, the consequence of cold stress is an imbalance between degradation and repair shifted toward the former. The application of heat treatments induces a shock response that is manifested in most fruits as induction or enhanced synthesis of heat shock proteins (HSPs). The increase in HSPs seems to confer tolerance to heat by protecting proteins from irreversible denaturation and breakdown (Ferguson et al., 2000). It is clear that there is a positive interaction between heat and low temperature storage of sensitive produce, although there is no general rule for the combination temperature-time and there is more than one mechanism involved in the amelioration of CI.

There are two principal ways to perform the heat treatment of fruit to decrease CI fruit susceptibility, either by heat application (hot water and hot air) or by intermittent warming (IW), which consists of a periodic disruption of the storage at low temperature and transfer of the fruits to short periods of warming (usually 20–27°C). The main problem with IW is the selection of the appropriate temperature, frequency of exits from cold rooms, and duration of warming. In addition, the interruption of cold storage should be carried out before the development of CI symptoms, usually within the first 48–72 hours of low-temperature storage.

For example, pomegranates are susceptible to CI if stored longer than 1 month at temperatures below 5°C. Upon transfer to 20°C to simulate market conditions, respiration and ethylene production rates increase and other CI symptoms such as skin browning, surface pitting, and higher susceptibility to decay manifest, and most of the time these symptoms reach the arils (pale coloration) and brown discoloration of the white locular septa, which depreciates both internal and external fruit quality (Mirdehghan et al., 2007b). The application of hot water dips (45°C, 4 minutes) led to significantly lower percentage of ion leakage as well as husk browning, which was correlated with lower color changes after 30 days of storage at 2°C plus 3 days at 20°C (Figure 5.4), and thus this heat treatment minimized the CI development. In addition skin from heat-treated pomegranates exhibited a significantly higher ratio of unsaturated/saturated than control husks over all storage, the degree of unsaturation of membrane lipids being described as a mechanism of acclimation to low temperatures, while control pomegranate was not able to develop this adaptation mechanism and CI occurred to a greater extent (Mirdehghan

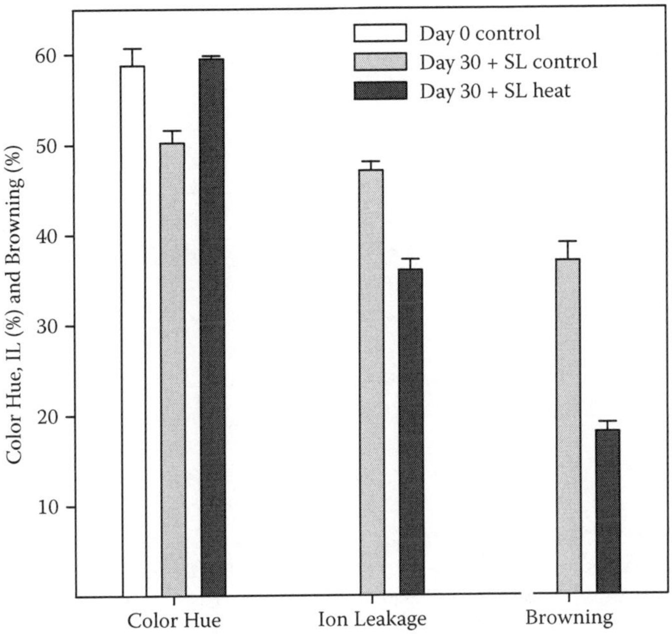

Figure 5.4 Color (Hue parameter), ion leakage (IL), and browning (%) of pomegranates at day 0 (harvest) and after 30 days of cold storage at 2°C + 3 days at 20°C (SL) in control and heat-treated (water dips at 45°C for 4 min) fruits.

et al., 2007b). Other effective treatments that alleviated CI in pomegranate were IW through cycles of 1 day at 20°C every 6 days and the returning to cold conditions for 12 weeks or curing (hot air 33°C for 3 days), and both methods led to lowest CI symptoms (husk scald and pitting, weight loss, and decay), the best way to maintain fruit appearance being achieved by IW (Artés et al., 2000).

In tomato harvested at mature-green stage the hot water treatment at 42°C for 60 minutes was effective in reducing CI, ion leakage, and decay (McDonald et al., 1999), and breaker tomatoes submitted to IW at 20°C for 1 day during 7-day interval showed a large prevention of CI based on reduced yellow discoloration and decay (Artés et al., 1998). In addition, hot water treatments at 45°C for 35 minutes or 50°C for 30 minutes were used to reduce CI and decay of Friar plum stored at 0°C, the primary symptoms of which being translucent skin and flesh and decay as brown rot by *Monilinia* sp. (Abu-Kpawoh et al., 2002). Curing of orange fruits at 48°C for 12 hours or at 53°C for 6 reduced the development of CI incidence at the end of the 6-month storage period, with the symptoms of CI appearing in control fruits in the form of small, discolored pitted areas and skin depressions irregularly distributed over the fruit surface (Erkan et al., 2005). These air-heat treatments were also more effective in reducing fruit decay compared with hot water dips at 48 or 53°C for 12 or 3 minutes, respectively. These authors postulated that high temperatures could increase the transcript levels of HSPs, which may act to protect other proteins from breaking down and thus maintain the integrity of cells and prevent the tissues from developing CI.

However, control peach fruit exhibited CI after storage for 3 weeks with occurrence of internal browning symptoms and flesh mealiness, and the air heated (38°C for 12 h) peaches showed no internal browning but enhanced pulp mealiness (Jin et al., 2009). Apart from these possible mechanisms by which heat can ameliorate CI incidence in sensitive fruits, it is generally accepted that PAs, multifunctional regulators of physiological processes, and stress-protective compounds could be involved or be mediators of chilling tolerance, these aspects being addressed in Chapter 7.

5.3.4 Reducing decay

Postharvest heat treatments were used at commercial level to control fungal diseases and pest infestation of horticultural commodities, but with the development of selective synthetic and systemic fungicides, heat treatment lost popularity since fungicides were more effective, easier to apply, and cost less. However, in recent years the development and implementation of environmentally friendly strategies have gained much more attention due to several factors including (1) the concern about using agrochemicals as a means of preservation, (2) the enhanced proliferation of resistant strains of fungi due to the abuse and prolonged use of synthetic fungicides leading to diminution of their efficacy, and (3) the legal restrictions for registering new fungicides (Ben-Yehoshua and Porat, 2005).

Decay is one of the major factors limiting the storage life of fresh horticultural products, with losses estimated to be 5 to 25% in developed countries and 20 to 50% in developing countries (Kader, 2002). One of the most important factors that influence fruit decay is temperature management, since low temperature (avoiding the CI incidence) can slow pathogen growth and in turn reduce decay incidence (Chapter 4). However, prestorage exposure of a fruit to high temperature for a short period of time and then low temperature storage can have beneficial effects in disinfecting the commodity and in reducing decay incidence during storage (Ben-Yehoshua and Porat, 2005). However, the inhibitory effect of heat treatment on pathogen growth does not last long, and the fungus may restart its growth shortly after the heat treatment.

There are some modes of action by which heat application can control fruit decay (Schirra et al., 2000):

1. Slowing pathogen growth or killing its germinated spores. The inhibition of pathogen growth is dependent on both the temperature and

duration of the heat treatment. Thus, spore germination of *P. digitatum* was only partially inhibited by exposure to 56°C for up to 20 s, but was completely inhibited by exposure to 59 or 62°C for 10 or 15 s. Moreover, the fungus type influences its tolerance to heat, with *M. fructicola, R. stolonifer,* and *B. cinerea* being sensitive and *P. expansum* tolerant (Barkai-Golan, 2001). These factors can be seen in Table 5.1, in which some fruits such as pear and mango needed temperatures in the range 46–52°C for a short period of time (10–20 minutes) to control fungal decay, and the time increased up to 60 minutes in tomato, while prolonged exposure (6–12 h) were necessary to control orange decay.

2. Enhancing the host pathogen-defense responses and thus rendering the commodity more resistant. The induction and enhancement of the host pathogen-defense response by heat treatment involves several mechanisms such as increased biosynthesis and accumulation of phytoalexins (which are specific plant antimicrobial compounds), increased lignification of cell walls in wound sites (providing mechanical barriers against pathogen invasion), and induction or enhancement of the level of pathogenesis-related proteins, including the accumulation of specific enzymes able to hydrolyze fungal cell walls (Ben-Yehoshua and Porat, 2005).
3. Melting the epicuticular surface of fruits or vegetables, and thus occluding and sealing microcracks and wounds that could serve as possible pathogen invasion sites. During the course of aging some types of fractures may develop on the epicuticular surface that could serve as possible invasion sites for wound pathogens. The application of heat treatments may eliminate these cracks, probably by partially melting the natural wax of the cuticle, with the consequent occlusion of these cracks and of other microwounds that develop in the cuticular surface in the course of aging or following mechanical damage. Possibly, the heat may change the physical status of the wax making it more plastic so that it may be stretched to occlude the microcracks.

5.4 Limitations: Heat damage

Although this chapter has focused on the beneficial effects of heat treatments on fruit quality after storage, there are some situations in which the application of inappropriate heat treatment leads to tissue damage. This is one of the main reasons that there are a vast number of researchers trying to find a time-temperature regime to reach the desired effects without damaging the commodity. Often, the difference between controlling the postharvest fruit quality and causing damage to the commodity under treatment is a matter of only a few degrees. Fruit damage can be both external, such as peel browning, pitting, yellowing, and decay development, and internal, such as poor color development, abnormal softening, lack of starch breakdown, flesh darkening, and development of internal cavities. These alterations, together with increased weight loss, can be confused with CI symptoms.

Tolerance to heat exposure is influenced by species, cultivar, harvest maturity, growing conditions, and handling between harvest and treatment. Tissue damage caused by heat will also result in increased decay development (Lu et al., 2007). In addition, antioxidant enhancement is an expected benefit of heat treatment; however, as long as the temperature is higher than the threshold temperature, other negative effects could accompany heating injury.

In summary, a better understanding of the physiology, biochemistry, and molecular process occurring in fruit during and following heat treatment will enable the development of more precise and effective hot treatment techniques to control fungal decay and to maintain fruit quality with attractive economic perspectives. The main problem for the scale-up of heat treatments is that the temperature tolerances between an effective treatment and heat damage can be as little as 1–2°C, and the duration at these temperatures also has an effect on produce quality.

chapter six

Calcium treatments

6.1 Introduction

Calcium is an essential plant nutrient, since the divalent Ca^{2+} is required for structural roles in the cell wall and membranes, as a counter-cation for inorganic and organic anions in the vacuole and as an intracellular messenger in the cytosol. Calcium readily enters the apoplasm and is bound in an exchangeable form to cell walls and to the exterior surface of the plasma membrane. Its rate of uptake into the cytoplasm is severely restricted and seems to be only loosely coupled to metabolic processes. Calcium deficiency is rare in nature, but may occur on soils with low base saturation and/or high levels of acidic deposition. Calcium shortage in plants is related to poor Ca uptake, its limited movement to above-ground plant parts, and the strong competition for Ca between leaves and generative plant parts, such as fruits and seeds. Thus, some Ca-deficiency disorders occur in horticulture when calcium is momentarily unavailable to developing tissues, the most important being tip burn and brown heart in leafy vegetables and blossom end rot in watermelon, tomato, and pepper fruit. Another important Ca-induced disorder is cracking in tomato, cherry, and apple fruit, which occurs in tissues lacking sufficient calcium upon hypo-osmotic shock following increased humidity or rainfall, presumably as a result of structural weaknesses in cell walls. These disorders occur because calcium cannot be mobilized from older tissues and redistributed via phloem. This situation forces the developing tissues to rely on the immediate supply of calcium in the xylem, which is dependent on transpiration, the main problem being that transpiration is low in young leaves and fruits, and competition for calcium between low-transpiring fruit and vigorously growing, highly transpiring leafy shoots occurs (White and Broadley, 2003).

Most calcium activity is related to its capacity for coordination by which it provides stable but reversible intermolecular linkages especially in the cell walls and the plasma membrane. These Ca-mediated linkages respond to local changes in environmental conditions and are part of the control mechanism of growth and developmental processes. Calcium is a nontoxic mineral nutrient, even in high concentrations, and is very effective in detoxifying high concentrations of other mineral elements in plants.

There are two distinct areas in the cell wall with high Ca^{2+} concentrations, the middle lamella and the extension surface of the plasma membrane. In both sites, Ca^{2+} has essential structural functions, namely, the regulation of the membrane permeability and related processes and the strengthening of the cell walls.

Calcium treatments represent a safe and potentially effective method for increasing the quality and storage life of a wide range of fruit species, since they reduce postharvest spoilage, softening, ethylene production, and senescence rate. Calcium applications may be performed by preharvest treatments in the irrigation system or by spraying the tree canopy with calcium solutions, although they are more effective when calcium is applied directly to the fruit surface, as little or no subsequent translocation of calcium occurs from leaf to fruit (Kadir, 2004). However, calcium may be applied as a postharvest treatment, by dipping fruits in solutions of calcium salts or by vacuum infiltration. However, some damage can occur if calcium is applied at high concentration (Valero et al., 1998c; Ferguson and Boyd, 2001; Serrano et al., 2004c; Bakshi et al., 2005).

6.2 *Calcium sources and pre- and postharvest methods for application*

Different calcium salts have been studied for pre- and postharvest treatments of fruits to increase fruit quality at harvest and during postharvest storage, to prevent fruit decay, and to enrich the nutritional value of the produce. The selection of the appropriate source depends on several factors, the most important being bioavailability and solubility, followed by flavor change and the interaction with food ingredients. Nevertheless, calcium chloride has been widely used as a preservative and firming agent in fruit and vegetable industries for whole and fresh-cut commodities, with satisfactory results in apples, strawberries, grapefruits, and fresh-cut cantaloupe and honeydew melons and peaches, among others. Other forms of calcium used with this finality are calcium carbonate, calcium citrate, calcium lactate, calcium propionate, calcium phosphate, and calcium gluconate (Martín-Diana et al., 2007).

Preharvest calcium treatments are performed in the irrigation systems and by foliar spray. In the irrigation system, the most used calcium sources are calcium chloride, followed by calcium nitrate and calcium thiosulphate at concentration of 3.5–4.0 mmol L^{-1} (Madrid et al., 2004; Johnstone et al., 2008; Serrano et al., 2002). In foliar spray treatments, the most used sources of calcium have been Cl_2Ca and $Ca(NO_3)_2$, followed by some calcium-chelated forms, such as amino acid–chelated calcium and mannitol-complexed calcium, which have been applied at different stages of fruit development, from flowering to 48 hours before harvesting and in a wide range of concentrations, from 0.5 to 10% (Agustí et al., 2004; Serrano et al., 2004b; Lester and Grusak, 2004; Manganaris et al., 2005b; 2006; Besada et al., 2008; Stückrath et al., 2008; Randhawa et al., 2009; Cronje et al., 2009).

For postharvest treatment two main ways of calcium application in fresh fruits and vegetables have been reported: dipping-washing and vacuum infiltration processes. Dipping treatments are commonly used for flesh perishable products and consist of the soaking of the produce, sometimes applying mechanical agitation, followed by the removal of excess washing solution. This method of calcium application favors the solution dispersion on the fruit and vegetable surface and has the extra benefit on minimally fresh-cut commodities of rinsing the enzymes and substrates released from the injured cells during the minimal procedure, avoiding oxidations that could lead to browning and off-flavors generation. The dipping time ranges from 5 to 120 min and the calcium concentration from 0.5 to 6%, the most used source of calcium being calcium chloride followed by calcium nitrate, calcium lactate, calcium propionate, and calcium gluconate (Suntharalingam, 1996; Lara et al., 2004; Manganaris et al., 2005a; 2007; Martín-Diana et al., 2007; Hernández-Muñoz et al., 2008; Mahmud et al., 2008).

Vacuum infiltration processes consist of the penetration of the calcium solution into the intracellular spaces by capillary and pressure gradients generated when the air is extracted from the tissue pores following the application of vacuum and restoration of the atmospheric conditions. Different calcium concentration (1.5–7.5%), pressure applied (2–33 kPa), and time (30 s–10 min) have been used in several experiments, with both whole and sliced fruits (Valero et al., 1998c; 2002b; Lara et al., 2004; Safizadeh et al., 2007; Mahmud et al., 2008; Pinheiro and Almeida, 2008; Eryani-Raqeeb et al., 2009). The partial substitution of the internal gas by the new liquid phase allows the reformulation of the food commodity by the modification of the solid matrix, leading to increases in textural properties and being a more effective method of getting calcium into the fruit than the dipping one (Gras et al., 2003; Martín-Diana et al., 2007).

6.3 *Pre- and postharvest calcium treatments and calcium fruit content*

As commented in the introduction section, calcium deficiency during fruit growth on plant can occur as a result of limited root uptake, and immobility within the plant and its essential structural functions in plant cell walls may be altered, causing many disorders on fruits, the most important being bitter pit in apples, blossom end rot in tomato, and water core or glassiness in melon (Bakshi et al., 2005). Thus, the incidence of glassiness or vitrescence in cantaloupe melon has been associated with calcium deficiency, this disorder being highly reduced when calcium concentration in the irrigation system was increased up to 4 mmol L^{-1} in the hydroponic system, using a soilless culture, since these treatments increased calcium in the rind and flesh of melon fruits (Madrid et al., 2004; Serrano et al., 2002). However, in experiments performed in California with honeydew and muskmelon plants different results have been obtained. Thus, amino acid–chelated calcium and mannitol-complexed calcium at calcium concentration of 6 and 10%, respectively, increased calcium content in skin and flesh of melon fruits, this effect being also evident after postharvest storage, although four spray applications from flowering to 3 days before harvesting were needed (Lester and Grusak, 2004). However, calcium application in the fertirrigation system as calcium nitrate, calcium chloride, or calcium thiosulphate, at similar concentrations, had no effect on melon fruit calcium concentration (Johnstone et al., 2008). The later results can be explained by the relatively high soil calcium concentration, around 12–13 meq L^{-1}.

Preharvest calcium spray over tree canopy or plant is one of the most important practices applied in the new production systems to increase calcium content in fruits, such as tomato (Dong et al., 2004), blueberry (Stückrath et al., 2008), litchi (Cronje et al., 2009), pomegranate (Ramezanian et al., 2009), and peach and nectarine (Serrano et al., 2004b; Manganaris et al., 2005b; 2006), with important effect on quality attributes at harvest and during postharvest storage. Thus, preharvest calcium sprays on peach and nectarine tress significantly increased calcium content in the skin of fresh fruits (Figure 6.1). Calcium from these foliar treatments uptakes through the fruit peel by natural openings such as stomata and lenticels. Additionally, cracks fuzz and surface discontinuities, which are more apparent during the late phase of fruit growth, seem to offer other sites for calcium penetration. At harvest time, calcium concentration was higher in the peel than in the flesh, and during storage calcium decreased in the peel and increased in the flesh, suggesting a movement of calcium from the peel to the flesh. The higher concentration of calcium at harvest in peach from treated trees was found in the insoluble pectic fraction of the cell wall. However, during cold storage and subsequent shelf life calcium increased in the water-soluble pectins (Manganaris et al., 2005b; 2006). In tomato fruit calcium concentration increased with both calcium treatments, in the irrigation system and foliar sprayed at anthesis, while no effect was obtained when calcium was applied on 3-week-old fruits (Dong et al., 2004). In addition, in plum trees it has been shown that calcium content in fruit increased when foliar preharvest calcium treatments were combined with titanium, the plum fruits being also more resistant to handling damages. These effects have been interpreted as a consequence of the beneficial effect of titanium on the calcium absorption and assimilation

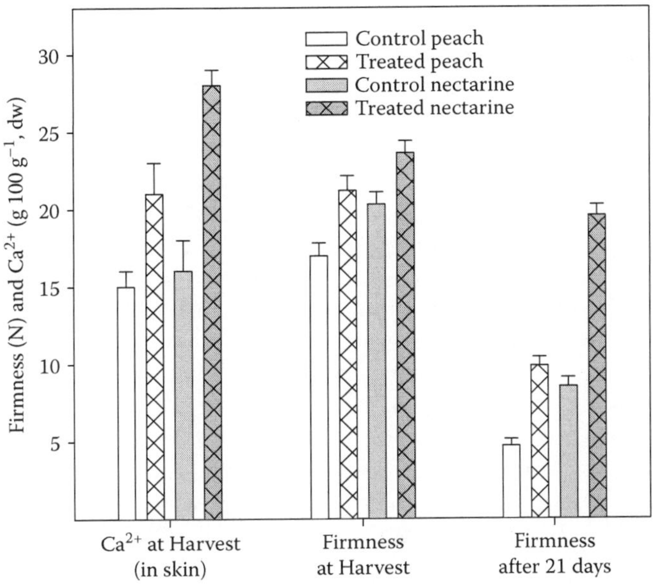

Figure 6.1 Calcium concentration in the skin and fruit firmness at harvest and after 21 days of cold storage in control and calcium-treated peach and nectarine (preharvest treatment with Ca^{2+} by foliar spray along fruit development according to Serrano et al., 2004b).

processes, since treatments were performed during the period in which calcium moves passively to fruit, thus permitting the calcium integration in the cell wall and consequently increasing the fruit firmness (Alcaraz-López et al., 2003).

Accordingly, postharvest dipping treatments increased calcium content in both peel and flesh of peach fruits, although calcium source (calcium chloride, lactate, or propionate) did not seem to affect calcium absorption (Manganaris et al., 2007). During peach cold storage an increase in cell wall calcium occurred, mainly due to the enhancement of calcium in the water-soluble pectin fraction, as well as in calcium infiltrated apples (Chardonnet et al., 2003), suggesting that soluble calcium was mobilized and integrated into the cell wall. The increase in cell wall–bound calcium of calcium-treated peaches was related to both calcium concentration and time of storage.

6.4 *Effect of preharvest treatment on fruit size*

The double application of 2% $CaCl_2$ to litchi at fruit set and 40 days after (fruitlet stage) increased total yield by enhancements in both fruit weight and size (Cronje et al., 2009). In peach and nectarine trees, preharvest treatments with calcium solutions increased fruit set and fruit size at harvest, leading to higher yield in terms of both fruit number and size (Serrano et al., 2004b). Similar results were observed in plum treated with three preharvest applications of 0.1 mmol of Ca^{2+} before harvest (Alcaráz-López et al., 2003). However, in honeydew or muskmelon fruit calcium fertirrigation had no effect on marketable yield, fruit size, or quality, regardless of the application times or calcium source applied (Johnstone et al., 2008). Pomegranates treated with Ca^{2+} at 2 or 4% one month after full blossom increased average fruit weight, but treatment was ineffective when performed earlier, at full blossom (Ramezanian et al., 2009). Moreover, in blueberry contradictory results have been found, since fruit weight was inversely proportional to the calcium level applied (Stückrath et al., 2008). This effect has been attributed to the high proportion of low-methoxyl pectins in these fruits, which interact through their carboxyl groups without esterification with calcium ions to form quelate-type unions. These unions occurring during fruit growth lead to a greater rigidity of the cell wall, thus limiting fruit expansion.

6.5 *Calcium treatments and fruit firmness*

Most of the reports on calcium treatments have been focused on their effect on fruit firmness. Calcium, as a constituent of the cell wall, plays an important role in forming cross-bridges among pectic substances, leading to stabilization of the plant cell wall and protection from the cell wall–degrading enzymes, specifically from the pectolitic enzymes (White and Broadly, 2003; Serrano et al., 2004c). The most important, PG, breaks the glycosidic links between units of nonesterificated galacturonic acids. If calcium interacts with these carboxylic groups without esterification, it reduces their number and thus the PG action decreases. In fact, calcium content in the nutrient solutions affected positively whole fruit firmness of cantaloupe and honeydew melons (Serrano et al., 2002; Lester and Grusak, 1999; Madrid et al., 2004). The softening process started 2 days early on melon treated with low calcium concentration and coincided with increases in β-GAL and PG activities, while in melon irrigated with high calcium concentration the softening process was lower and delayed on time and no PG activity was detected (Serrano et al., 2002). However, in other experiments performed in California, calcium fertirrigation had no effect on firmness losses during honeydew or muskmelon postharvest storage and was not correlated with calcium concentration in fruit tissue (Johnstone et al., 2008). Thus, these contradictory results could be attributed to different soil characteristics or to other cultural or environmental factors.

Preharvest calcium sprays provided peaches and nectarines with increased firmness at harvest and during storage (Serrano et al., 2004b) or only during storage (Manganaris et al., 2005a). Accordingly, preharvest spray with calcium solution increased calcium concentration and firmness in litchi and blueberry fruits, with a strong positive correlation being found between these two parameters (Stückrath et al., 2008; Cronje et al., 2009). Additionally, preharvest calcium sprays have been useful in delaying softening after harvesting of some fruits such as pears (Gerasopoulos and Richardson, 1999), ber fruits (Randhawa et al., 2009), persimmon (Agustí et al., 2004; Besada et al., 2008), and strawberries (Chéour et al., 1990). Nevertheless, the applied calcium concentration is critical in the calcium chloride formulation, since high concentration can damage the leaves (Serrano et al., 2004b; Manganaris et al., 2005a; 2006).

Figure 6.1 shows that fruit firmness at harvest in peach and nectarine fruits was higher in fruits from calcium-treated trees than in those from control ones. In addition, during postharvest storage, the softening process was delayed on time in those fruits from calcium-treated trees, which showed higher levels of fruit firmness than controls after 21 days of storage.

Postharvest calcium treatments have also been effective in retaining firmness during storage in a wide range of fruits, such as apple (Conway et al., 1994; Chardonnet et al., 2003), mango (Suntharalingam, 1996), kiwifruit (Hopkirk et al., 1990), peach (Manganaris et al., 2007), plum (Valero et al., 2002b), blueberry (Hanson et al., 1993), strawberry (García et al., 1996; Lara et al., 2004), nectarine (Manganaris et al., 2005a), lemon (Valero et al., 1998c; Martínez-Romero et al., 1999; Safizadeh et al., 2007), tomato slices (Artés et al., 1999; Pinheiro and Almeida, 2008), cantaloupe and honeydew melon cylinders (Luna-Guzman et al., 1999; Saftner et al., 2003), and zucchini slices (Izumi and Watada, 1995). In other experiments, calcium lactate has been more effective in increasing texture and crispness of fruits and vegetables than calcium chloride (Martín-Diana et al., 2007).

Figure 6.2 shows the changes in fruit firmness during storage of lemon, and the plum cultivars Black Star and Santa Rosa. The postharvest application of Ca^{2+} led to significantly higher firmness levels in Ca-treated lemons and Black Star plum, this effect being still evident after 7 days of storage, whereas in Santa Rosa plum cultivar calcium treatment only delayed firmness loss. In addition, calcium treatment makes the fruit less susceptible to mechanical damage during processing, handling, and packaging, as has been shown in lemon (Martínez-Romero et al., 1999) and plum fruits (Serrano et al., 2004a). Accordingly, in papaya dipping or vacuum calcium treatments increased storage life and diminished the softening process, the effect being greater, with calcium chloride concentration increased up to 2.5%, with the vacuum treatment (Mahmud et al., 2008).

The reasons for calcium increasing fruit and vegetable firmness has been attributed to its role in cross-linking pectic substances in the cell wall

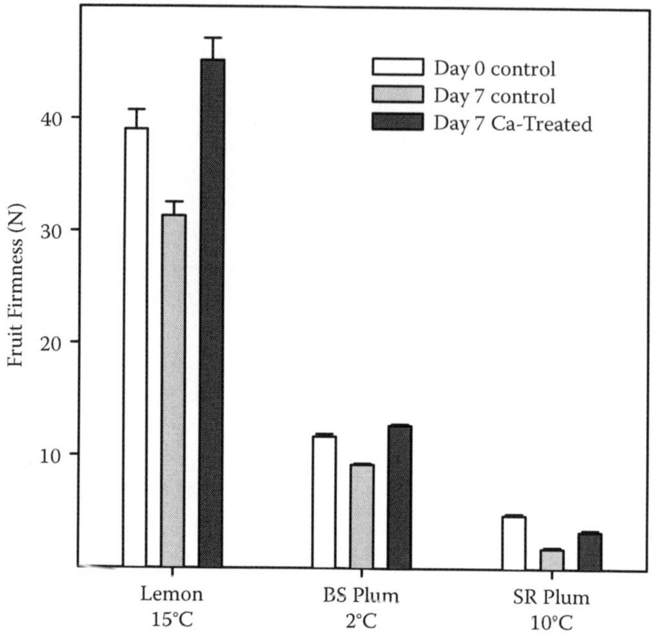

Figure 6.2 Levels of firmness in lemon and Black Star (BS) and Santa Rosa (SR) plums at harvest (day 0) and after 7 days of storage at 15, 2, and 10°C, respectively, of control and calcium-treated (postharvest 1 mM by pressure infiltration) fruits.

and middle lamella, resulting in the formation of calcium pectate by the calcium binding to free carboxyl groups of polygalacturonate polymer, stabilizing and strengthening the cell wall, this effect being detectable immediately after calcium treatments (Valero et al., 1998c; 2002b; Serrano et al., 2004a; 2004c). This effect of calcium treatments on reinforcing and consolidating the cell wall has been recently proved by light microscopy in fresh-cut apples and pears after storage. In control fruits, the cell walls were irregularly stained because of the loss of the cellular package, some cell walls were broken, the cell-to-cell contacts were lost, and the plasmalemma had retracted toward the center of the cell. However, in treated fruit the plasmalemma remained close to the cell wall and the cell walls were homogeneously stained, since cellulose fibrils were closely packed together (Quiles et al., 2007; Alandes et al., 2009).

It has been also proposed that calcium can affect some hydrolytic enzymes of the cell wall, such as PME (Javeri et al., 1991), and a possible role for calcium in reducing the expression or activity of PG and the production of pectic oligomers, which induce ripening, has been addressed (Mignani et al., 1995). Preharvest treatment of ber fruit with $CaCl_2$ and $Ca(NO_3)_2$ at color break stage leads to slower rise in PME activity during cold storage as compared to nontreated fruits (Randhawa et al., 2009). Calcium treatments may also activate the synthesis of several cell wall compounds, resulting in higher accumulation of noncellulosic polysaccharides such as lignin and an inhibition of cellulose deposition. This *de novo* synthesis led to increases in the extractable cell wall compared to controls. Thus, the degradation rate would be much lower than the synthesis rate, and the cell wall solubilized more slowly (Conway et al., 1999).

An additional effect on fruit firmness has been observed when combined treatment of calcium and mild heat (40–70°C for 5 minutes or less) was applied to strawberry and melon. Heat can be applied with the calcium treatment by increasing the temperature of the calcium solution or prior to the calcium treatment. This effect has been explained in terms of PME activation by the increase in temperature. Thus, PME cleaving the methoxyl groups from methylated galacturonic acid residues in pectin generates free pectic acids, which contain newly available carboxyl groups to bind with more endogenous or added Ca^{2+}, thus increasing tissue firmness (Martín-Diana et al., 2007; Aguayo et al., 2008). Accordingly, the addition of calcium-gluconate to chitosan to be applied as edible coating on strawberry, leads to higher fruit firmness levels during storage, compared to fruit coated with chitosan alone (Hernández-Muñoz et al., 2006; 2008).

6.6 Calcium treatments and color, soluble solids, and total acidity

Preharvest foliar spray treatments of apples, persimmon, and litchi trees led to an increase in the skin redness color of the fruits at harvest time, with a positive correlation between color value a* and skin calcium concentration (Kadir, 2004; Besada et al., 2008; Cronje et al., 2009). However, in peach and nectarines no differences were found in color a* parameters at the time of harvest between fruits from control and calcium-sprayed trees, although the evolution of this color parameter during postharvest storage was delayed in treated fruits with respect to nontreated ones (Figure 6.3), showing a delay on the postharvest ripening process in fruits from calcium-treated trees. Accordingly, the characteristic color evolution of papaya (Mahmud et al., 2008) and mango fruits (Suntharalingam, 1996) was delayed on postharvest infiltrated fruits with calcium solutions.

With respect to the effect of calcium treatment on TSS and TA, different and somewhat contradictory results have been obtained. Thus, foliar spray of pomegranate trees with 2 or 4% of calcium chloride increased total TSS in the arils at harvest time, with no significant effect on TA (Ramezanian et al., 2009). Contrarily, TSS and TA were lower in tomato

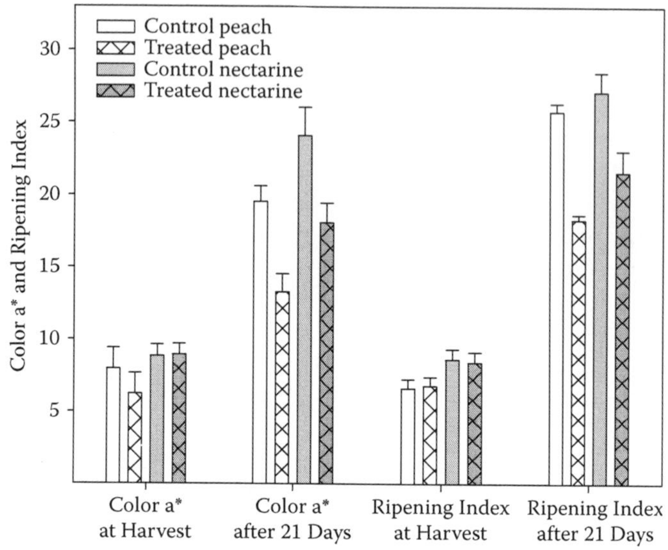

Figure 6.3 Color (a* parameter) and ripening index (TSS/TA) at harvest and after 21 days of cold storage in control and calcium-treated peach and nectarine (preharvest treatment with Ca^{2+} by foliar spray along fruit development according to Serrano et al., 2004b).

from calcium-treated plants (Dong et al., 2004; Fanasca et al., 2006). However, TSS and TA concentration at harvest in peach and nectarines were not affected by preharvest foliar sprays of calcium solutions, and similar ripening indexes were found in fruits from control and treated trees (Figure 6.3). However, their evolution during postharvest storage was influenced by the preharvest calcium sprays, especially the decrease in total acidity, leading to a lower value of the ripening index after 3 weeks of cold storage in fruits from treated trees than in those from control ones. In addition, the increase in TSS was delayed by postharvest infiltration calcium treatments on papaya, due to slower changes from carbohydrates to sugars, as well as the decrease in TA in papaya and strawberry, by reducing the enzymatic reactions of respiration (Lara et al., 2004; Mahmud et al., 2008), showing a delay on the ripening process in these treated fruits.

The relationship between calcium treatments and aroma volatile production is of interest, although only a few works on this subject have been published. For example, prestorage apple treatments with $CaCl_2$ caused enhanced emission of some impact compounds and improved the aroma quality after middle-term storage. In addition, sensory analysis by means of a consumer panel indicated higher acceptance scores for calcium-treated fruits (Ortiz et al., 2009). After middle-term storage the effect of calcium treatment on increasing production of volatiles probably arises from enhanced supply of precursors for ester production as a consequence of increased pyruvate decarboxylase and alcohol dehydrogenase activities, while after long-term storage, the enhancement of alcohol-acyltransferase activity might also contribute. Thus, postharvest calcium treatments have the potential to improve aroma quality of cold stored apple.

6.7 Calcium treatment and bioactive compounds

The effect of calcium treatments on bioactive compounds with functional properties has been addressed in only a few reports and in very recent years. Thus, in apple and litchi fruits increased anthocyanin concentration in the skin was found in fruits from sprayed calcium trees at fruit set and fruitlet stage, the concentration of anthocyanin being correlated with the calcium concentration of the skin (Kadir, 2004; Cronje et al., 2009). In pomegranate arils this treatment induced an increase in ascorbic acid (Ramezanian et al., 2009). Accordingly, in tomato from calcium-treated plant, in the irrigation system and foliar sprayed, an increase in ascorbic acid was also found by Dong and colleagues (2004), but no effect was detected by Fanasca and colleagues (2006). In contrast, carotenoid and provitamin A contents were lower when Ca^{2+} was increased from 2 to 8 mmol L^{-1}, but the content of total phenolics was enhanced (Marín et al., 2009).

Moreover, Fanasca and colleagues (2006) also reported a decrease in lycopene content as a consequence of the increase of the calcium concentration in the nutrient solution, due to an antagonism between Ca and K, which is involved in the carotenoid biosynthesis by its action on the activity of enzymes that regulate carbohydrate metabolism, such as pyruvate kinase and phosphofructokinase as well as on precursors of pyruvate and glyceraldehyde 3-phosphate.

With respect to postharvest treatments, calcium treatments of papaya fruit led to maintenance of higher ascorbic acid concentration during storage as compared with nontreated fruits, this effect being greater with vacuum infiltration treatment than with dipping treatment (Mahmud et al., 2008).

Thus, due to the antioxidant properties of the anthocyanins, ascorbic acid and lycopene, these results would lead to a contradictory conclusion: Calcium treatments possibly increase and decrease the functional properties of both in fruits, and thus more research is needed to clarify this issue. Recently a great potential has been shown of the fresh-cut fruit and vegetables industry for developing high-quality fresh-cut commodities that are fortified with vitamin E and minerals. Thus, by using vacuum impregnation technology and solutions with the desired component, the fresh-cut fruit can be fortified by vitamins and minerals, leading to an increase of these nutraceuticals in human diets (Park et al., 2005; 2006).

6.8 *Calcium treatment, cell membrane stability, and CI reduction*

Other beneficial effects of calcium infiltration on postharvest quality of fruit are probably mediated through the stabilizing influence of Ca^{2+} on cell membranes leading to a delay in membrane protein and phospholipid catabolic processes and to a reduction of ion leakage during postharvest storage of fruit (Picchioni et al., 1998). These effects of calcium ions on increasing membrane integrity as a consequence help maintain or enhance cell turgor pressure, which contributes to a delay in fruit softening and weight loss during postharvest storage, as has been shown in papaya fruits (Eryani-Raqeeb et al., 2009), and could also be attributed to the effect of calcium on decreasing water vapor diffusivity through the cell wall structure.

In addition, a role of calcium on maintaining membrane stability under stress conditions, such as low temperature storage, has been also addressed. This calcium effect could explain the fact that pre- and postharvest calcium treatments have a positive effect on reducing CI as has been observed in mandarins (D'Aquino et al., 2005) and lemons (Safizadeh et al., 2007). In postharvest treatments, 1.5% $CaCl_2$ was the most effective concentration in reducing CI symptoms when applied by vacuum infiltration, the effectiveness becoming more negative as $CaCl_2$ concentration increased up to 7.5%. Accordingly, postharvest calcium dips of peaches decreased flesh browning after cold storage, which is a symptom of CI associated with low calcium content (Manganaris et al., 2007). In addition, an effect of calcium on reducing browning, which occurs as a result of oxidation of membrane phospholipids and polymerization of polyphenols, has been observed, with special interest in fresh-cut fruits such as apples, pears, and melons (Martín-Diana et al., 2007; Alandes et al., 2009). Thereafter, a reduction of other fruit disorders such as sour core, watercore, and internal breakdown was reported (Yuen, 1994). Calcium chloride added to the irrigation water of mushrooms was also effective in reducing postharvest browning by maintaining vacuolar membrane integrity and thereby reducing the opportunity for tyrosinase to react with its substrates and develop browning (Kukura et al., 1998).

However, combined treatments of hot water and calcium infiltration had no advantage compared with hot water alone in reducing CI in lemon. Moreover, at too high calcium concentration a negative result, increased CI and weight loss, was found mainly due to a cytotoxic effect of the overload calcium concentration acting as physiological transducer of cell injury or death (Safizadeh et al., 2007).

6.9 *Effects of calcium treatment on postharvest decay*

The increase of calcium in fruits is another means of suppressing storage disease by maintaining or enhancing the natural resistance of fruits and vegetables to pathogens. In this sense, calcium treatment was effective in controlling postharvest decay caused by *Penicillum expansum*, *Botrytis cinerea*, *Glomerella cingulata*, and *Gloeosporium* in apple and strawberry, as well as on papaya fruit, the effect being higher when calcium treatment was performed by vacuum infiltration compared to the dipping treatment (García et al., 1996; Lara et al., 2004; Mahmud et al., 2008). Additional reduction of decay has been reported by combined heat and calcium treatments in Golden Delicious (Conway et al., 1994) and Gala apples (Conway et al., 1999), in cactus pear (Schirra et al., 1997), and in fresh-cut melon (Aguayo et al., 2008), showing that these combined treatments may be a useful alternative to the chemical fungicides in controlling postharvest decay. Calcium chloride infiltration was also effective in reducing anthracnose (*Colletotrichum gloeosporioides*) disease incidence on papaya fruits, in a dose-dependent manner from 1.5 to 3.5%, this effect being increased by the combined treatment chitosan-calcium (Eryani-Raqeeb et al., 2009). In addition, different calcium salts have been shown to inhibit bacterial and yeast growth, this effect being the highest by calcium propionate. The antimicrobial properties of organic acid salts, such as calcium propionate, are dependent upon their ability to form disassociated acids in solution and to uncouple microbial substrate transport and oxidative phosphorylation from the electron transport system (Aguayo et al., 2008).

The mechanisms by which exogenous calcium reduces fruit decay and increases fruit firmness are closely related, and are attributed to the increased calcium bound to the cell wall. Most of the calcium that penetrates into the host tissue seems to accumulate in the middle lamella region of the cell wall. The calcium-induced resistance of storage fruits to postharvest pathogens has been attributed to an interaction between the cell wall pectins and Ca ions. By binding to pectins in the cell wall, Ca ions contribute to maintaining the structural integrity of the cell wall. Thus, calcium enhances tissue resistance to fungal attack by stabilizing or strengthening cell walls, thereby making them more resistant to harmful enzymes produced by fungi, and also delays aging of fruits (Conway et al., 1994; 1999; Lara et al., 2004; Eryani-Raqeeb et al., 2009). Although prolongation of storage life as a result of calcium application is thought to be due mainly to the role of calcium in ameliorating physiological disorders and thus indirectly reducing pathogen activity, direct effects of calcium on the pathogen, such as interfering with spore germination and germ tube elongation of *P. expansum* and *B. cinerea*, have also been recognized (Barkai-Golan, 2001).

6.10 Calcium treatment and ethylene production and respiration rate

High calcium content in fruits has been related to longer postharvest life as a result of reduced rates of respiration and ethylene production, delayed ripening, increased firmness, and reduced incidence of physiological disorders and decay. Thus, preharvest treatments with calcium solution have shown an effect on delaying ethylene production and ripening process in climacteric fruits, such as tomato (Wills et al., 1997), persimmon (Agustí et al., 2004), pears (Gerasopoulos and Richardson, 1999), and peach and nectarines (Serrano et al., 2004b). In addition, apple tree treatments with calcium chloride by foliar sprays decreased ethylene production and respiration rate in apple fruits at harvest and after postharvest storage under controlled ultralow oxygen atmosphere conditions, both physiological parameters being correlated with fruit calcium content (Recasens et al., 2004). However, contradictory results have been found in melons, since the increase of calcium concentration in the irrigation system of melon plants increased ethylene production rate, although the time course of the climacteric peak was not affected (Madrid et al., 2004) or was delayed with high calcium concentration (Serrano et al., 2002). Since calcium has a positive effect on stabilizing cell membranes, the lower ethylene production of melons irrigated with low calcium solutions might be due to low activity of ACO, which is located at the external face of the plasma membrane.

In addition, postharvest calcium treatment can inhibit ethylene production and fruit ripening of climacteric fruits, such as apple and plum, ethylene production being more reduced with increasing calcium concentrations. This effect has been attributed to a decrease in the activity of ACO (Serrano et al., 2004c). In tomato discs, ethylene production was inhibited by $CaCl_2$ treatments in a dose-dependent way, in both the wildtype and the ethylene receptor mutant tomato (*Nr*), showing that the ethylene inhibition by calcium is independent of ethylene perception. However, ACS was not affected by calcium treatment, while ACO activity increased, as did calcium chloride concentrations. Based on these results Wang and colleagues (2006b) have proposed that the membrane strengthened by calcium should inhibit the translocation of endogenous ACC from synthesis sites (cytosol) to the external face of the plasma membrane where the ACO is located. Nevertheless, an effect of calcium inhibiting the expression of the *Le*ACO1 gene, which reduced the amount of ACO protein, was also found. However, a contrary effect was observed when bananas were dipped in $CaCl_2$ with or without vacuum treatment, where time to ripening was markedly reduced (Serrano et al., 2004c). In addition, different results have been found in mango, depending on the $CaCl_2$ concentration applied in postharvest treatment, since 4 and 6% decrease of color evolution and softening was detected, leading to increased shelf life (Suntharalingam, 1996), while by using calcium chloride at 2% an increase on the ripening process was found (Singh et al., 2007).

Figure 6.4 shows a net increase of ethylene production rate in Black Star plum a few hours after mechanical damage. This ethylene production is so-called wound-inducible ethylene and it seems to be a general response of plant tissues to injury through an activation of ACS and ACO (Kato et al., 2000). However, in calcium infiltrated plums before the application of mechanical damage, the increase in wound ethylene was significantly lower. Similarly, respiration rate increased as a consequence of the mechanical damage, this response being reduced in calcium-treated plums (Figure 6.4). In addition, during prolonged storage, the climacteric peak of both ethylene production and respiration rate occurred earlier and reached higher values in damaged control fruits. However, in those plums that were treated with calcium before mechanical damage, ethylene and respiration rates were even lower than in nondamaged control fruits, showing a net effect of calcium treatment on protecting fruit tissues against mechanical damage (Serrano et al., 2004a). Lower respiration rates have also been observed in calcium chloride–treated melon

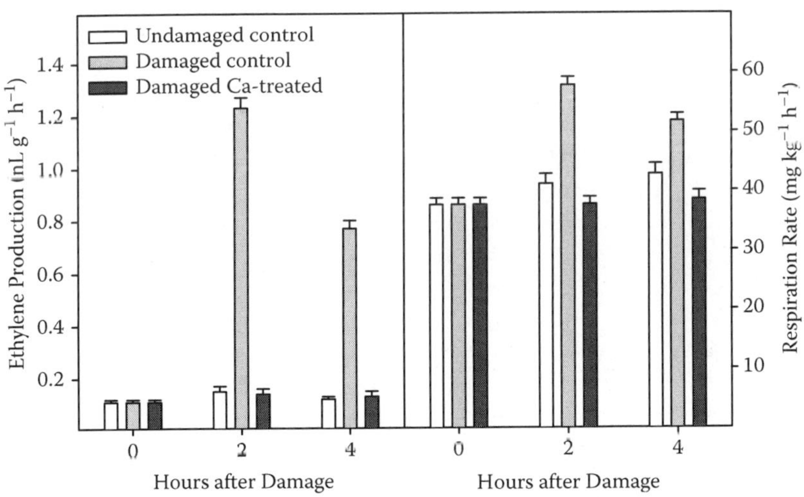

Figure 6.4 Effect of mechanical damage (50 N load) on ethylene production and respiration rate in control and Ca-treated plum (Black Star) within a few hours after damage.

slices (Luna-Guzman et al., 1999) and in apples, although with very high calcium concentrations, respiration rate increased (Serrano et al., 2004c). In addition, calcium propionate and calcium lactate have shown also to be effective in decreasing both ethylene production and respiration rate in fresh-cut melon (Luna-Guzman and Barret, 2000; Aguayo et al., 2008).

6.11 *Undesirable effects of calcium treatments*

As explained above, in general pre- and postharvest calcium treatments have positive effects on fruit quality and lead to longer storage periods. However, undesirable effects of calcium treatments have also been reported, especially when calcium concentration is not adequate. Thus, one of the major problems with using calcium infiltration to reduce decay has been the inability to predict the amount of calcium absorbed and the resulting surface damage, such as discoloration, if too much is absorbed (Conway et al., 1994). In addition, some fruits do not tolerate calcium treatments, which may induce peel injuries. Thus, calcium treatment did not suppress the occurrence of oleocellosis in Kiyomi tangerine, while in papayas and grapefruits $CaCl_2$ treatments promoted CI, as well as in cactus pear when calcium treatment was combined with hot water (Schirra et al., 1997; Serrano et al., 2004c). Postharvest nectarine dipping with high concentrations (187.5 mM) of calcium salts resulted in surface damage, leading to undesirable characteristics during fruit ripening (Manganaris et al., 2005a). In berries, the use of vacuum infiltration or dips in solutions of $CaCl_2$ is not recommended because of their sensitive texture (García et al., 1996).

Finally, sensory analysis of minimally processed fruits has revealed the occurrence of bitterness and salty taste as side effects of the calcium treatment in fruits such as blackberries dipped in 2 and 4% calcium chloride (Hanson et al., 1993) and melons dipped in 2.5% calcium chloride, which are avoided when calcium lactate or calcium propionate instead of calcium chloride were used (Luna-Guzman and Barret, 2000) or with lower calcium concentration (Aguayo et al., 2008).

In conclusion, calcium treatments may improve fruit quality during storage and increase shelf life through maintaining fruit firmness, reducing the rate of fruit ripening, reducing decay, and eliminating specific calcium-related disorders if appropriate concentrations are applied to avoid occurrence of detrimental side effects.

chapter seven

Polyamine treatments

7.1 Introduction

Polyamines (PAs) are organic cations containing amino groups that are present in all eukaryotic cells (both animal and plant) and intimately involved in, and required for, distinct biological functions. An increasing body of evidence indicates that the regulation of cellular PAs is a central convergence point for the multiple signaling pathways driving various cellular functions. Over the last decade, considerable progress has been made in understanding the molecular functions of cellular PAs (Wang and Casero, 2006). PAs are essential for cell growth and differentiation and their intracellular concentrations increase during periods of rapid cell proliferation, though their explicit role in these cellular processes is mostly unknown.

In plant organs, PAs are positively implicated in plant growth and differentiation as well as in stress responses. In plant tissues, the main PAs (Figure 7.1) are putrescine (Put, 1,4-diaminobutane), spermidine (Spd, *N*-3-aminopropyl-1,4-diaminobutane), and spermine (Spm, [bis(*N*-3-aminopropyl)-1,4-diaminobutane]). The three PAs are present ubiquitously as polycationic compounds and are found in significant amounts in vegetable cell types (nanomolar to micromolar concentrations) to support a wide variety of cellular functions.

Anton Leeuwenhoek was the first to observe crystals of Spm phosphate in human semen as early as 1678. Put was identified more than two centuries later while Spd was discovered only in 1927 (Mattoo and Handa, 2008). Improved knowledge of the physiology of PAs during fruit development and ripening can be achieved not only by analyzing endogenous PA levels and biosynthesis, but also through experimental protocols aimed at manipulating fruit PA levels. These include exogenous PA supply under field and postharvest conditions, isolation of mutants, and genetic engineering of PA biosynthetic genes. The present chapter examines various aspects of the involvement of PAs in the regulation of fruit growth, ripening, and postharvest behavior. Therefore, the next sections focus on the current advances in the dietary PAs, the knowledge of PA

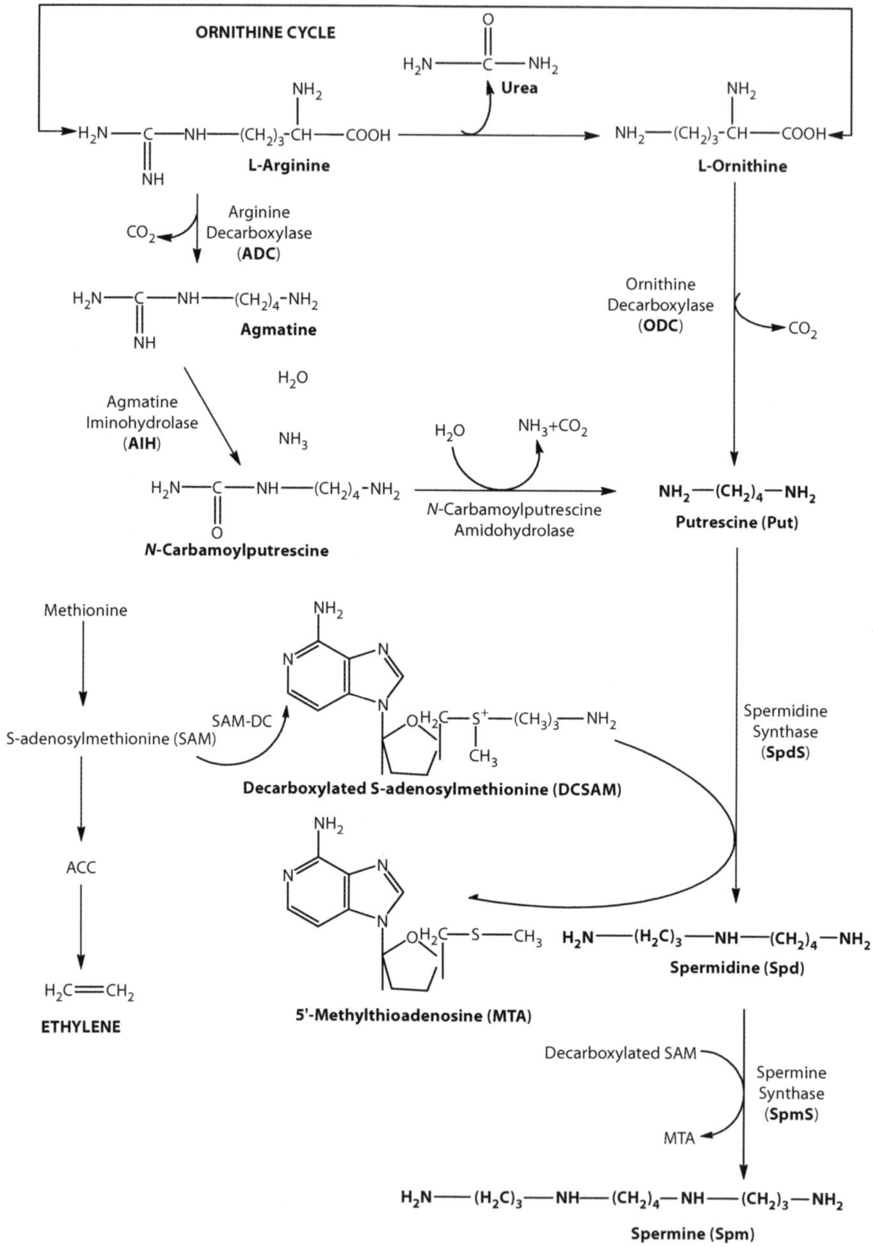

Figure 7.1 Polyamine biosynthetic pathway. Connection with ethylene biosynthesis (schematic) is also provided. Full ethylene biosynthesis is shown in Figure 2.11 (Chapter 2).

biosynthesis and metabolism, endogenous significance, and exogenous applications related to fruit quality as well as their relation with CI and mechanical damage in fruits.

7.2 Polyamine biosynthesis and regulation in plant tissues

The biosynthesis and catabolism of the PAs (Put, Spd, and Spm) are carefully controlled processes in plant and animal cell types. In plants, the PA biosynthetic pathway is shown in Figure 7.1, in which connection with the ethylene biosynthesis is also provided. The biosynthesis pathways for PAs are well established in many organisms: mammals, fungi, bacteria, and plants (Kumar et al., 1997; Valero et al., 2002a; Kusano et al., 2007). In mammals and fungi, Put is produced by a single pathway catalyzed by ornithine decarboxylase [EC 4.1.1.17, ODC]. In contrast, plant-Put is usually produced by two alternative pathways. One is the ODC-catalyzed reaction, as in mammals; the second is from arginine, as a result of the action of arginine decarboxylase [EC 4.1.1.19, ADC] via agmatine. A few plant species, including *Arabidopsis thaliana*, lack the ODC pathway. Conversion of agmatine into Put requires two enzymes, agmatine iminohydrolase [EC 3.5.3.12, AIH] and *N*-carbamoylputrescine amidohydrolase [EC 3.5.1.53]. Put is converted into Spd, and then into Spm by symmetrical addition of an aminopropyl residue from decarboxylated S-adenosylmethionine (DCSAM), which results from decarboxylation of SAM by SAM decarboxylase [EC 4.1.1.50, SAMDC]. These reactions are sequentially catalyzed by two closely related but distinct enzymes, Spd synthase [EC 2.5.1.16, SpdS] and Spm synthase [EC 2.5.1.22, SpmS]. SAM is also known as AdoMet. The genes encoding the PA biosynthetic enzymes have been isolated from a variety of plant species (Kusano et al., 2007).

The existence of two alternative routes (ADC/ODC) for the synthesis of Put could be explained by the differential compartmentalization of the two enzymes (ADC is chloroplast-localized and ODC is generally considered to be cytoplasmic), resulting in the specific regulation of different plant processes. The enzymes ADC and ODC can be inhibited by the reversible inhibitors DL-α-difluoromethylarginine (DFMA) and DL-α-difluoromethylornithine (DFMO), respectively. It has been demonstrated that Put and Spd levels inhibit ODC mRNA translation. Methylglyoxal-bis-guanylhydrazone (MGBG) and cyclohexylamine are irreversible inhibitors of SAMDC and Spd synthase activities, respectively. SAM is an important metabolic crossroad in the regulation of nitrogen metabolism, since it is also a precursor of ethylene via ACC (Chapter 2, Section 2.3.7). Furthermore, in some plants, the methyl moiety of SAM can be transferred to Put via Put-*N*-methyl-transferase, to form *N*-methyl-Put, which serves as a precursor of nicotine and other alkaloids.

As in the case of any plant growth regulators, the intracellular free PA pool depends not only on its synthesis but also on several other processes including degradation, conjugation, and transport. Cellular PA content is also controlled by catabolic pathways (Cona et al., 2006). Copper containing diamine oxidases (DAO) and flavine-containing PA oxidases (PAO) catalyze the oxidative de-amination of PAs. The first enzyme oxidizes Put whereas the second oxidizes Spd and Spm, producing 4-aminobutanal and N-(3-aminopropyl)-4-aminobutanal, respectively, in addition to 1,3-diaminopropane and H_2O_2. Finally, conjugated PAs are amides of hydroxycinnamic acid (soluble) and associated to cell wall (cell wall–bound PAs) and could serve as pool of free PAs (Martín-Tanguy, 1997; Valero et al., 2002a).

Since ethylene and PA (Spd and Spm) biosynthesis share the common precursor SAM and are known to exert opposite effects with respect to fruit ripening and senescence, a large number of research papers attest to the role of ethylene and PAs as modulators of plant senescence. Thus, it has been shown that the balance between the two opposite growth regulators is crucial to retard or to accelerate both processes (Pandey et al., 2000; Valero et al., 2002a). Usually, the concentration of PAs decreased during tissue senescence, this decline being likely a cause of the initiation or acceleration of ethylene production through the induction of ACS and/or the increase of the sensitivity of the tissue to the action of ethylene. Conversely, it is possible that PAs (probably in conjunction with other growth-promoting substances) are required for reducing the expression of ACS gene(s) and thus for the inhibition of ethylene production in developing tissues (Yahia et al., 2001). In this sense, tomato fruit cultivars with high levels of PAs produced low levels of ethylene and had a long shelf life (Dibble et al., 1988; Martínez-Madrid et al., 1996). Although this relationship does not seem a general mechanism for all fruits, these two groups of plant growth regulators act in opposite directions and often play a crucial role in either suppressing the onset of fruit ripening or triggering and promoting this process.

7.3 Polyamine and human diet

The PAs are part of a class of proteins called *biogenic amines* and are present in low concentrations in all human, animal, and plant cells. PAs are essential for maintenance of the high metabolic activity of a normal functioning and healthy body. In addition to the intestine, all other organs of the body require polyamines for their growth, renewal, and metabolism. So the first thing to realize when we consider the role of PAs in the body is that they are widespread, ubiquitous, and essential in proper amounts for health and wellness. They are also critical to the healthy function of the nervous system and the growth of young children (Bardocz et al., 1995). All cell growth requires certain amounts of PAs and the concentration of PAs inside the cell is tightly regulated, since the range of cellular PA concentration is determined at the lower limit by their absolute requirement for cell growth and at the upper limit by their potential toxicity. Basically, PAs make things grow, with kids having higher PA content than adults, although just exactly how PAs stimulate growth is far from clear (Larqué et al., 2007). It is believed that they have a profound stabilizing effect on a cell's genetic material (DNA). One mechanism for their involvement in growth processes may be via their influence on the activity of growth-promoting genes. The size and electrical charge of the PAs permit them to interact with huge molecules such as DNA and RNA, and pass through phospholipid membranes and compartments with ease. There appears to be an intimate relationship between PAs and RNA, in which PAs seem to stabilize and amplify the message contained in messenger RNA, which serves to increase the protein produced from it.

It was believed that most of the PAs needed for growth were synthesized in the gut. However, a recent work has shown that PAs accumulated in the small bowel are largely obtained from the food consumed in our diet and thus dietary PAs contribute to the total body PA pool. As PAs are important in health and disease, it is of interest to obtain information on the food PA content, making it possible to calculate and manipulate the PA intake. Uptake of PAs by intestinal cells has been suggested to be an important regulatory mechanism of the intracellular PA concentration (Eliassen et al., 2002).

Many sources refer to the PAs as *dead flesh proteins*, since when living tissue is shocked or dies its protein structure cracks open. Bacteria or enzymes contained in the food itself subsequently convert many of the protein fragments into PAs. This is why PAs are found in very high amounts in the tissues of severely injured trauma patients and in food that has been morphologically shocked by excessive processing, such as rapid freezing (Kalač and Krausová, 2005).

Some evidences have shown that the diet can theoretically supply sufficient amounts of PAs to support the cell growth. This pool of PAs comes from intracellular PA *de novo* synthesis and uptake of extracellular primarily dietary PAs. The normal adult diet provides a daily supply of several micromoles of PAs. The PA content of foods is extremely wide, ranging from a few nanomoles to a few micromoles per gram, with cheese, owing to microbial fermentation, being particularly rich in PAs. In addition, the distribution of the different PAs varies according to the food type, and generally meat is rich in Spm, while foods of plant origin contain mostly Put and Spd (Moinard et al., 2005).

Estimates of PA intake have been made for several countries, including the United Kingdom, Italy, Spain, Finland, Sweden, and the Netherlands. The average estimated polyamine intakes for adults in countries surveyed to date are 211,910 nmol/day Put, 86,959 nmol/day Spd, and 54,704 nmol/day Spm (Bardocz et al., 1995), while average daily PA intakes in the United States were: 159,133, 54,697, and 35,698 nmol/day for Put, Spd, and Spm, respectively (Zoumas-Morse et al., 2007). The major sources of Put were fruit juices, cheese, and nongreen vegetables. All foods contributed similar amounts of Spd to the diet, although levels were generally higher in green vegetables, and meat was the richest source of Spm. The importance of the significant contribution of milk dietary PAs to the PA body pool with an essential function in organ growth during infant nutrition has also been reported (Löser, 2000). This author observed that human and cow milk contained high PA levels, although they differed in the concentration and type of PA. Thus, human's milk had higher PA contents than cow's milk, with mainly Spd and lower amount of Put being found in the milk from humans, while cow's milk had Spd and Spm but absence of Put was observed.

In general, most fruits and vegetables normally contain lower levels of PAs than meat products or fresh fish, but it must taken into account that PA concentration in fish increases rapidly upon storage and/or processing (Eliassen et al., 2002; Kalač et al., 2002; 2005; Cipolla et al., 2007). Table 7.1 summarizes the average content of Put, Spd, and Spm in a wide range of fresh fruits harvested at commercial maturity stage. Among fruits, *Citrus* species (orange, mandarin, lemon, and grapefruit) and their juices have considerably high Put level (>450 nmol g^{-1}). In addition, Spd content in plant-derived foods is commonly higher than Spm (Kalač and Krausová, 2005), for which absence or nondetectable concentration is usually found.

A balanced diet with respect to nutrients, low or high in PAs, should be possible to compose from food items with known concentrations of PAs. However, it must be borne in mind that storage, transport, and handling will influence to some extent the PA type and concentration. However, when calculating the contribution of PAs from the diet, one should consider that only a limited fraction of the dietary PAs are absorbed from the intestinal tract, as they can also be metabolized during the passage through the intestinal wall. Furthermore, the degree of absorption will be partly determined by the presence of other amines, e.g., histamine and cadaverine, as they compete with Put for the degrading enzyme DAO (Eliassen et al., 2002). Recently, agmatine has been identified as PA, which is derived from arginine and considered a neurotransmitter with health implications as antiproliferative effects (Moinard et al., 2005). Although it has been reported that PAs are preferentially taken up by tumors developing tissues, most authors have postulated that the

Table 7.1 Average Range of Polyamine Contents (nmol g^{-1} Fresh Weight) of Selected Fresh Fruits at Commercial Ripening Stage

Fruit	Put	Spd	Spm	Reference
Apple	181–300	620–2000	35–100	Kalač et al., 2005.
Grapefruit, lemon, orange, mandarin	70–400	7–34	5–10	Shiozaki et al., 2000; Kalač et al., 2005; Kalač and Krausová, 2005.
Orange (skin)	1000–1733	3–80	0–7	Eliassen et al., 2002; Cipolla et al., 2007.
Lemon (skin)	40–80	50–70	ND	Valero et al., 1998b; 1998c; Martínez-Romero et al., 1999; Cipolla et al., 2007.
Mandarin (skin)	180–220	30–110	40–110	Valero et al., 1998a.
Green pepper	18–90	2–30	0–5	Pretel et al., 1995; Kalač et al., 2005; Serrano et al., 1997.
Tomato	14–375	15–37	0–7	Martínez-Madrid et al., 1996; Eliassen et al. 2002; Cipolla et al., 2007.
Cucumber	23–99	2–65	1	Moret et al., 2005; Cipolla et al., 2007.
Peach	7–70	18–40	10	Valero et al., 1997; Martínez-Romero et al., 2000; Liu et al., 2006b.
Avocado	15	60	40	Kushad et al., 1988.
Pear	0–4	18	0–2	Cipolla et al., 2007.
Strawberry	18	40	14	
Melon	23	78	5	
Banana	4	45	1	

biogenic amine content of fresh fruits and vegetables does not represent a risk for healthy consumers (Kalač and Krausová, 2005; Larqué et al., 2007; Nishibori et al., 2007).

7.4 *Polyamine and fruit development*

PAs are involved in the overall physiological process from floral development to fruit growth and ripening. Involvement of PAs in floral development has been reported in a wide range of crops based on several lines of evidence. First, increase in total PAs or in a single PA type accompanies floral development. Second, inhibitors of polyamine biosynthesis cause a strong inhibition of flowering, whereas the inhibitory effect is abolished by applying Spd exogenously. Third, PAs promote flowering of some plants under noninductive conditions and some mutant plants deficient in polyamine metabolism demonstrated aberrant morphology in anthers and ovules (Liu et al., 2006a). For example, a clear relationship has been reported between the concentration of free PAs (mainly Spd and Spm) in the apricot ovary and the ovule development, its viability, and fruit set (Alburquerque et al., 2006). Accordingly, a large accumulation of free PAs occurs concomitantly with flower development in damson plum, which is closely related to the onset of ovarian development (De Dios et al., 2006). PAs are also related to flower genders or fertility as well as to the pollen germination and pollen tube growth (Liu et al., 2006a). In addition, fruit set in grape vine is positively influenced by the increase in free and soluble-conjugated Spd in the floral organs (Aziz et al., 2001) and Put directly applied to the cluster 2 days before full bloom increased fruit set in Japanese pears (Franco-Mora et al., 2005b). However, in some citrus species, PAs have been proposed to act as a nitrogen source rather than as a regulator of fruit set (Arias et al., 2005).

The changes in free PA levels during the growth and ripening have been investigated in a wide variety of fruit, both climacteric and nonclimacteric ones. Table 7.2 shows some examples of the main changes of free PAs during growth and ripening phases. Most of these studies reported a fundamentally similar observation, that is, peak levels of PAs during the early phase of fruit growth, followed by decline with fruit development process, as occurred in pepper (Pretel et al., 1995), tomato (Martínez-Madrid et al., 1996; Yahia et al., 2001), strawberry (Ponappa and Miller, 1996), peach (Valero et al., 1997; Kushad, 1998; Liu et al., 2006a), plum (Zuzunaga et al., 2001), and apricot (Paksasorn et al., 1995), among others. The high PA concentration soon after full bloom may be related to the high growth rate and active cell division. However, avocado mesocarp cells are unique, since they continue to divide as long as the fruit remains attached to the tree and PAs nevertheless also decreased during fruit growth (Kushad et al., 1988).

In addition, the decrease in PAs at late stages of fruit growth has been regarded as a signal for fruit ripening. In fact, in a wide range of fruits PA concentration also decreased during fruit ripening on tree, although a few exceptions exist. Thus, Put increased during ripening in long-keeping tomato (Dibble et al., 1988; Martínez-Madrid et al., 1996; Yahia et al., 2001) and both Put and Spd levels raised in Golden Japan plum (Zuzunaga et al., 2001), a suppressed climacteric plum phenotype. The high levels of PAs in these mature fruits may be responsible for the long keeping quality and low ethylene production of these tomato and plum cultivars. Moreover, since ethylene and PAs share a common precursor, it is normally accepted that they compete with each other during fruit development and ripening, and thus diminution of Spd and Spm during fruit ripening may be a

Table 7.2 Changes in PA Contents during Fruit Growth and Ripening Phases

Fruit	During growth phase			During ripening phase			References
	Put	Spd	Spn	Put	Spd	Spn	
Nonclimacteric							
Pepper	↓	↓	↓	↓	↓	↓	Pretel et al., 1995; Yahia et al., 2001.
Long-keeping tomato	↓	↓	↓	↑	↓	↓	Martínez-Madrid et al., 1996; Yahia et al., 2001.
Golden Japan plum	↓	↓	ND	↑	↑	ND	Zuzunaga et al., 2001.
Strawberry	↓	↓	↓	↓	↓	↓	Ponappa and Miller, 1996.
Lemon (skin)	NA	NA	NA	↓	↓	ND	Valero et al., 1998c.
Grape	↓	↓	≅	≅	≅	≅	Shiozaki et al., 2000.
Climacteric							
Tomato	↓	↓	↓	↓	↓	NA	Martínez-Madrid et al., 1996; Valero et al., 2002a.
Santa Rosa plum	↓	↓	ND	↓	≅	ND	Zuzunaga et al., 2001.
Damson plum	↑	↑	↑	↑	↑	≅	De Dios et al., 2006.
Muskmelon	↑	↑	NA	↑	↓	NA	Lester, 2000.
Paraguayo	↓	↓	ND	↑	↓	ND	Martínez-Madrid et al., 2000.
Peach	↓	↓	↓	↑	≅↑	≅	Valero et al., 1997; Kushad, 1998; Liu et al., 2006b.
Apricot	↓	↓	↓	↓	↓	↓	Pakasorn et al., 1995.
Cherimoya	NA	NA	NA	↑	≅	≅	Escribano and Merodio, 1994.
Avocado	↓	↓	↓	↓	↓	↓	Kushad et al., 1988.

Note: ↓ = Decreases, ↑ = increases, ≅ unchanged, ND = no detectable, NA = not available.

consequence of SAM diversion to ACC for ethylene biosynthesis, concomitantly with the increase of Put (Valero et al., 2002a). In agreement with this proposal, an inverse relationship has been found between PA content and ethylene production and ACC concentration during ripening of seven pear cultivars, ranging from low to moderate and high ethylene production rates at ripening (Franco-Mora et al., 2005a).

However, increase in Put concentration during ripening has been also found in some climacteric fruits, such as muskmelon (Lester, 2000), paraguayo (Martínez-Madrid et al., 2000), peach (Valero et al., 1997; Kushad, 1998; Liu et al., 2006b), and cherimolla (Escribano and Merodio, 1994), as well as increases in Put, Spd, and Spm in the climacteric damson plum (De Dios et al., 2006). Moreover, the introduction of the yeast SAM-decarboxylase gene into a commercial variety of tomato led to increased levels of Spd and Spm, although these transgenic tomatoes produced more ethylene than did the parental line (Mehta et al., 2002). Thus, it seems that the two metabolic pathways can operate simultaneously *in vivo*, suggesting that the levels of the precursor, SAM, are not limiting for either partway.

7.5 Preharvest polyamine application and fruit ripening

Ethylene and PAs exhibit opposite effects on fruit ripening and senescence, since reduced levels of PAs have been correlated with increased ethylene production, fruit ripening, and senescence, while high endogenous concentrations of PAs are associated with a delay in these processes. Thus, a balance between these two opposite growth regulators is crucial to retard or accelerate ripening and senescence (Pandey et al., 2000; Valero et al., 2002a). In this sense, several experiments have shown that exogenous application of PAs during the growing season (preharvest) can decrease ethylene production and delay the ripening process in apricot (Paksasorn et al., 1995), peach (Bregoli et al., 2002), mango (Malik et al., 2003; Malik and Singh, 2006), nectarine (Torrigiani et al., 2004), and plum (Khan et al., 2008).

In fact, foliar spray treatments of peach trees 19 days before fruit harvest with Put (10 mM), Spd (0.1, 1 and 5 mM), or Spm (2 mM) strongly reduced or even nullified ethylene production during peach on-tree ripening, Spd being more efficient than Put or Spm. All PA treatments markedly slowed down the softening process, while only Spd affected the accumulation of TSS, leading to lower levels at harvest as compared with control fruits (Bregoli et al., 2002). Similar results about the efficacy of PAs on modulating ethylene production were obtained in nectarine during on-tree fruit ripening, in which PA treatments decreased flesh softening and acidity losses and increased TSS (Torrigiani et al., 2004). However, at harvest, endogenous levels of Put and Spd in the mesocarp of treated fruits were comparable with those of control. In addition, Put treatments led to a lower accumulation of ACO and ACS transcripts at harvest, in accordance with their effect on inhibiting ethylene production, and to their lower levels of SAMDC and ADC transcripts. On the contrary, Spd applications, which also decreased ethylene biosynthesis, did not result in changes in ACS, ACO, SAMDC, or ADC transcripts. The differential effects of the two amines could be due to a different uptake rate or to a different mechanism of action. Moreover, it has been reported that SAMDC and ADC transcript levels were initially depressed by Spd treatment, as well as ACO and ACS transcript, and later, at harvest time, recovered up to control levels, while the effect of Put treatments on ACO and ACS were still evident at harvest, in which an increase of ethylene receptors mRNA was also found (Ziosi et al., 2006). Thus, both Put and Spd treatments increased temporally the endogenous pool of PAs and strongly interfered, both at a biochemical and at a biomolecular level, with the temporal evolution of the ripening syndrome. These results support the proposal that PA effect on delaying fruit ripening on tree is mediated by inhibition of ethylene biosynthesis and confirm the capacity of PAs to exert their antisenescence effects under field conditions.

However, preharvest treatments with PAs have been shown also to be effective in delaying the postharvest ripening process. Thus, an early report on apricot showed that preharvest treatments of apricot trees with 0.1 mM of Put, Spd, or Spm 20 days before harvest decreased postharvest ethylene production (Paksasorn et al., 1995). In addition, treatments of mango trees with Put (0.5, 1 or 2 mM) 7 days prior to harvest led to higher levels of firmness and TSS and lower fruit rot index after 20 days of storage at 20°C as compared to fruit from nontreated trees (Malik et al., 2003), although sugar content was at lower concentration, probably due to a slower conversion of starch to sugars, and the evolution of color development was delayed (Malik and Singh, 2006). Accordingly, preharvest treatment by foliar spray of plum trees with Put delayed and inhibited both ethylene production and respiration rate during postharvest storage, these effects being higher as Put concentration increased from 0.1 to 2 mM and also evident after a 6-week period of cold storage. Put treatments also decreased fruit softening, maintained TA at higher levels, diminished the increase in TSS, and delayed the color evolution during postharvest storage as compared to control fruits, showing a delay in ripening evolution and leading to a net extension of plum shelf life (Khan et al., 2008). However, the levels of total antioxidants after postharvest storage were lower in treated plum than in controls, which could be due to the effect of Put on delaying the ripening process, since the bioactive compounds with antioxidant activity have been recently reported to increase during plum fruit ripening on tree and during postharvest storage (Díaz-Mula et al., 2008; 2009b).

7.6 Postharvest polyamine application and fruit quality

Most of the research about the effect of PAs on fruit ripening has been performed with postharvest treatments and their effects are similar to those addressed in the previous section about preharvest treatments. Thus, postharvest application of PAs, by immersion or vacuum infiltration, has been reported to delay fruit ripening and extend shelf life in some fruits, including Golden Delicious and McIntosh apple (Kramer et al., 1991); Kesington Pride mango (Malik and Singh, 2005); Baby Gold 6 peach (Martínez-Romero et al., 2000); Mauricio apricot (Martínez-Romero et al., 2002); blueberry (Basiouny, 1996); and Golden Japan, Black Diamond, Black Star, Santa Rosa, and Angelino plum (Pérez-Vicente et al., 2002; Serrano et al., 2003; Khan et al., 2008) and Mollar de Elche pomegranate (Mirdehghan et al., 2007a). Other fruit commodities in which PA application induced beneficial effects in terms of maintenance postharvest quality were reviewed by Valero and colleagues (1999; 2002a).

These effects could be attributed to the fact that Put treatments led to increases in endogenous Put and Spd in a wide range of fruits, such as lemon (Valero et al., 1998c), peach (Martínez-Romero et al., 2000), apricot (Martínez-Romero et al., 2002), plum (Pérez-Vicente et al., 2002; Serrano et al., 2003), and pomegranate (Mirdehghan et al., 2007a), the increased PA concentration being evident after treatment and remaining during postharvest storage. Some examples are shown in Figure 7.2, in which Put and Spd concentrations in lemon skin and in the pulp of peach, apricot, and plum after 7 days of treatment and storage at 20°C were significantly higher in Put-treated fruits than in control ones. The increase in Spd concentration as a result of Put treatments shows an active metabolism from Put to Spd in the biosynthetic pathway.

7.6.1 Ethylene production

The effect of 1 mM Put treatments by vacuum infiltration (pressure of 0.2 bar for 8 min) on ethylene production in several *Prunus* species, such as apricot, peach, and four plums cultivars, is shown *in Figure* 7.3. Control fruits exhibited rises in the ethylene production during storage at 20°C with climacteric peaks after 14 days for Black Diamond plum, after 7 days for Black Star plum, after 5 days for peach, and after 4 days for Santa Rosa plum and apricot, while in Golden Japan plum no increase in ethylene production was observed, since this cultivar has a suppressed climacteric phenotype (Zuzunaga et al., 2001). However, exogenous Put treatment led to a reduction and/or delay of the ethylene production, which was inversely correlated with the maximum ethylene production at the climacteric peak and was dependent on the fruit type. Thus, at the day

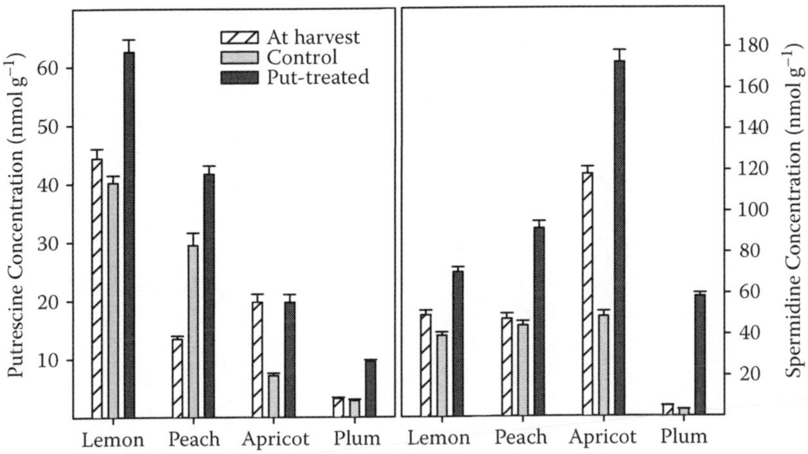

Figure 7.2 Putrescine and spermidine concentration at harvest and after 7 days of storage at 20°C in control and 1 mM putrescine-treated fruits (by pressure infiltration) in lemon skin and in the pulp of peach, apricot, and plum.

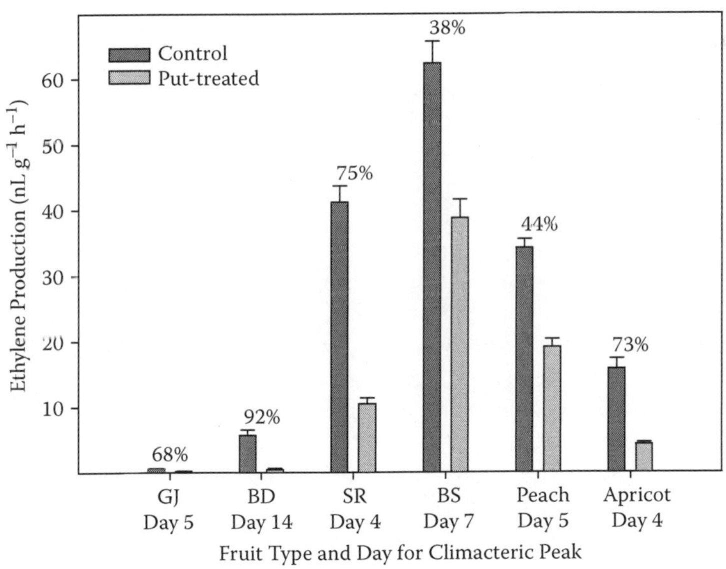

Figure 7.3 Effect of postharvest putrescine treatment (1 mM pressure infiltrated at 0.2 bar for 8 minutes) on ethylene production at the maximum climacteric peak of the control fruits of four plum cultivars (GJ, Golden Japan; BD, Black Diamond; SR, Santa Rosa; and BS, Black Star), peach (Baby Gold 6), and apricot (Mauricio). Percentages of ethylene inhibition are shown on the bars.

of climacteric peak, fruits with the lowest ethylene production, Black Diamond plum, showed the highest percentage of ethylene inhibition (92%) by Put treatment, while in those with the highest ethylene levels, Black Star plum, the lowest percentage of ethylene inhibition was detected (38%). These results are in agreement with previous reports on several fruits, such as avocado, mango, pepper, kiwifruit, tomato, and Angelino plum cultivar (Valero et al., 1999; 2002a; Petkou et al., 2004; Malik and Sing, 2005; Khan et al., 2008).

The inhibitory effects of exogenous PAs in ethylene production may be ascribed to both the competitive biosynthesis mechanism between ethylene and PAs and to the inhibition of ACC synthase and ACC oxidase. However, in apples Put treatment did not decrease ethylene production through the normal course of ripening during storage (Kramer et al., 1991; Wang et al., 1993). Since ethylene inhibition by Put treatment has been shown to be inversely correlated to the maximum level at the climacteric peak (Valero et al., 2002a; Serrano et al., 2003), the failures of ethylene inhibition reported in some fruits may be due to their high levels of ethylene production.

7.6.2 Fruit quality parameters

As stated in Chapter 3 (Section 3.5), fruit softening is a common process during postharvest storage, and can be seen in Figure 7.4 for some plum cultivars, apricot and peach, in which fruit firmness, expressed as force-deformation ratio, rapidly declined during storage at 20°C in all the *Prunus* species and cultivars, the magnitude of the softening being affected by fruit type and even cultivar. The application of Put prior to storage induced a delay of the softening process through maintenance of firmness significantly higher in Put-treated than in control fruits. Accordingly, postharvest Put application markedly slowed softening during ripening at ambient temperature of Angelino plum, this effect being higher as Put concentration increased from 0.1 to 2 mM (Khan et al., 2008). Put treatment at 10 mM was also effective in delaying softening in blueberry, while no effect was observed with 1 mM Spd treatment (Basiouny, 1996). Several mechanisms have been postulated to explain the increased fruit firmness after Put treatment. One is supported by decreased activity of ethylene biosynthetic enzymes by PA, ACS, and ACO, as well as cell wall–related enzymes, such as the inhibition of the action of endo- and exo-PG, EGases, and PME involved in softening. Another mechanism would involve the PA capacity to cross-link pectic substances in the cell wall, producing rigidification (Valero et al., 1999; Martínez-Romero et al., 2002; Pérez-Vicente et al., 2002). This binding also blocks the access of such degrading enzymes reducing the rate of softening during storage (Valero et al., 2002a, and citations therein).

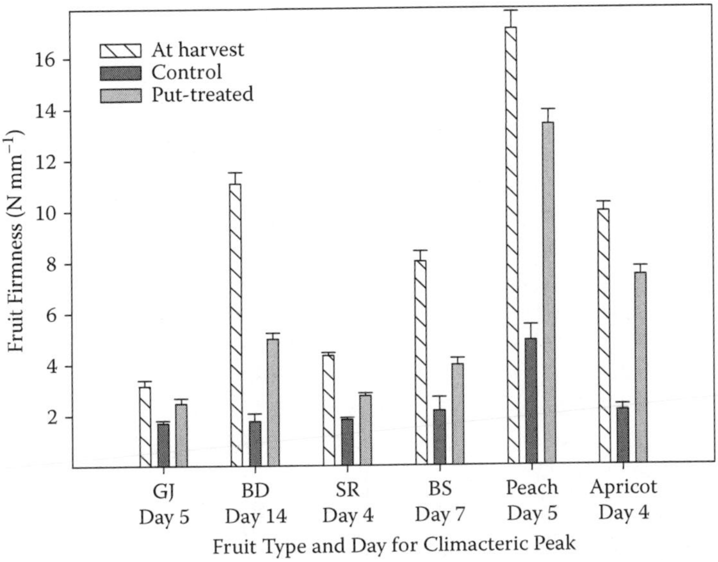

Figure 7.4 Effect of postharvest putrescine treatment (1 mM pressure infiltrated at 0.2 bar for 8 minutes) on fruit firmness in four plum cultivars (GJ, Golden Japan; BD, Black Diamond; SR, Santa Rosa; and BS, Black Star), peach (Baby Gold 6), and apricot (Mauricio). For each fruit type the period of storage at 20°C is indicated.

It is also true that exogenous PAs can fail in maintaining fruit firmness, since Redhaven peaches and Stark Red Gold nectarines at two different ripening stages (based on fruit firmness) were subjected to treatments with 10mM Put or 1mM Spd, and neither PA substantially affected ethylene production or firmness of peaches, but Put showed effects on nectarines (Bregoli et al., 2005). The efficacy of these treatments was higher in firmer than in softer nectarines, suggesting that the former are less permeable or sensitive to Put, or that a pathway exists that actively degrades the diamine such as DAO. Nevertheless, the higher efficacy of PAs in nectarines than in peaches may be due to the fact that Put is taken up to a higher extent in nectarines than in peaches. Thus, in order to optimize experimental conditions and results, the extent of PA uptake, which is inversely proportional to the number of positive charges, should be taken into consideration (Torrigiani et al., 2008).

Another effect of PA infiltration is to ameliorate chlorophyll breakdown in several plant organs, including fruit, such as lemon and apricot, since Put treatment delayed the color change during storage, which is an indicator of reduced senescence rate (Martínez-Romero et al., 2002; Valero et al., 1998c). Also, exogenous PAs retarded chlorophyll loss in muskmelon by reducing the hydrolytic activities acting on chloroplast thylakoid membranes (Lester, 2000). Similarly, Put-treatments reduced color a* value after

3 and 6 weeks of low temperature storage in Angelino plum, the effect being also attributed to lower chlorophyll degradation and delay in the senescence process (Khan et al., 2008).

Most of the reports about PA postharvest treatments have shown to have little or no effect on TSS evolution during fruit postharvest storage, while they significantly delay the diminution in TA that normally occurs in a wide range of fruits (see Chapter 3, Section 3.6). Thus, as can be observed in Figure 7.5, TA decreased after several days of storage at 20°C in control fruits of four plum cultivars and pomegranate, while in Put-treated fruits TA did not change or remained at higher concentration than in controls. Accordingly, postharvest Put applications to Angelino plum maintained TA at higher level as compared to control fruits, and fruits exhibited a linear reduction in TSS/TA in the range of the Put-treatment concentration from 0.1 to 2 mM after 3 and 6 weeks of cold storage (Khan et al., 2008). Exogenous application of Put or Spd also delayed the increase in the ratio TSS/TA in pomegranate arils during storage (Mirdehghan et al., 2007a). However, 10 mM Put application was also effective in delaying acidity loss on blueberry, while in blueberry treated with 1 mM of Spm losses of acidity were even greater than in controls (Basiouny, 1996).

Taking into account data of the commented parameters related to fruit quality (firmness, color, TSS, and TA), as well as the visual appearance of

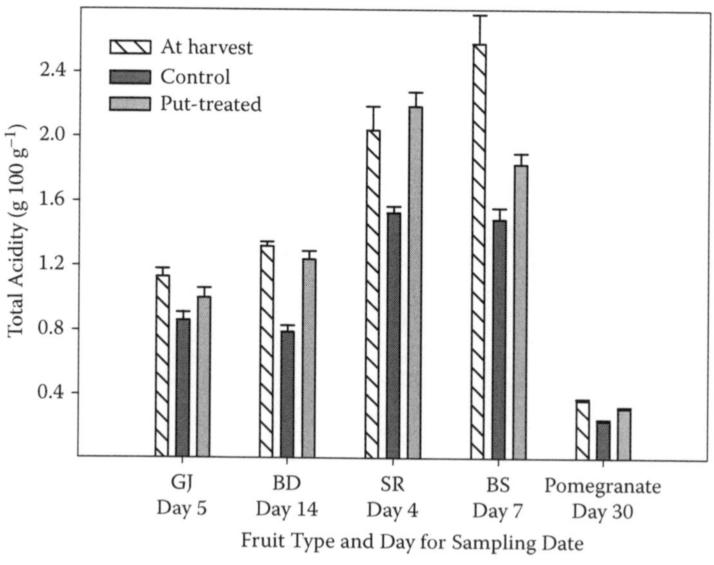

Figure 7.5 Effect of postharvest putrescine treatment (1 mM pressure infiltrated at 0.2 bar for 8 minutes) on total acidity in four plum cultivars (GJ, Golden Japan; BD, Black Diamond; SR, Santa Rosa; and BS, Black Star) and pomegranate. For each fruit type the period of storage at 20°C is indicated.

these fruits, it could be concluded that Put treatment increased the fruit shelf life 2 days in Golden Japan plum and apricot, 3 days in Santa Rosa plum and peach, and 5 days in Black Star and Black Diamond plums. In addition, in the different plum cultivars, the effect of Put treatment on increasing shelf life was highly correlated with the fruit firmness at harvest, that is, the higher the plum firmness at harvest the longer the increase in shelf life (Martínez-Romero et al., 2000; 2002; Serrano et al., 2003).

7.6.3 *Bioactive compounds with antioxidant activity*

There is little information about the effect of PA treatment on the concentration of bioactive compounds in fruits. The first evidence of the *in vivo* role of PAs in the fruit ripening process was obtained with transgenic tomatoes. Engineering of tomato fruit with the yeast SAMDC1 gene under a fruit-specific promoter led to both Spd and Spm accumulation at the expense of Put throughout the fruit growth cycle (Mehta et al., 2002). In the two transgenic lines examined, this led to prolonged vine life, enhanced fruit juice quality, and two–threefold higher levels of lycopene than cultivated tomatoes, although the rates of ethylene production were enhanced compared with the parentals. The results showed that red ripe transgenic tomatoes accumulated 200–300% more lycopene than did the red fruits from the parental lines. This is of special significance as tomato fruits are an important source of lycopene for human consumption. Lycopene, as stated in Chapter 2, Section 2.3.5, is a biologically important carotenoid with natural and high antioxidant activity. This work also confirms that PA and ethylene biosynthesis pathways can act simultaneously during tomato fruit ripening.

Recently, it has been reported that in pomegranate arils, the application of 1 mM of Put or Spd, either by pressure infiltration or immersion, was effective in maintaining the concentration of total anthocyanins and total phenolics compounds as well as the H-TAA at higher levels than in control fruits during storage (Mirdehghan et al., 2007c). As can be observed in Figure 7.6, after 45 days of cold storage plus 3 days at 20°C, the concentration of total phenolics and the H-TAA in pomegranate arils had increased as compared to values at harvest, although these increases were higher in the arils of PA-treated pomegranates, in which increases in total anthocyanins were also found, these effects being similar in Put- and Spd-treated fruits, independently of the method of application. The mechanism by which Put and Spd induce these effects is still known, although they may be related to their antisenescence effects (Valero et al., 2002a).

However, the enhancement of H-TAA found in the arils after PA treatments could be attributed to the PA capacity to act as effective scavengers of free radicals, as even to their role on the SOD/ascorbate-glutathione cycle, as has been recently reported (Kim and Jin, 2006). On the contrary,

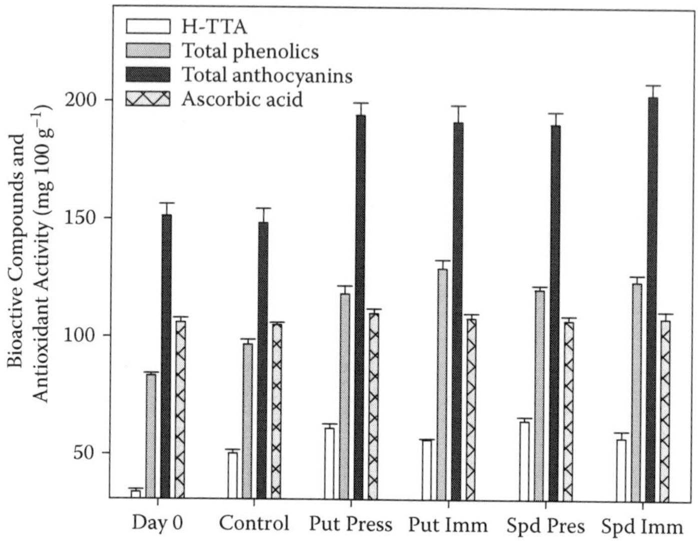

Figure 7.6 Total phenolics, total anthocyanins, ascorbic acid concentration, and total antioxidant activity in the hydrophilic fraction (H-TTA) of pomegranate arils at harvest and after 45 days of storage at 2°C plus 3 days at 20°C in control and putrescine-(Put-) or spermidine-(Spd-)treated fruits (by immersion, Imm, or pressure infiltration, Pres).

pre- and postharvest Put application to Angelino plum led to a linear reduction in the levels of ascorbic acid, carotenoids, and TAA during postharvest storage, which were more pronounced with increased concentrations of Put and storage periods, these effects being ascribed to increased ascorbate oxidase activity (Khan et al., 2008), according to a previous report on pepper and tomato (Yahia et al., 2001). Thus, more research is needed to clarify the effects of PA treatments on fruit functional compounds. Finally, it is interesting to point out that although most papers dealing with PA postharvest treatments in fruits have been carried out by pressure infiltration in order to ensure the PA intake, Mirdehghan and colleagues (2007c) showed that the immersion method could be considered lower cost and easier to handle than pressure infiltration and could be incorporated as a continuous process at the horticultural industry.

7.7 Polyamines and chilling injury

PAs may associate with anionic components of the membrane such as phospholipids, and this interaction serves to stabilize the bilayer surface and may thus retard membrane deterioration. Thus, given the relationship between CI and membrane damage and PAs and membrane protection, the possible connection between PAs and CI is of great interest. In this sense, increases in Put concentration have been found in several fruits suffering CI, such as lemon, orange, lime, grapefruit, pepper, and zucchini (Serrano et al., 1996; 1997; 1998; González-Aguilar et al., 2000a). Thus, as shown in Figure 7.7 for pepino fruits at ripe yellow-green stage, free, conjugate-soluble and cell wall–bound Put forms increased sharply in pepinos stored at 1°C, with respect to values at day 0, while in pepinos stored at 10°C these increases were slower and no changes were found in pepinos stored at 20°C. Also, a close correlation could be established between the scores given for CI symptoms and the increases in the three forms of Put during storage at chilling temperatures, which occurred in ripe yellow green pepinos but not when fruits were harvested at more immature stage, such as green and light green ones (Martínez-Romero et al., 2003c).

In addition, in peach fruit it has been shown that wooliness (a CI symptom) occurred during storage at 5°C and subsequent shelf life at 20°C in fruit harvested at an advanced ripening stage, but not in fruits harvested at less mature stage, this disorder being associated with an increase in Spd concentration (Valero et al., 1997). Such results support the proposal that accumulation of Put and/or Spd or Spm in tissues seems to be a general response of fruit to chilling temperatures, although they do not indicate whether the increase in Put or Spd is a protective response to CI or Put or Spd themselves are the result of the stress-induced injury.

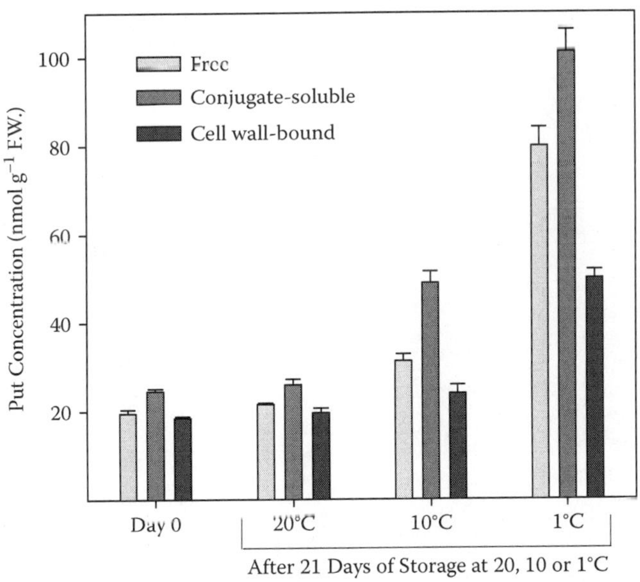

Figure 7.7 Free, conjugated-soluble, and cell wall–bound putrescine concentration in pepino (*Solanum muricatum*), in ripe yellow-green stage, at harvest and after 21 days of storage at 20, 10, or 1°C.

However, some prestorage treatments that reduce CI are related to enhancement of PA concentration. Thus, CI could be reduced in zucchini fruits by conditioning treatments, such as storing them at low but not-chilling temperatures before storage at chilling ones (Wang, 1994). This low temperature conditioning increased polyamine levels and SAMDC activity and reduced CI. Accordingly, pretreatment at 25°C for 2 days before cold storage reduced CI in peach by elevating PA levels (Xu et al., 2005). In Fortune mandarins, temperature pretreatments for 3 days above 20°C also increased progressively Put and Spd levels in flavedo, as did the temperature treatment and reduced CI (González-Aguilar et al., 2000b). Another type of prestorage manipulation that has been demonstrated to decrease CI is heat treatment, which induced high Spd and Spm levels in skin tissue of zucchini squash (Wang, 1994). Likewise, in plum fruits, CI symptoms were reduced by prestorage treatment at 45 and 50°C for 35 and 30 min, respectively, which also maintained increased PA levels (Abu-Kpawoh et al., 2002), as well as in pepper fruit treated with hot water at 53°C for 4 minutes (González-Aguilar et al., 2000a). Accordingly, the application of heat treatment to pomegranate fruit led to both decrease in CI and increase in Put and Spd concentration in the skin during cold storage, their concentration being always higher in heat-treated pomegranates than in control ones (Mirdehghan et al., 2007b). Thus, as shown in Figure 7.8, Put and Spd concentration

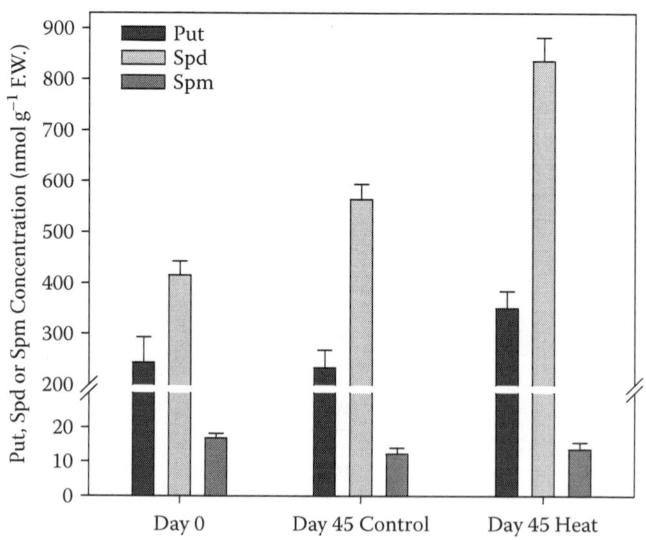

Figure 7.8 Putrescine (Put), spermidine (Spd), and spermine (Spm) concentration in pomegranate skin at harvest and after 45 days of storage at 2°C plus 3 days at 20°C in control and heat-treated fruits (hot water at 45°C for 4 minutes).

after 45 days of storage at 2°C plus 3 days at 20°C was higher in the skin of heat-treated pomegranates than in controls and they had increased with respect to values at harvest. However, it is not understood if the increase in PAs induced by high temperature treatments is only a consequence of the heat stress or if it is related to the beneficial effect of this conditioning treatment.

Overall, these results indicate that PAs may be involved in reducing CI due to their ability to preserve membrane integrity, both by lowering the membrane phase transition temperature fluidity and by retarding lipid peroxidation, resulting in increased cell viability, due to their membrane-binding capacity and/or antioxidant properties. This hypothesis is supported by the fact that exogenous PA treatments after harvest but before cold storage decreased CI in chilling sensitive fruits, such as apple (Kramer et al., 1991), zucchini (Martínez-Téllez et al., 2002), and mango (Kondo et al., 2003; Nair and Singh, 2004).

Prestorage treatments of pomegranate with Put or Spd (1 mM), by immersion or pressure infiltration, decreased significantly the occurrence of CI after cold storage at chilling temperatures (Figure 7.9), since the percentage of skin browning was close to 50% in control fruits after 45 days of storage at 2°C plus 3 days at 20°C and ≈20–25% in treated ones, without significant differences among Put and Spd treatments or the way of application. Moreover, the application of Put led to an increase in Put and Spd concentration in the skin, these concentrations being three- and twofold higher, respectively, in treated than in control fruits. The reduction

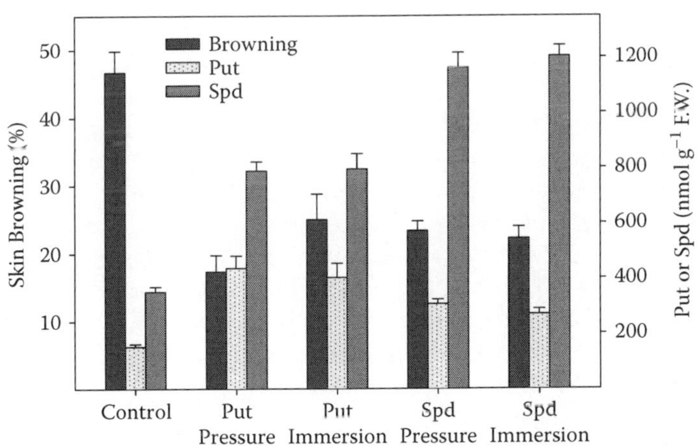

Figure 7.9 Skin browning and putrescine (Put), spermidine (Spd), and spermine (Spm) concentration in pomegranate skin at harvest and after 45 days of storage at 2°C plus 3 days at 20°C in control and Put- or Spd-treated fruits (1 mM pressure infiltrated at 0.04 bar for 4 minutes).

of CI symptoms was correlated with increased PA endogenous levels, especially Spd concentration after Put treatment. This evidence suggests an activation of the PA biosynthesis pathway, with part of the exogenous Put being transformed to Spd using DCSAM, while the conversion of Spd to Spm did not occur, since no significant increase in Spm was found (Mirdehghan et al., 2007a). The increased concentration of Put after Spd treatment could be attributed to an up-regulation of ADC, a key enzyme of one of the routes for Put biosynthesis.

These results support the hypothesis that the PA treatments could induce acclimation of fruits to low temperature, and in turn protect them from CI, by maintaining membrane integrity, this effect being greater as the number of positive charges per molecules increases, that is, Spm > Spd > Put (Valero et al., 2002a; Nair and Singh, 2004). Thus, the increase of PAs in chilling injured fruits could be a natural defense mechanism of fruit tissues against this stress, although this effect itself may not be totally accurate if the increase in PAs is not high enough.

7.8 Polyamines and mechanical damage

Mechanical damage as a consequence of inappropriate harvest, manipulation, and transport techniques is considered a type of stress that occurs during the postharvest manipulation of fruits (see Chapter 3, Section 3.9). This stress is accompanied by physiological and morphological changes that affect the fruit commodity, such as increased respiration and ethylene production rates, bruising, cell rupture, and ion leakage (Martínez-Romero et al., 2004). In addition, mechanical damage has been shown to modify PA concentrations in fruit tissues. Thus, in Fortune mandarin, the application of mechanical damage led to an increase of Put concentration in the peel, the magnitude of this increase being force-dependent from 10 to 30 N and evident just a few hours after the mechanical damage was performed. This mechanical damage also increased Spd concentration although without significant differences among the applied forces (Figure 7.10). However, in Clementine mandarin no significant changes in PA concentration were observed as a consequence of mechanical damage. These differences could be attributed to the different peel characteristics of these two cultivars, since Clementine peel has great thickness and sponginess, while Fortune peel is thinner and tightly adheres to the segments. Thus, Fortune is more susceptible to bruising than Clementine. In fact, the application of 10, 20, and 30 N forces caused a higher deformation of fruit peel in Clementine than in Fortune mandarins, and observation of the damaged sections using magnifying lens (10×) revealed that only Fortune mandarin showed mechanical damage consisting of breakdown and disruption of the albedo tissue (Valero et al., 1998a).

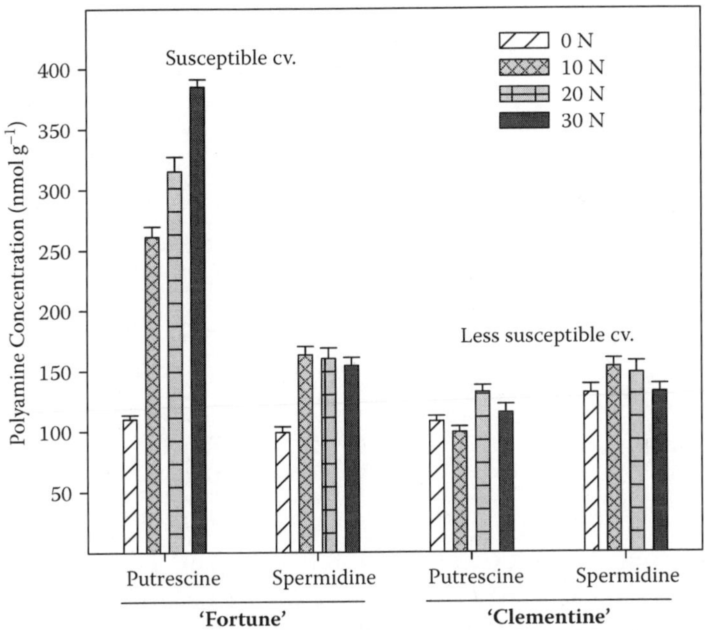

Figure 7.10 Effects of mechanical damage, with force load of 10, 20, and 30 N, on polyamine concentration of two mandarin cultivars, Fortune (susceptible to mechanical damage) and Clementine (less susceptible to mechanical damage), after 6 h of mechanical damage application.

Similarly, in damaged peach, apricot, and plum (Martínez-Romero et al., 2000; 2002; 2004; Pérez-Vicente et al., 2002) an increase in Spd levels was found, which could be the result of an active transformation of Put to Spd, because Put concentration was lower in the damaged areas than in nondamaged fruits. However, mechanically damaged lemons (Martínez-Romero et al., 1999) showed a significant increase in levels of both Spd and Spm. These results showed direct effects of the mechanical stress on the metabolism of PAs, and consequently an increase in PA concentration could act as a physiological marker of mechanical stress, one of the less known types of stresses in fruits and vegetables.

Moreover, exogenous application of Put could protect the fruits against mechanical damage. Thus, as can be observed in Figure 7.11, the volume and surface of the fruit damaged area were significantly lower in peaches and apricots treated with Put before being mechanically damaged than in control fruits. This protective effect has been proposed to be mediated by an increase in endogenous levels of PAs in lemons (Martínez-Romero et al., 1999), peaches (Martínez-Romero et al., 2000), apricots (Martínez-Romero et al., 2002), and plums (Pérez-Vicente et al., 2002).

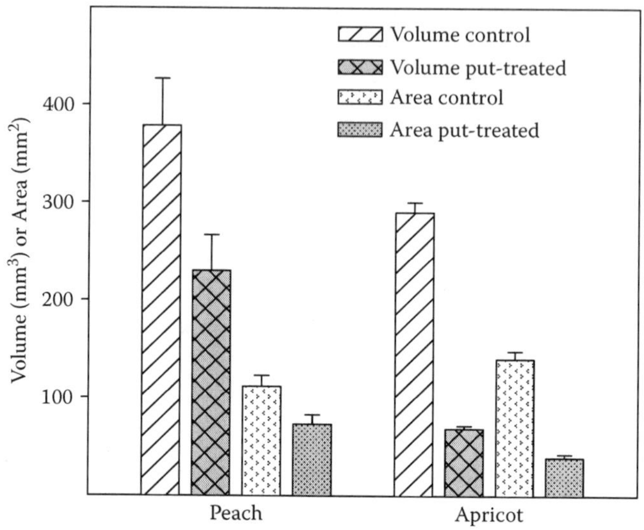

Figure 7.11 Effects of putrescine treatment (1 mM pressure infiltrated at 200 mm Hg for 8 minutes), in volume and area of damaged surface of peach and plum fruits, 24 hours after application of a force load of 20 N.

7.9 Future trends

The beneficial effects of the exogenous PAs in fruits are numerous, but the commercial application is nowadays limited, although in the United States a patent was filled many years ago (Law et al., 1988) for the use of PAs as a method of extending shelf life and enhancing keeping quality of fruits. However, no specific regulations exist about the use of exogenous PAs in Europe. The latest advances into fruit ripening and PAs reviewed here have put the field in a good position to develop significant advances in coming years. Research needs emerge from the requirement to better understand the role of exogenous PAs on the improvement of fruit quality during storage. The known biochemistry of the enzymes involved in the PA pathway and their interrelation with ethylene, along the occurrence of molecular probes to the genes encoding the enzymes, should finally assure of the role of PAs in fruit ripening.

Considering that PAs are naturally occurring molecules, their application as postharvest treatment could be considered an environmentally compatible tool as they can be metabolized by fruit cells.

Although exogenous application of PAs enhances their endogenous levels, the concentrations remain far lower than the toxic ones. Finally, more extensive metabolic profiling is needed to gain deeper insight into the nutritional attributes of PA-enriched/-treated fruit. We are only now beginning to understand their role in growth, development, and senescence through molecular genetics and modern biochemical approaches, and the elucidation of PA roles in modulating pre- and postharvest biology will contribute to the development of functional foods using modern biotechnology. Thus, modern agriculture, which is searching for effective biological molecules with well-known metabolic and without toxicological effects, may have the answer in PAs.

chapter eight

1-Methylcyclopropene treatments

8.1 Introduction

The discovery that some olefin compounds counteract ethylene action was carried out in 1972 (Sisler and Pian, 1973). It was first noted that 2, 5-norbornadiene seemed to counteract ethylene, acting as competitive inhibitor of ethylene responses as does silver ion. Trans-cyclooctene and diazocyclopentadiene were also ethylene action inhibitors, the ring strain being the primary factor for this effect, while the last chemical structures having this action were cyclopropenes (Sisler, 2006). Then, the discovery of 1-methylcyclopropene (1-MCP) as an ethylene inhibitor began in the late 1980s with research by Blankenship and Sisler as reported in the review of Blankenship and Dole (2003). In those years, little was known about how ethylene reacted with its receptors or receptor characterization. In order to improve extraction and purification of the receptor molecules, Blankenship and Sisler decided to look for a compound, other than ethylene, that would bind tightly to the receptor site and serve as a "tag" during extraction and purification procedures (Sisler, 2006). The scientific research on this compound has shown that is a powerful inhibitor of ethylene action and is capable of maintaining postharvest quality in many fresh horticultural products, and thus an exciting new strategy for controlling ethylene production and thus ripening of climacteric fruits as well as senescence of vegetative tissues has emerged with the discovery and commercialization of the inhibitor of ethylene perception, 1-MCP. This compound has been applied commercially as a stable powder that is easily released as a gas when the powder is dissolved in water. 1-MCP was approved by the Environmental Protection Agency (EPA) in 1999 for use on ornamentals and marketed as Ethylbloc® and under the trade name SmartFresh™ for edible horticultural products with global use rights of Rohm and Haas and now transferred to Agrofresh Inc., which is the company in charge of commercializing 1-MCP at the industrial level worldwide. Very recently (2005), the European Union approved the use of 1-MCP within the Member States as a plant growth regulator and established a maximum residue limit (MRL) as 0.01 mg kg^{-1}, since 1-MCP has a nontoxic mode of action and negligible residue and is active at very low concentrations.

During the last decade research about the application of this compound has increased progressively with more than 400 research papers on the topic of 1-MCP and fruit (Figure 8.1, inner graph) and 50 papers on vegetables. The most studied fruit has been apple followed by banana, tomato, pear, and plum (Figure 8.1). Other important fruits with contrasted 1-MCP efficacy are avocado, peach, nectarine, apricot, papaya, melon, and kiwifruit. Nowadays, the effects of 1-MCP on maturity stage, fresh-cut produce, bioactive compounds, storage conditions, and the expression of the genes responsible for the biosynthetic pathway of ethylene are the most important topics under study. However, time for treatment and applied doses still must be studied in different fruits and vegetables. Thus, the impact of 1-MCP on postharvest science and technology has two approaches: (1) It provides the potential to maintain fruit and vegetable quality after harvest, and (2) 1-MCP provides a powerful tool to gain insight into the fundamental processes that are involved in ripening and senescence. Professor Chris Watkins and his colleagues at Cornell University maintain and update a Web page (http://www.hort.cornell.edu/mcp/) with a summary of physiological processes or disorders in fruits, vegetables, and ornamental plants that are delayed or decreased, increased, or unaffected by application of 1-MCP (Watkins and Miller, 2005).

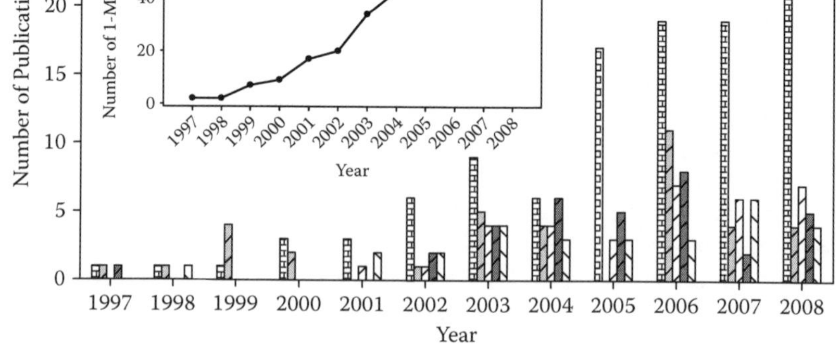

Figure 8.1 Number of publications per year about 1-MCP on the fruits in which 1-MCP has been most studied in the last 20 years. Insert graph shows the total number of publications per year about the use of 1-MCP in fruits and vegetables.

In the present chapter the latest knowledge about 1-MCP and ethylene receptor interaction as well as the main effects of 1-MCP on fruit ripening and quality will be provided.

8.2 1-MCP as blocking ethylene receptors

The biosynthesis pathway of ethylene has been provided in Chapter 2 (Section 2.3.7, Figure 2.11), and once synthesized the first step in ethylene signaling occurs when ethylene binds to the receptors via a copper cofactor, which is probably delivered by the copper transporter (Guo and Ecker, 2004). Phenotypic changes in response to ethylene are determined by three general steps: (1) the perception of the hormone, (2) the transduction of the signal through gene expression regulators, and (3) the expression of genes and synthesis of proteins sensitive to the received ethylene signal.

To study the ethylene perception and signal transduction researchers have used two plant species: *Arabidopsis* for getting insights into the molecular regulation at the early steps of fruit formation and development, and tomato which has been adopted as a model for studying fleshy fruits and ripening. In *Arabidopsis,* ethylene is perceived by a family of five membrane-localized receptors that are homologous to bacterial two-component histidine kinases involved in sensing environmental changes. The system typically consists of two proteins: a histidine kinase as the sensor that autophosphorylates an internal histidine residue in response to environmental signals, and a response regulator that activates the downstream components upon receiving a phosphate from the histidine residue of the sensor on its aspartate residue (Wang et al., 2002). The ethylene receptors in *Arabidopsis* can be divided into two subfamilies based on structural similarities: subfamily 1 includes ETR1 and ERS1; subfamily 2 includes ETR2, ERS2, and EIN4 (Bleecker and Kende, 2000). The ETR1-like subfamily features three membrane-spanning regions at the N-terminal region, where ethylene binding occurs, and a well-conserved histidine kinase domain at the C-terminal part of the protein. The ETR2-like subfamily is predicted to have four hydrophobic extensions at the N terminus and a degenerate histidine kinase domain that lacks one or more elements considered necessary for catalytic activity, implying that these receptors may function differently. The fact that members of a family of photoreceptors, the phytochromes, have a histidine kinase domain related to two-component systems but exhibit serine/threonine kinase activity supports the notion that the ETR2 class of receptors may function not as histidine kinases but possibly as serine/threonine kinases.

Tomato (*Solanum lycopersicon*) is emerging as another important system to study ethylene receptor function. In tomato there are six receptor isoforms, five of which have been tested for ethylene binding and found to bind ethylene with high affinity (Binder, 2008). Three of these are subfamily I receptors (LeETR1, LeETR2, and NR, never ripe or LeETR3) while the remainder (LeETR4, LeETR5, and LeETR6) resemble subfamily 2 receptors. The expression of the tomato ethylene receptors has been detected in all tissues analyzed, but they present distinct expression patterns throughout development and in response to differing environmental stimuli. LeETR1 and LeETR2 are expressed at constant levels in all tissues throughout development, while NR, LeETR4, LeETR5, and LeETR6 are highly expressed in reproductive tissues (flowers and fruits) with a significant increase of NR, LeETR4, and LeETR5 in ripening fruits (Cara and Giovannoni, 2008). A cumulative body of genetic and biochemical evidence led to a proposal for a model for ethylene perception and metabolism (Klee and Tieman, 2002). As the receptor also acts as a negative regulator of downstream responses, in the absence of ethylene, receptors actively suppress expression of ethylene responsive genes. Consistent with this model, a reduction in the overall level of receptor increases ethylene responsiveness of a tissue, while higher expression of receptor decreases ethylene sensitivity.

The mode of action of 1-MCP is mediated through the inhibition of ethylene perception of plant tissues by interacting with the receptor and competing with ethylene for binding sites (Sisler and Serek, 1997) and thereby preventing the ethylene-dependent responses. In addition, the effectiveness of inhibiting fruit ripening is a function of the 1-MCP concentration applied, up to saturation of the binding sites. The affinity of 1-MCP for the receptor is approximately 10 times greater than that of ethylene. Compared with ethylene, 1-MCP is active at much lower concentrations. 1-MCP also influences ethylene biosynthesis in some species through feedback inhibition (Blankenship and Dole, 2003). Depending on the product it can be desirable for the inhibition of ethylene-mediated responses to persist indefinitely, especially in the case of leafy vegetables, but for fruit, recovery from 1-MCP–induced inhibition of ripening is often essential to provide a ripened product that is acceptable to the consumer (Watkins, 2006). This is the main reason that the concentration of 1-MCP necessary to block the ethylene receptors varies largely depending on plant species, from 0.1 nL L^{-1} to 100 μL L^{-1}. The extent and longevity of 1-MCP action is affected by species, cultivar, tissue, and mode of ethylene biosynthesis induction. A concentration × time effect is apparent with longer exposure periods required for lower 1-MCP concentrations to obtain the same physiological effects (Sisler and Serek, 1997). Research with yeast has shown that ETR1 and ERS1 genes encoding the ethylene binding proteins show equal sensitivity to 1-MCP, but little research on expression of these genes in fruit and vegetables is yet available. Accumulation of transcripts for the genes encoding ERS decreased in treated apple (Defilippi et al., 2005), while 1-MCP did not affect transcription of the gene PP-ETR1 but down-regulated that of ERS1 (Rasori et al., 2002).

In some fruits such as apple, banana, melon, and pear, 1-MCP application induced a lower expression of the genes encoding the two key enzymes of the ethylene biosynthetic pathway (ACO and ACS) and lower activity of their respective enzymes (Lelièvre et al., 1997; Defilippi et al., 2005). In tomato, transcript accumulations of ACO, phytoene synthase 1 (PSY1), and expansin 1 (EXP1), used as indicators of treatment effects on ethylene biosynthesis, color, and softening, respectively, were decreased by 1-MCP (Hoeberichts et al., 2002). Increases in transcript abundance of LE-ACS2, LE-ACS4, and LE-ACO1 mRNAs in ripening fruit were inhibited by 1-MCP, but ethylene production, ACC content, and ACS and ACO activities were not inhibited to the expected levels, suggesting involvement of negatively regulated genes in ethylene biosynthesis.

However, it has been assumed that 1-MCP binds permanently to receptors present at the time of treatment and any return of ethylene sensitivity is due to appearance of new sites, although plant tissues vary greatly in their ability to regenerate sites. Thus, the receptor regeneration might explain the differences in response of 1-MCP to the assayed horticultural products, as well as the necessary 1-MCP doses to gain effectiveness in delaying the ripening process.

8.3 Postharvest 1-MCP application

Extensive literature exists about the effects of 1-MCP in many horticultural produce, in which beneficial effects have been obtained following the application of 1-MCP postharvest in terms of delaying and/or inhibiting the ripening process through the blockage of the ethylene receptors. Thus, the main studied fruits are those within the climacteric ripening group due to dependence of ethylene in controlling the ripening process. A summary of the metabolic changes, reduction, delay, or unaffected, after 1-MCP treatment is given in Table 8.1. The overall effect in reducing ethylene production and respiration rate is noticeable for most fruits, which in turn modulates the quality parameters dependent on ethylene. In order to be used commercially, 1-MCP is complexed with α-cyclodextrin to produce a stable water-soluble powder. The method of application is to generate 1-MCP as a gas by mixing the soluble powder in water and then dispersing it around the product. The commercial application has been increasing in recent years, although registration of 1-MCP for a specific country is strictly necessary. In this section, the main effects of 1-MCP on the plant hormone ethylene and respiration rate, as well as the parameters related to fruit quality, will be provided.

Table 8.1 Effect of 1-MCP on Metabolism and Fruit Quality Parameters

Fruits	1-MCP reduce or delay	Unaffected by 1-MCP
Apple (*Malus sylvestris*) Apricot (*Prunus armeniaca*) Plum (*Prunus salicina*, *P. domestica*) Tomato (*Lycopersicon esculentum*)	Ethylene production, respiration, softening, loss of titratable acidity, color change, and aroma volatiles. Reduced weight loss in apricot, plum, and tomato.	Soluble solids content and titratable acidity in several cultivars.
Banana (*Musa* L.) Mango (*Mangifera indica*)	Ethylene production, respiration, softening, loss of titratable acidity in banana, color change, and aroma volatiles.	Soluble solids content in both fruits and titratable acidity in mango.
Peach (*Prunus persica* Batsch) Nectarine (*Prunus persica*)	Ethylene production, respiration, softening, loss of titratable acidity.	Respiration in some nectarine cultivars. Loss of titratable acidity in low acid cultivars.
Pear (*Pyrus communis*) Kiwifruit (*Actinidia deliciosa*) Avocado (*Persea americana*)	Ethylene production, respiration, softening, color change.	Soluble solids content and titratable acidity in pear and kiwifruit.
Persimmon (*Diospyros khaki*) Strawberry (*Fragaria x ananassa*)	Ethylene production, softening, color change, soluble solids content in strawberry.	Decay and respiration in both fruits. Soluble solids content in persimmon.

Source: Adapted from Guillén, 2009.

8.3.1 *Ethylene production, respiration rate, and 1-MCP*

1-MCP is thought to interact with ethylene receptors and thereby prevent ethylene-dependent responses. A few review papers have emerged in the last few years describing the effects of 1-MCP on fruit commodities (Blankenship and Dole, 2003), in which apple, banana, pear, tomato, and stone fruits (especially plums) are the most studied at both research and commercial levels (Watkins, 2006, Figure 8.1). Table 8.2 shows 1-MCP concentration, duration for treatment, and temperature application with positive effects in retarding the ripening process in a wide range of fruit commodities, as well as the main observed adverse effects that sometimes occur. From Table 8.2 it can be inferred that for a particular fruit the

Table 8.2 Fruit Types, 1-MCP Concentration, Duration for Treatment, and Temperature with Positive Effects in Retarding the Ripening Process, as Well as the Main Adverse Effects

Fruit	1-MCP ($\mu L\ L^{-1}$)	Duration (h)	Temperature (°C)	Adverse effects
Apple	0.5–10	12	20	Reduced volatiles
Banana	0.01–1	6–24	20	
Pear	0.1–4	12–24	0, 20	
Tomato	0.1–100	1–24	0–25	
Peach	0.02–0.5	18–24	20, 24	Internal browning
Apricot	0.05–0.75	6–48	3, 5, 20, 22	
Nectarine	0.2–1	12–24	20, 24	Flesh woolliness
Plum	0.1–40	6–24	2, 20	
Mango	1–100	6–14	20	Decay
Avocado	0.1–25	6–48	20–24	
Kiwifruit	0.5–5	16–20	20	
Papaya	0.5–10	4–24	20	

Source: Data obtained from Blankenship and Dole, 2003; Watkins, 2006; Guillén, 2009.

appropriate 1-MCP concentration, duration of treatment, and temperature need to be established to get positive results in terms of reducing the ripening process by inhibiting the ethylene production.

In apple, 1-MCP dramatically inhibits fruit ripening, the increase in ethylene production, and internal ethylene concentration associated with the climacteric ripening stage, the extent of these inhibitions being related to cultivar, temperature for 1-MCP application, type of storage, temperature, and duration of storage. In fact, 1-MCP has been assayed in a wide range of apple cultivars including Gala, Fuji, Golden Delicious, McIntosh, Granny Smith, Red Chief Delicious, Law Rome, Jonagold, and Empire. The results obtained with early-, mid-, and late-season apple cultivars from the postharvest application of 1-MCP under air storage conditions revealed that a dose response of internal ethylene concentrations to 1-MCP existed in McIntosh and Law Rome, while Red Chief Delicious and Empire ripening was generally prevented by all 1-MCP concentrations; moreover the effectiveness of 1-MCP was not related to harvest time of different cultivars (Watkins et al., 2000). Respiration rates in 1-MCP–treated apple have been less commonly reported, although some reports have found reduction in respiration rate to levels close to that found at preclimacteric stages (Watkins, 2006).

Banana has also been another fruit with good results in terms of ethylene inhibition during postharvest storage, especially in the Cavendish subgroup, with the cultivar Williams being the most studied. The banana is typically harvested at the green stage of maturity, transported, and then ripened artificially with ethylene before being sent to market in the United States, while in Europe this is not a typical procedure since banana reaches the ripe stage at the supermarket or at homes. The earliest report of banana and 1-MCP established that the increased green life after 1-MCP was a function of concentration × exposure time (Golding et al., 1998), in which 1-MCP doses (0.45 μL L^{-1}) were applied at several intervals. Both ethylene production and respiration rates were lower in 1-MCP–treated fruits than in nontreated ones even in those fruits treated with propylene to stimulate the ripening process, and thus 1-MCP can disrupt the normal sequence of biochemical changes associated or dependent on ethylene. On a general basis, concentration over 0.30 μL L^{-1} is necessary to inhibit the ethylene production, since lower concentrations just show a delay in the onset of the ethylene climacteric peak.

In the case of pears, the interaction between 1-MCP and shelf life has also been studied. Pear is considered an exception within the fruit type since it requires exposure to chilling temperatures to ripen properly, with winter pears requiring as long as 8 weeks. In addition, postharvest cold treatment is required to induce endogenous ethylene production and subsequent ripening of green fruits. Among pear cultivars, Conference, d'Anjou, Blanquilla, and Bartlett have been the most studied. d'Anjou pears treated with 1-MCP (0.1–1 μL L^{-1}) extended preclimacteric period with low ethylene production and respiration rates, although total inhibition was not observed (Argenta et al., 2003). A dose response of 1-MCP for delaying ethylene production was also evident. Fruit treated with 0.1 or 1 μL L^{-1} 1-MCP began to produce ethylene 2 and 4 months later than controls, respectively, and fruit treated with 1 μL L^{-1} had ethylene production lower than controls at 6 and 8 months after treatment. In Bartlett pears, the degree and duration of the effects of 1-MCP on CO_2 and ethylene production at 20°C were related to the treatment concentration (Ekman et al., 2004). Ethylene production during ripening was inhibited by exposure to 0.1 μL L^{-1} 1-MCP compared with untreated fruits when stored for 6 weeks at –1°C, but not when the fruits were stored for longer periods. Similarly, treatment with 0.5 or 1 μL L^{-1} reduced CO_2 and ethylene production in ripening fruit stored for 0, 6, or 12 weeks. However, after 18 weeks of storage, mean ethylene production was no longer affected by 1-MCP application, and only fruit treated with 1 μL L^{-1} 1-MCP respired more slowly than the untreated controls during ripening. Thus, the effects of 1-MCP treatment at harvest declined with duration of storage, and repetition of the treatment during storage was not effective.

Stone fruits comprise several species (peach, apricot, nectarine, and plum) in which the efficacy of 1-MCP has been assayed. In a survey on several stone fruits 1-MCP applied at 0.5 μL L^{-1} was observed to be effective in reducing the ethylene production compared with control non-treated fruits (Figure 8.2), although the extension in ethylene inhibition was dependent on fruit species and even cultivar. Thus Reina Claudia plum and Currot apricot showed the lowest percentages of ethylene inhibition compared with Golden Japan and President plums. Moreover, it is interesting to point out that the percentage of ethylene inhibition by 1-MCP was correlated inversely to the maximum value of ethylene production at the climacteric peak of each particular fruit (Figure 8.2, insert). Thus, fruit with the lowest ethylene production (Golden Japan plum, <0.5 nL g^{-1} h^{-1}) showed the highest rate of ethylene inhibition (over 95%). Conversely, in Currot apricot, which had a climacteric peak production rate of >40 nL g^{-1} h^{-1}, an inhibition below 40% was observed. Since treatments were performed under the same conditions (24 hours at 0°C), the fruit type, the cultivar, and the maximum ethylene production at the climacteric peak should be taken into account to explain the different effect of 1-MCP on ethylene production inhibition (Martínez-Romero et al., 2007a). In stone fruits, the effects of 1-MCP are generally dose dependent, with maximum responses occurring at the highest 1-MCP concentration

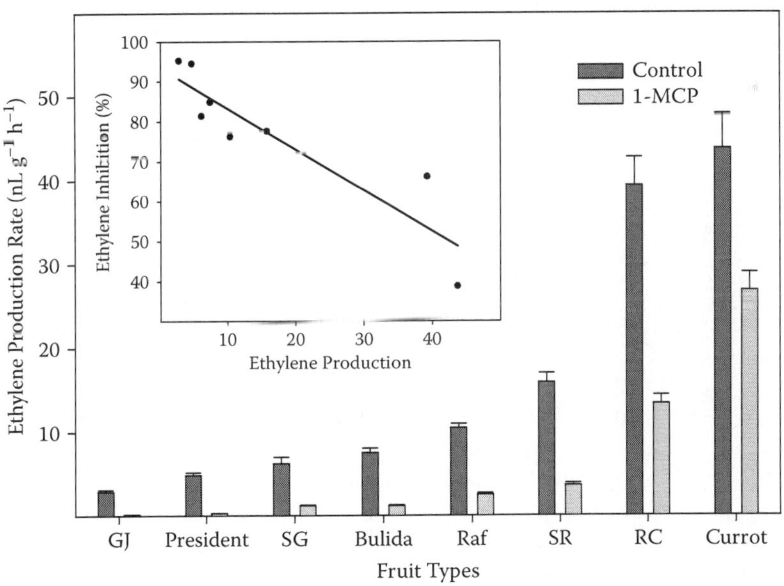

Figure 8.2 Ethylene production at the climacteric peak in control plums (GJ, Golden Japan; President; SG, Songold; SR, Santa Rosa; and RC, Reina Claudia), apricots (Bulida and Currot), and tomato (Raf), and those obtained in their 1-MCP (0.50 μL L^{-1} for 24 hours) corresponding treated fruits. Insert graphic shows the relationship between ethylene production at the climacteric peak and the inhibition caused by 1-MCP.

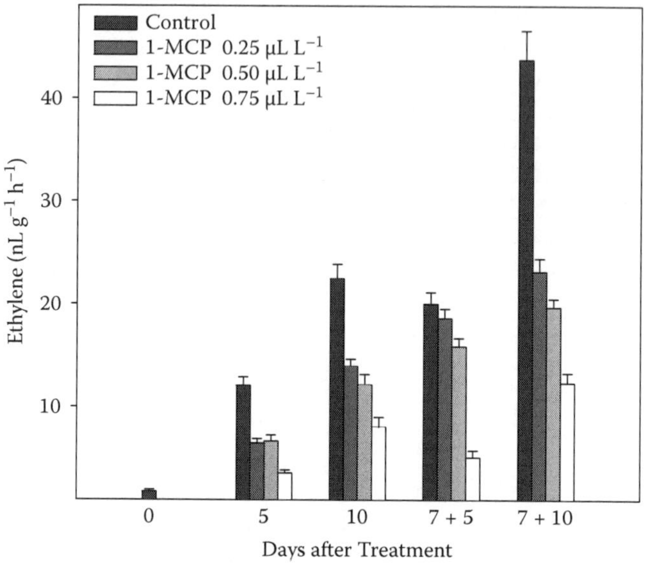

Figure 8.3 Ethylene production in apricot as affected by 1-MCP dose applied (0.25, 0.50, and 0.75 μL L^{-1} for 24 hours) at harvest (Day 0), after 5 or 10 days of storage at 20°C (5 and 10, respectively), and after 7 days of cold storage + 5 or 10 days of storage at 20°C (7 + 5 or 7 + 10).

applied, as can be observed in Figure 8.3 for Currot apricot, in which the ethylene inhibition was higher at 0.75 than 0.5 or 0.25 μL L^{-1} doses.

Among stone fruits, reviewed literature confirms that plums behave better than others to 1-MCP action in terms of delaying the ripening process and maintaining fruit quality during prolonged storage. Peaches stored 0, 3, and 5 days and treated at 0.02 μL L^{-1}, either in a single application or multiple treatments, showed that 1-MCP used as a single dose had little effect on ethylene biosynthesis and the abundance of PP-ACS1 mRNA, but pulse treatment with 1-MCP delayed significantly the induction of ethylene biosynthesis and PP-ACS1 and PP-ACO1 genes (Mathooko et al., 2001). Sisler and Serek (1997) proposed that plants are able to overcome the inhibition caused by 1-MCP through the synthesis of new receptors. Therefore, the small response of peach fruit to a single treatment with 1-MCP with respect to ethylene biosynthesis and the expression of ACS and ACO genes could imply that the ethylene receptors are regenerated within a short time, such that the fruits need continuous or intermittent exposure to 1-MCP for complete and continuous suppression of the expression of these genes. Nectarines treated with 1-MCP (1 μL L^{-1}) showed lack of efficacy after cold storage at 4°C but delayed ethylene production when fruit were stored at 20°C, which is attributed to stress imposed by the combination of cold and 1-MCP (Bregoli et al., 2005).

An early report on plum (Abdi et al., 1998) revealed that application of 1-MCP to the climacteric cultivars (Gulfruby and Beauty) slightly delayed the onset of the climacteric ethylene in a dose-dependent mode, and contrarily in suppressed-climacteric varieties absence of ethylene production or a clear respiratory climacteric was observed after 1-MCP treatment, although fruits became over-ripe and rotted. A later work with climacteric and suppressed-climacteric plum cultivars showed a complete inhibition of the ethylene production, the extension of inhibition being dose-dependent in the climacteric type (Santa Rosa) and independent in the nonclimacteric Golden Japan (Martínez-Romero et al., 2003a). The inhibition of ethylene by 1-MCP in these cultivars was attributable to the fact that the treatment was performed at 0°C, while most of the previously mentioned assays were carried out at 20°C or higher temperatures, and thus a fewer number of receptors could be present at time of application. Thus, effectiveness of 1-MCP treatments is dependent on temperature, and to gain more inhibition on ethylene production, treatment with 1-MCP should be carried out in cooled fruits and at low temperature.

The ripening stage at harvest was also studied in plums (Valero et al., 2003), in which 1-MCP was equally effective at inhibiting the ethylene production in plums harvested at commercial ripening stage or in those picked 10 days later, although in the more mature ones a slight increase in ethylene was detected after 5 weeks of storage, which could be associated with some kind of ethylene receptor generation. Moreover, for commercial purposes, the effect of 1-MCP applied to plum packaged in small cardboard boxes or in bulk revealed that when 1-MCP was applied to fruit handled and packaged in perforated cardboard boxes, ethylene production was totally inhibited during all storage periods, while in those plums treated with 1-MCP in bulk (before handling and packaging), ethylene production increased after 3 and 4 weeks of cold storage plus 7 days at 20°C, the differences being attributed to the higher gas diffusion around the fruit when they are packaged in small-perforated boxes (Valero et al., 2004).

As stated previously, the applications were achieved by mixing the product with water to release the 1-MCP gas in enclosed areas. However, the availability of the proper facilities to treat the fruit could be a limitation under certain commercial situations. For this reason, alternatives, such as sprays or dips, are being developed, and in the case of plums a novel 1-MCP immersion formulation delayed and reduced ethylene production in a dose-dependent manner, reaching the saturation points at 1000 ng kg^{-1} (Manganaris et al., 2008).

Ripening of green tomatoes held at 20°C in air containing 0.1 $\mu L\ L^{-1}$ ethylene was substantially delayed by exposure to 1-MCP in the concentration range 0.1–100 $\mu L\ L^{-1}$ with the extent of the delay being directly related to the concentration of 1-MCP and exposure time, while ripe tomatoes needed over 20 μL L^{-1} to extend the shelf life (Wills and Ku, 2002). Another positive effect of 1-MCP has been shown in cherry tomatoes harvested as bunches, in which limitations for marketing are due to abscission, and the application of 1-MCP delayed the abscission through a drastic repression of the genes responsible for EGases activity (Beno-Moualem et al., 2004). For commercial purposes, different combinations of 1-MCP doses (0.5 or 1 μL L^{-1}) and duration (3, 6, 12, or 24 h) were used on tomatoes harvested at the mature-green stage, with the main conclusion being that 0.5 μL L^{-1} for 24 hours induced the maximum benefit in terms of ethylene inhibition and retarding the ripening process (Guillén et al., 2007a). Based on this result, these authors studied the effect of tomato cultivar and ripening stage at harvest and concluded that for both stages 1-MCP treatment blocked the tomato receptors and absence of sharp increase in ethylene production or respiration rate was obtained, indicating that typical autocatalytic ethylene biosynthesis was also inhibited in tomatoes at both ripening stages (Guillén et al., 2006). The inhibition of both ethylene production and respiration rate by 1-MCP was negatively correlated with the maximum ethylene value reached for each of the cultivars and ripening stage assayed.

8.3.2 Effect of 1-MCP on fruit quality parameters

According to the delay and/or inhibition of ethylene production in climacteric fruits, all the quality parameters that are dependent on ethylene, such as firmness, color, soluble solids concentration, and loss of acidity, are retarded, together with the reduced weight loss.

Fruit softening is prevented or delayed by 1-MCP, the effects of treatment often being closely associated with the inhibition of ethylene production. Accordingly, Figure 8.3 showed that the inhibition of ethylene production in apricot was dependent on 1-MCP concentration, and results of firmness confirm that the degree of reducing the softening process also shows dose-dependence, since apricot treated with 0.75 μL L^{-1} had higher fruit firmness than those treated with 0.25 or 0.5 μL L^{-1} (Figure 8.4). This effect has been observed for most of the studied fruits (apple, pear, tomato, plum, banana, avocado, etc.), although the components of texture that are affected by 1-MCP have not been adequately investigated. In this sense, studies of 1-MCP on cell wall changes of treated fruit are limited, but a number of investigations on cell wall enzymes are available. Decreased softening in 1-MCP–treated bananas is associated with lower expression of an ethylene-induced expansin (MaExp1) gene, and lower activities of PME, PG, EGase, and PL activities (Lohani et al., 2004). Effects of 1-MCP on softening of pears were associated with decreased β-GAL activity and differential effects on expression of its genes (Mwaniki et al., 2005). In

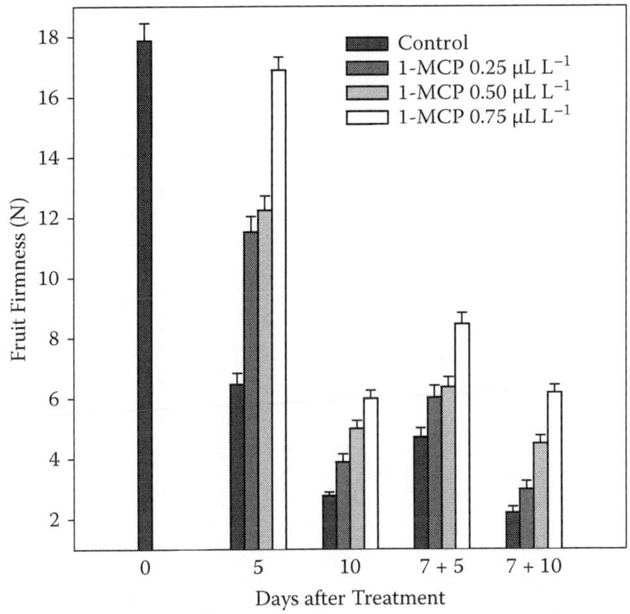

Figure 8.4 Fruit firmness in apricot as affected by 1-MCP dose applied (0.25, 0.50, and 0.75 μL L^{-1} for 24 hours) at harvest (Day 0), after 5 or 10 days of storage at 20°C (5 and 10, respectively) and after 7 days of cold storage + 5 or 10 days of storage at 20°C (7 + 5 or 7 + 10).

plums, the activities of exo-PG and EGase were lower in 1-MCP treated than in nontreated fruit, but treatment did not affect activities of endo-PG and PME (Watkins, 2006).

Color change is another fruit attribute whose evolution is retarded following the application of 1-MCP, although little is known about the effects of 1-MCP on pigment metabolism. It has been found that 1-MCP prevents or delays chlorophyll degradation and various types of color changes in a wide range of crop species including apple, pear, green plum, kiwifruit, and avocado. Accordingly, apricots (Bulida and Currot) and red plums (President) harvested at two ripening stages (S1 or S2) and treated with 1-MCP exhibited less color changes than controls (Figure 8.5). Thus, color a* decreased from day 0 (harvest) to 28 days of storage at 1°C plus 7 days at 20°C in control plums, showing the typical skin darkening of red plums, while in 1-MCP–treated plums no significant changes were found. However, in the two apricot cultivars color a* parameter increased in control fruits showing color changes from yellow to dark orange, which were also delayed by 1-MCP application. In addition, in apricot this effect was dose dependent, since fruits treated with 0.5 μL L^{-1} remained more yellow than those treated with 0.3 μL L^{-1} after 21 days

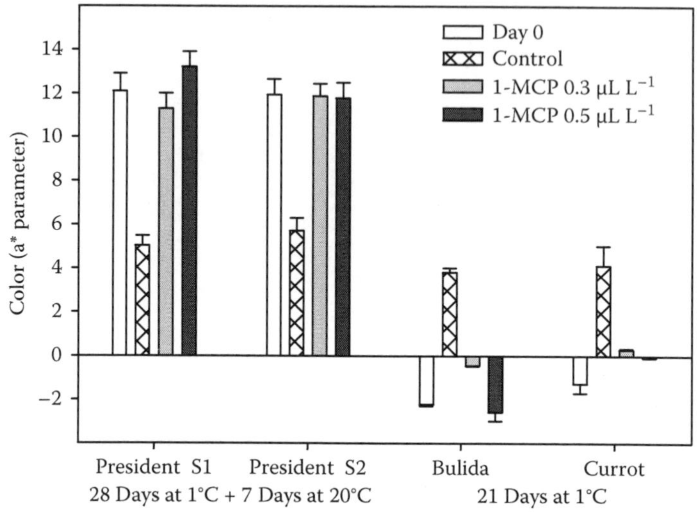

Figure 8.5 Color changes from values at harvest in President plum harvested at two ripening stages (S1, commercial harvest, and S2, 10 days later) and two apricot cultivars (Bulida and Currot) to those obtained after storage in control and 1-MCP–treated fruits (0.3 and 0.5 μL L^{-1} for 24 hours).

of cold storage. On the contrary, other researchers found that plum color changes were not affected by 1-MCP (Abdi et al., 1998) and concluded that ethylene was not necessary for color development in climacteric and suppressed climacteric plums. However, the 1-MCP concentration could not be considered alone, since studies combining applied dose and duration show that for any particular dose (e.g., 0.5 μL L^{-1}), the efficacy in retarding color changes in tomato is increased as duration of treatment is higher, as shown in Figure 8.6, although the application of greater dose (1 μL L^{-1}) does not enhance the delay in color. This could be explained by the higher inhibition of both ethylene production and respiration rate detected after 24 hours at 0.5 μL L^{-1} compared with those obtained using 1 μL L^{-1} for 3 or 6 hours of treatment. Nevertheless, successful 1-MCP use requires a delay, but not irreversible inhibition, of the processes involved in pigment metabolism, since consumers demand fruits with their typical color associated with ripening.

One clear effect of 1-MCP has been the acidity retention during postharvest storage, as reported for most of the fruits assayed, while the effect of 1-MCP on TSS is unclear. In general, 1-MCP delays loss of TA in apricot, plum, avocado, pear, tomato, and others (Watkins, 2006). Moreover, TA was maintained after prolonged storage at levels close to those found at harvest in plum (Martínez-Romero et al., 2003a; Valero et al., 2003) and tomatoes (Guillén et al., 2006). However, TSS concentration

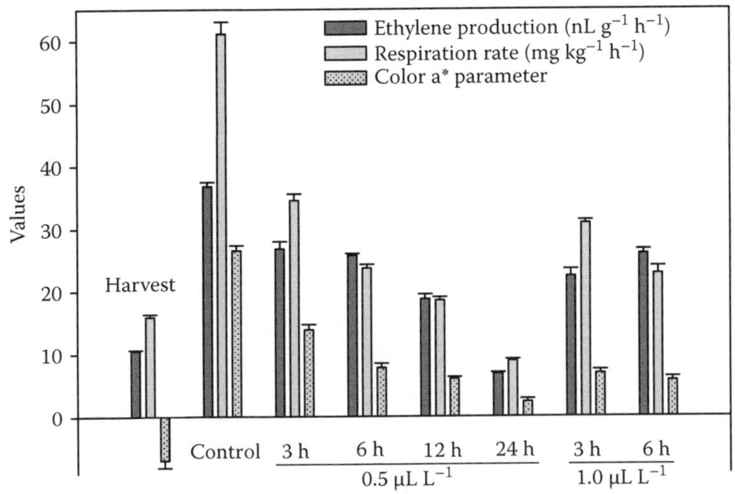

Figure 8.6 Effect of 1-MCP dose concentration and duration of treatment on ethylene production, respiration rate, and color a* parameter in tomato after 7 days of cold storage (10°C) plus 4 days at 20°C (shelf life) with respect to control fruits.

in 1-MCP–treated apple can be higher, lower, or the same as those in untreated fruit. These contrasting results with apples are notable and may be due to different cultivars or other experimental conditions used. Watkins and colleagues (2000) found differences in responses of apple cultivars to 1-MCP treatment, with McIntosh and Law Rome fruit having lower TSS than controls, and Delicious and Empire having higher soluble solids than untreated fruit. In peaches and nectarines, 1-MCP treatment either did not affect or resulted in lower TSS (Bregoli et al., 2005). In stone fruits, such as apricots and plums, the TSS/TA ratio was lower in 1-MCP-treated than in nontreated fruits after postharvest storage (Figure 8.7), although for this parameter no dose dependence was observed, mainly due to the fact that TSS was not affected by 1-MCP. In this sense, TSS in treated products might be expected to be higher than in untreated products because of lower respiration rates, but can be higher, lower, or the same as in untreated fruit depending on the product and the storage conditions (Watkins, 2006).

One of the poorly studied effects of 1-MCP is fruit weight loss, although this parameter has great influence on both produce quality and economic issue (Chapter 3, Section 3.3). Thus, 1-MCP–treated avocado had lower weight loss than untreated fruit, but the contrary occurred in pear with increase in weight loss followed by 1-MCP application (Watkins, 2006), and thus a potential risk of 1-MCP treatment is that weight loss may be greater because of the extension of the ripening period. In the case of

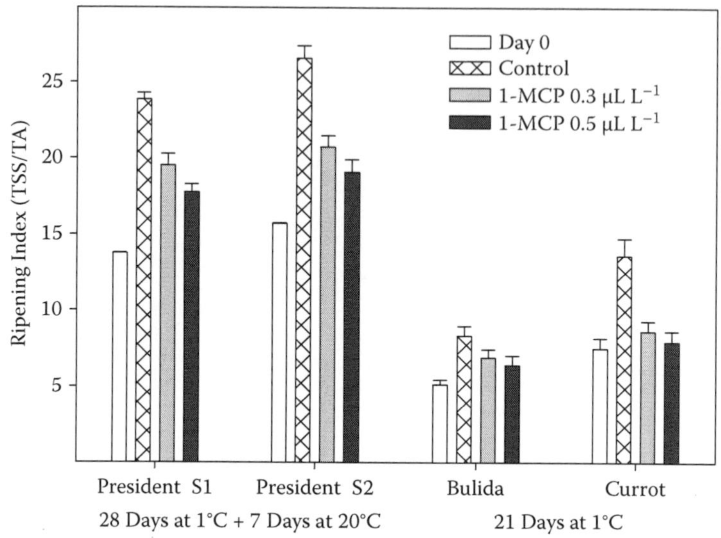

Figure 8.7 Ripening index changes from values at harvest in President plum harvested at 2 ripening stages (S1, commercial harvest, and S2, 10 days later) and two apricot cultivars (Bulida and Currot) to those obtained after storage in control and 1-MCP–treated fruits (0.3 and 0.5 μL L^{-1} for 24 hours).

plums (Valero et al., 2003) and tomatoes (Guillén et al. 2006), significant reductions in weight loss have been reported independently of the ripening stage at harvest or the climacteric-suppressed climacteric pattern (Martínez-Romero et al., 2003a). There is no a known mechanism by which 1-MCP delays the transpiration process, but the lower weight loss could be related to the lower respiration rate found in 1-MCP fruits, although weight loss is not ethylene dependent (Valero et al., 2003; Guillén et al., 2007a). It is well known that RH control is more important at warm than at cold storage temperatures. Even if the RH is maintained, the vapor-pressure deficit is greater at higher storage temperatures. Some products are more susceptible to moisture loss than others (Sozzi and Beaudry, 2007), and thus, for example, apples and kiwifruit have a low moisture loss rate, while postharvest water loss can cause rapid deterioration and reduction in the marketable quality of a range of other tree fruit crops that respond to 1-MCP and have a high moisture loss rate, such as persimmons, plums, mangoes, and guavas. To reduce moisture loss, products must be effectively precooled, and RH during transit and storage must be kept as high as possible.

As stated in Chapter 2 (Section 2.3.4), aroma compounds are important components of fruit flavor and influence consumer's acceptance of fresh fruits. During normal ripening of apples, the largest changes in volatile compounds are increased esters followed by alcohols, the enhancement of esters being responsible for the development of characteristic flavor and aroma of apple fruit. The application of 1-MCP at 10 μL L^{-1} was able to inhibit totally ethylene production in Fuji apples during 15 days of storage at 20°C, but also decreased the concentration of total esters by preventing the conversion of some alcohols to esters as well as the production of some alcohols, since these compounds also decreased during storage (Fan and Mattheis, 1999), indicating that the ester volatile production requires continuous ethylene action.

In banana, alcohol and esters are also the main volatile groups contributing to flavor, and the application of 1-MCP significantly delayed and suppressed the onset and magnitude of fruit respiration and volatile production. The 1-MCP treatments also caused a quantitative change in the composition of the banana aroma volatiles, resulting in a substantial increase in the concentration of alcohols and a decrease in their related esters (Golding et al., 1999), suggesting that the processes providing enzymes, enzyme activation, or critical substrates to volatile production are dependent on the continuous presence of ethylene. The large increase in the concentrations of alcohols and the concomitant decrease in esters followed by 1-MCP treatment suggests that the final step in ester formation, the esterification of the alcohol and the acyl CoA catalyzed by the enzyme alcohol acyl transferase, is disrupted by 1-MCP.

In pears, esters and alcohols are also the predominant volatiles, but their occurrence depends on length of storage, since esters were the most abundant volatiles produced after 2 or 4 months, while alcohols were the most abundant volatiles after 6 or 8 months. In these fruits, as a consequence of the 1-MCP–induced inhibition of ethylene action, the emanation of esters and alcohols was also reduced, but when 1-MCP–treated fruit began to ripen at 20°C after cold storage, the ripening process proceeded normally, and qualitative volatile production was similar to those untreated fruits (Argenta et al., 2003).

In conclusion, flavor is a composite of taste and odor, and volatile production can be greatly affected by ethylene. Therefore, decreased and/or altered volatile production in 1-MCP–treated fruits compared with untreated ones may impact product acceptance by consumers. In those situations in which reduced aroma is associated with 1-MCP treatment, the commercial implications are likely to vary by product type, being more critical for products and cultivars where aroma is a quality characteristic expected by the consumer. For some fruits, certain aromas are associated with over-ripening and therefore their inhibition is desirable, or aroma concentrations may be less important than texture and acid/sugar levels.

8.3.3 1-MCP, bioactive compounds, and antioxidant activity

The nutritional importance of the horticultural products focused on the human health aspects related to their content in bioactive compounds such as vitamin C and E, carotenoids, flavonoids and anthocyanins was provided in Chapter 2 (Section 2.3.5). However, there is little information about how 1-MCP can modulate the content of the bioactive compounds and antioxidant activity during postharvest storage of the produce. Recently, Guillén (2009) reviewed the effect of 1-MCP on nutritive quality and bioactive compounds in a wide range of fruits and vegetables (Table 8.3). Generally, 1-MCP slowed the decrease of ascorbic acid (vitamin C) in peach, pineapple, quince, and tomato, but ascorbic acid in apple showed lower content in 1-MCP–treated than in control fruits (Vilaplana et al., 2006). With respect to TAA, both H-TAA and L-TAA, the effect of 1-MCP is to increase the antioxidant capacity in sweet cherry by increasing the content of total phenolics or flavonoids, although hydroxycinnamic acids and anthocyanins were unaffected (Mozetiĉ et al., 2006). Conversely, 1-MCP delayed the increase in total phenolics

Table 8.3 Effect of 1-MCP on Nutritive and Bioactive Compounds

Product	Effect of 1-MCP on nutritive quality and bioactive compounds
Apple	↑ H-TAA, total phenolic, flavonoids, chlorogenic acid only in peel extracts (cv. Empire).
	↑ H-TAA. ↔ Flavonoids and anthocyanins (cv. Red Delicious).
	↑ Vitamin C (cv. Golden Smoothee).
Peach	↑ Vitamin C (cv Jiubao).
Pineapple	↑ Vitamin C (cv. Queen).
Strawberry	↓ Total phenolic content and anthocyanins (cv. Everest).
Apricot	↑ H-TAA and total carotenoids (cv. Bulida).
Pear	↓ Vitamin C (cv. Blanquilla).
Cherry	↔ Hydroxycinnamic acids and anthocyanins (cv. Bing, Rainier and Lambert).
Mango	↑ Vitamin C (cv. Zihua).
Quince	↑ Vitamin C (cv. Ekmek).
Tomato	↓Lycopene, H-TAA (cv. Rapsodie).
	↑ L-TAA (cv. Raf y cv. De la Pera).
	↑ Vitamin C (no cultivar mentioned).
Cherry tomato	↑ Lycopene and total carotenoids (cv. Cerasiforme).
Lettuce	↑ Vitamin C (cv. Baby Butterhead).

Note: ↑: Increase ↓: Decrease ↔: Unaffected.

Source: Adapted from Guillén, 2009.

and anthocyanins occurring during ripening of strawberry, which was associated with lower PAL activity (Jiang et al., 2001). In tomato cultivars, it seems that 1-MCP induces a clear effect on reducing lycopene and total carotenoids but TAA either increased or decreased (Guillén, 2009). In mango, 1-MCP inhibited the production of H_2O_2 and maintained higher ascorbic acid during storage (Wang et al., 2009). These authors also found that 1-MCP inhibited activities of antioxidant enzymes including CAT, SOD, and ascorbate peroxidase, suggesting that 1-MCP could play a positive role in regulating the activated oxygen metabolism balance. In air-stored apple fruit, total phenolic concentration was higher in the peel of 1-MCP–treated fruit than in the controls but slightly lower in the flesh of 1-MCP treated fruit. On the contrary, in CA-stored fruit, few consistent trends were observed, although flavonoid concentrations were higher in the flesh of 1-MCP–treated than untreated fruit kept in 2 kPa O_2 while anthocyanin concentrations, only measured in the peel, were not affected by 1-MCP treatment (Fawbush et al., 2009). However, these authors did not find correlations between antioxidant activity and total phenolics and/or ascorbic acid. Thus, further research is warranted on the effects of 1-MCP on various nonenzymatic and enzymatic antioxidant systems to better understand how 1-MCP can enhance TAA.

8.4 1-MCP in nonclimacteric fruits

It is clear that there are more studies about 1-MCP effects in climacteric fruits than about nonclimacteric fruits, since ethylene is not responsible for controlling the ripening process of these products (Chapter 2, Section 2.3.7), and thus in general 1-MCP is unlikely to be of postharvest benefit. However, literature exists about 1-MCP application on several nonclimacteric commodities such as sweet cherry, citrus, and strawberry, although there are no commercial applications. In fact, strawberries treated with 1-MCP (0–1000 nL L^{-1}) tended to maintain fruit firmness and color (Jiang et al., 2001), but disease development was accelerated in fruit treated at high 1-MCP concentrations (over 500 nL L^{-1}). In addition, 1-MCP inhibited PAL activity, which was reflected in lower increases in both anthocyanin and phenolics during storage. In sweet cherry, 1-MCP transiently stimulated ethylene evolution but did not have impact on respiration rate, softening, or color changes (Gong et al., 2002). In many cases, 1-MCP maintains, or delays, loss of greenness of a range of nonclimacteric citrus including orange, mandarin, and lime. In the latter, this is of special importance since maintenance of the green skin is desirable during storage for better commercialization, while as the green color fades, fruit acceptance gradually decreases. Therefore, ethylene seems to be involved in some maturation-related events in nonclimacteric fruits, such as chlorophyll degradation of the citrus skin, and it is possible that the skin green coloration loss in some citrus cultivars can be delayed by the application of 1-MCP, because of its influence on the ethylene action (Jomori et al., 2003). Accordingly, 1-MCP effectively inhibited ethylene responses in Shamouti oranges as indicated by its inhibition of the degreening process, the most effective concentrations of 1-MCP being 50–100 nL L^{-1} (Porat et al., 1999), while 1-MCP had no effects on the loss of fruit weight and firmness.

8.5 Preharvest 1-MCP application

As stated in Section 8.3, many horticultural commodities have shown benefits from postharvest use of 1-MCP, while the potential for commodity improvements with preharvest applications of this plant growth regulator are now only being addressed. Progress in this area has been limited by the difficulty in successfully applying gaseous 1-MCP to plants in the field. However, AgroFresh Inc. recently introduced its Harvista™ technology by 1-MCP application as foliar-spray preharvest treatment that enhances fruit quality and yields. Over the past 2 years, research trials using this new preharvest 1-MCP in apples and pears have been conducted demonstrating the benefits of the Harvista™ technology, although it is not yet commercially viable or registered for field use.

Commodities that may benefit most from preharvest 1-MCP applications are those negatively impacted by ethylene exposure but do not have the desired response to compounds that stimulate ethylene biosynthesis, such as the use of ethephon (Burns et al., 2006). Thus, combining preharvest 5 mM 1-MCP with 400 mg L^{-1} ethephon in the spray tank reduced ethephon-induced defoliation in oranges, but did not impact the desirable ethephon-induced fruit abscission to facilitate the mechanical harvesting (Burns, 2008). However, a sprayable formulation of 1-MCP was applied to mature Bartlett pear trees 1 week prior to first harvest, and fruits were harvested at 1 (optimum), 2, and 3 weeks after spray application. Results revealed that fruit drop, ethylene production, firmness loss, and color change (green to yellow) were delayed by preharvest sprayable 1-MCP treatment (DeEll, 2007), suggesting that sprayable 1-MCP applied at preharvest provided similar or better benefits to Bartlett pear quality than postharvest treatment with gaseous 1-MCP. This author also assayed preharvest 1-MCP in stone fruits (plums, peaches, and nectarines), showing that plums treated with 1-MCP were firmer, retained green color longer, and turned yellow-gold more slowly than nontreated fruit. In addition, TSS was significantly higher in 1-MCP–treated plums than in those not treated, these effects being attributed to the reduced ethylene production and respiration rate. However, treated peaches and nectarines exhibited higher firmness but the remaining parameters were unaffected.

8.6 1-MCP on physiological and pathological disorders

During storage of fresh horticultural commodities some disorders may occur and can be separated into several categories: physiological, mechanical, and pathological. Storage disorders are, by definition, disorders that are expressed after harvest, but there can be an overlap between pre- and postharvest expression, especially those that are related to mineral contents such as calcium (see Chapter 6). In addition, preharvest factors including climate, maturity at harvest, nutrition, and field management methods can markedly affect susceptibility and tolerance of harvested crops to postharvest stresses (Watkins, 2007). The disorders are usually manifested as visible symptoms of cell death in the susceptible plant part, but may also be manifested as non-necrotic symptoms such as water soaking and accumulation of undesirable metabolites (Watkins, 2008). Physiological disorders are distinct from other undesirable postharvest changes in quality, such as water loss, softening, degreening, and other ripening-related events associated with normal ripening and senescence. However, physiological disorders induce altered metabolism and disruption of normal ripening and senescence processes, often in response to imposition of stresses. They are also distinct from a number of direct postharvest injuries that occur as a result of mechanical damage, such as bruising (see Chapter 3, Section 3.9). Pathological disorders are also distinctly different, but it is common for diseases to be associated with physiological disorders as secondary infections.

In this section, we will focus on the physiological disorders related to ethylene action that can be alleviated by 1-MCP. For this reason, physiological disorders could be subclassified within 3 categories: (1) related directly to ethylene exposure, (2) senescence- and ripening-related, and (3) chilling and low temperature-related.

1. Physiological disorders induced by ethylene affect more vegetables than fruits and include russet spotting of lettuce; increased bitterness in carrots; inrolling of flower petals; fading, wilting, and abscission of many flowers; gummosis, bud necrosis, and flower blasting in flowering bulbs; and epinastic responses in ornamental plants (Watkins, 2007). In fruits, water soaking of watermelon is induced by ethylene in which the endocarp and placental tissues become liquefied with softening, enhancing solute leakage, degradation of pectic polymers, cell separation, and loss of cell wall rigidity. The prevention of this disorder by 1-MCP was evident in watermelon and was associated with lower lipid peroxidation and a reduction in the

activities of membrane-degrading enzymes such as phospholipases C and D and lypoxygenase (Mao et al., 2004).

2. Senescence- and ripening-related disorders are usually manifested by tissue browning, superficial scald, and internal breakdown, and have been especially studied in apple, in which 1-MCP inhibited or delayed the development of these disorders but increased the sensitivity to other disorder such as external carbon dioxide injury (Watkins et al., 2000).
3. The role of 1-MCP in reducing CI symptoms is perhaps the best studied disorder due to the economic repercussion. In this sense, there are some chilling-related disorders that are prevented by the inhibition of ethylene production by 1-MCP, such as superficial scald and brown core in apple, internal flesh browning in avocado, and soft scald in apple and pear (Fan and Mattheis, 1999; Woolf et al., 2005). The inhibition of these disorders by 1-MCP indicates that ethylene is required for their expression, although the mechanism of CI inhibition by 1-MCP is not known. Some evidence shows that electrical conductivity, and polyphenol oxidase (PPO) and peroxidase (POX) activities were lower in 1-MCP–treated avocado than in untreated fruit, suggesting that membrane stability was maintained by treatment.

However, it has been reported that other chilling-related disorders are enhanced by the inhibitory effect of 1-MCP on ethylene production, such as internal breakdown and wooliness in peaches and nectarines (Girardi et al., 2005) and CI incidence in citrus (Porat et al., 1999) and banana (Golding et al., 1998). The physiological basis for increased sensitivity to CI is not known, but is clear that occurrence of these disorders appears to be enhanced if ripening is inhibited, and thus ethylene-mediated responses may be required to alleviate the chilling-associated stresses, in the same way that a certain level of endogenous ethylene may be required to maintain disease resistance (Jiang et al., 2001). Increased CI of 1-MCP–treated bananas has been associated with reduced ethylene binding capacity of the tissues, while in stone fruits, flesh wooliness is thought to result from inhibition of PG activity.

According to Watkins (2008), pathological disorders can be separated into those that are increased, decreased, or unaffected by 1-MCP application. Although relatively little information exists about 1-MCP effects on disease incidence, most of these studies involve inoculation of the fruit with the pathogen and results are inconsistent. Thus, disease incidence in strawberry was lower at low 1-MCP concentrations and increased at higher 1-MCP concentrations (Jiang et al., 2001). Interactions between products and pathogens can be complex and are affected by the environment. 1-MCP may affect the product susceptibility to the disease complex simply by influencing factors such as skin integrity and firmness. Interestingly, ethylene can be an important component of product resistance because it regulates defense genes (Marcos et al., 2005), and these defenses may be compromised by 1-MCP treatment (Jiang et al., 2001). Accordingly, 1-MCP increased disease susceptibility of avocado (Woolf et al., 2005) and increased mold rots caused by *P. digitatum* and *P. italicum* in citrus (Porat et al., 1999). Thus, factors that influence the effects of 1-MCP on disease development are likely to be specific to the product and its interaction with the specific pathogen and the environment. For commercial purposes, delayed ripening associated with reduced ethylene production may increase product resistance to infection and lesion development. However, sensitivity can be beneficial against some pathogens but deleterious to resistance against other pathogens. Small amounts of endogenous ethylene may be necessary to maintain basic levels of resistance to environmental and pathological stress because of its involvement in regulation of plant defense genes (Marcos et al., 2005). Host-pathogen-environment interaction may be extremely complex, but postharvest technologies play significant importance in any disease control program, and, therefore, this area merits further research, under both laboratory and industry conditions, since 1-MCP may act at different levels within the intricate physiology of the host and the host-pathogen complex (Sozzi and Beaudry, 2007). Finally, mechanical damage can induce structural damage and loss of integrity that usually facilitates the pathological disorder, since most postharvest pathogens penetrate the host tissues through wounds, cuts, or bruises (Chapter 3, Section 3.8). Control of fruit ripening by 1-MCP is a successful technology that continues to be explored for a useful commercial application in many countries. 1-MCP is used in most cases as a supplement to proper temperature and relative humidity management, and can replace or be utilized in combination with controlled atmosphere (CA).

chapter nine

Storage in modified atmosphere packaging

9.1 Introduction

An important fact when dealing with vegetables is that they are still living structures and continue to respire as long as there are nutrients and gases available. Thus, respiration and transpiration continue after harvest. Since the produce is detached from its source of water, photosynthates and minerals, it is entirely dependent on its own food reserves and moisture content, which is the basis of the modified atmosphere (MA) storage. That is, modified atmosphere packaging (MAP) consists of sealing a certain quantity of fruit or vegetables through the use of plastic films with a particular permeability to gas diffusion. Then respiration of commodities increases CO_2 concentration and decreases O_2 concentrations inside the package, while transpiration rate increases vapor pressure.

These modifications on atmosphere composition inside the packaging films lead to a reduction in respiration rate produce, and consequently reduced losses in stored energy reserves occur in plant products. In addition, fruit stored under MAP conditions show a prevention or retardation of the ripening process and associated biochemical and physiological changes and growth inhibition of many spoilage microorganisms; thus, significant increases in fruit and vegetable shelf life can be achieved. Nevertheless, the most important use actually of MAP technique is for packaged salads and fresh-cut vegetables, and to a lesser extension for fresh-cut fruits, such as cantaloupe melons, pineapple, and apple (Kader et al., 1989; Kader and Watkins, 2000; Al-Ati and Hotchkiss, 2003; Artés et al., 2007). In addition, it is necessary to take into account that MA packages should be carefully designed for each particular commodity, otherwise it may be ineffective or it may even shorten the shelf life of the produce.

9.2 Films used in MA packaging

The commercial expansion of MAP has become possible because of the recent development of plastics polymers having the following required characteristics: selective permeability to CO_2 and O_2, transparency and brightness, slight weight, nontoxic, able to guarantee food safety, resistant to burst strength and stretching, facility to be sealed by heat at relatively low temperature, nonreacting with the product, resistance to heat and ozone, adapted for commercial use, attractive to consumer and a reasonable price, among others. Thus, the flexible films more frequently used for MAP are polyethylene (PE), polypropylene (PP), polyvinyl chloride (PVC), and polystyrene (Lange, 2000; Artés et al., 2006; Rai and Paul, 2007).

PE is classified by its density in medium, low, and ultra low, which indicates increasing resistance to water transmission. Low-density PE (LDPE) has a high selectivity toward CO_2 and O_2, allowing a reduction in the O_2 level without an excessive increase in CO_2 within the package. Recent trends are toward the use of linear PE of low and ultra low density, which have a more uniform density, higher O_2 permeability, greater clarity and thermal transparency, and better sealing, compared with conventional ones, although its cost is still elevated.

The chemical nature of PP is similar to that of PE, although it is up to tenfold less permeable to air gases and water vapor. It is easily sealable by heat and it could be oriented or not oriented, which is related to its molecular structure and manufacturing. Thus, when molecules are oriented in a longitudinal way it is called *oriented*, and if they are also oriented in a transverse way, it is called *bi-oriented*. The orientation increases film strength and reduces gas permeability. PP films commonly receive a treatment to avoid formation of water droplets by condensation, usually by covering their inner face with a thin layer of vinylidene polychlorure.

PVC films have moderate levels of permeability to water vapor and can be soft, clear, durable, and resistant to mist. Some of them have high CO_2 permeability, which is especially appropriate for MAP; recently, however, the commercial use of PVC has met progressive difficulties because it is not recyclable, due to the use of additives in its manufacture, which can be undesirable for food use, and that it has chlorine in its molecule, which is released by its degradation, harming the ozone layer.

Polystyrene is a polymer with a high permeability to O_2 and CO_2, which allows it to be used for very specific conditions, such as for products that cannot tolerate low O_2 levels. It is practically inert from the chemical point of view and shows a great transparency.

All these plastic films have certain permeability to CO_2, O_2, and N_2 diffusion, as well as different water vapor transmission (Artés et al., 2006; Sandhya, 2010), which is affected by temperature. However, oxygen and carbon dioxide permeation rates through these continuous films are often below the product respiration rate and the product headspace evolves toward a zero-oxygen atmosphere. Besides this effect, the permeability through a specific polymer differs with the permeant gas. Thus, for most common plastics, carbon dioxide permeates 4–8 times faster than oxygen, resulting in atmospheres below 1 bar or in a package collapse, this ratio between CO_2 and O_2 permeation coefficients being a limiting factor for certain MAP applications (Al-Ati and Hotchkiss, 2003). In the last few years, the use of porous packaging materials (with microperforations ranging from 40 to 200 μm) has become a widespread solution for the preservation of fresh produce, especially for those fruit and vegetables with a very high respiration rate, although they have also been used for slow-respiring products in large-volume packages. In these films, the flow through the pore is proportional to the pore surface and the permeation through film surface is a function of the pore number, providing high to very high mass exchange rates, irrespective of the chemistry of the material used to their performance. Perforated films have a permeability quotient close to 1 (Brody, 2005), and this allows the required concentration of CO_2 to be reached without anaerobiosis, taking into account that the respiration coefficient of the product can fluctuate between 0.7 and 1.3. However, at present their use is limited as they are quite expensive (Rai and Paul, 2007). Finally, mass transport through such films cannot be described using conventional permeability equations (Henry's plus Fick's laws) and other expressions such as Knudsen's law, gas diffusivities, or Poiseuille's hydrodynamic flow should be applicable (Del-Valle et al., 2003). Thus, recently good models have been proposed for describing the evolution of the gas composition in packages with microperforated films with constant volume, taking into account the permeation through the microperforation and the respiration rate of the packaged product (Fonseca et al., 2002; González-Buesa et al., 2009). These mathematical models are useful tools for defining the characteristics that a package should have and for predicting the evolution of the gas composition during conservation of the product.

9.3 Generation of the steady-state or equilibrium atmosphere

The reduction in O_2 partial pressure and the increase in CO_2 partial pressure, as a consequence of commodities respiration rate, create gradients that, according to Fick's law, cause O_2 to enter and CO_2 to exit the package until the steady state is reached. Thus, steady-state O_2 levels are achieved in the package when the O_2 uptake by the product is equal to that permeating into the package, a situation that exists only when the respiratory rate is constant. As for O_2, the steady-state CO_2 levels in the package are achieved when CO_2 production by the product equals CO_2 escape from the package. The steady-state levels for both O_2 and CO_2 are dependent on the interaction of respiration of the produce (respiration rate and mass of product in the package) and the size and permeability properties of

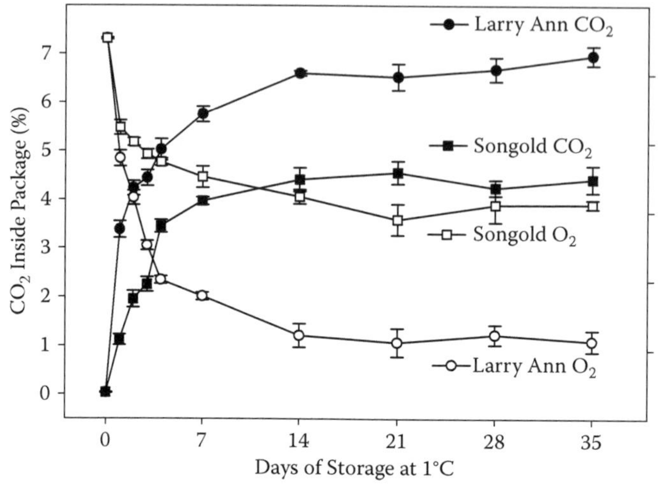

Figure 9.1 Evolution of CO_2 and O_2 concentration during cold storage of two plum cultivars (Larry Ann and Songold) inside MAP with microperforated polyester/polypropylene (12/60 µm thickness) films.

the packaging film (Kader et al., 1989). Thus, as it is shown in Figure 9.1, for Larry Ann and Songold plum cultivars during storage under similar MAP conditions, the atmosphere composition of the steady state was dependent on the respiration rate of each plum cultivar. The atmosphere inside the packages reached higher concentration of CO_2 (around 7%) and lower of O_2 (next to 12%) for Larry Ann plums, which had an initial respiration rate of 34.98 ± 2.56 mg CO_2 kg^{-1} h^{-1}, while for Songold these concentrations were 4 and 16%, respectively, and its initial respiration rate was 20.84 ± 0.47 mg CO_2 kg^{-1} h^{-1}.

For continuous film, since the permeability of CO_2 is usually 2–8 times higher than that for O_2, the decrease in O_2 inside the package is higher than the increase in CO_2, and the sum of CO_2 plus O_2 is lower than 20–21%, unless the respiration quotient (RQ) is of the same magnitude or greater than the ratio of CO_2 to O_2 permeability. However, for perforated films, since the permeability of perforations to CO_2 is only 20% less than to O_2, the sum of O_2 and CO_2 concentration is usually only slightly less than 21%, unless RQ is significantly greater than 1, and in that case the sum will be larger than 21%. This effect of film type on MA composition is displayed in Figure 9.2 for broccoli stored at 1°C in film packages of continuous and microperforated polypropylene, in which the concentration of CO_2 at the steady state was 2.0–2.5% in microperforated film and ca. 6% in the continuous one, while those concentrations for O_2 were ca. 14% and 5%, respectively.

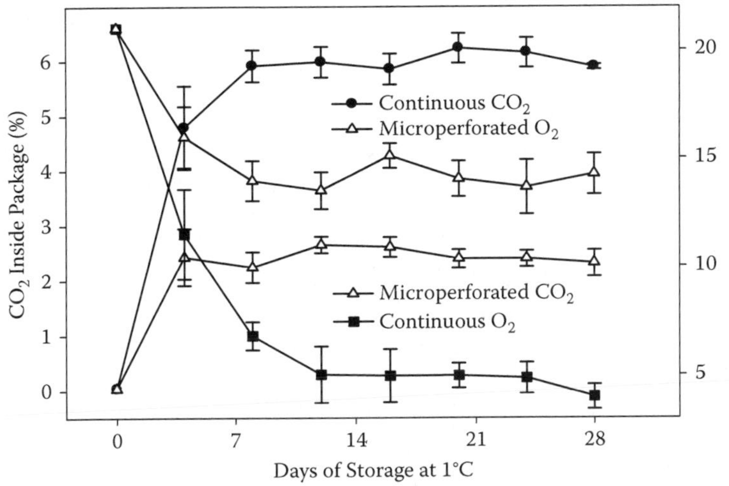

Figure 9.2 Evolution of CO_2 and O_2 concentration during cold storage of broccoli inside MAP with continuous and microperforated polypropylene (20 μm thickness) films.

Finally, RH within a pack is influenced by the rate at which the product loses water vapor and by the water vapor transmission rate (WVTR) of the packaging film. In general, plastic films used in MAP limit water vapor diffusion, generating a water vapor pressure inside the package which reduces transpiration rate leading to very low weight loss of commodities during storage compared to those stored in open air (Wang and Qi, 1997; Martínez-Romero et al., 2003b; Serrano et al., 2006).

Thus, MAP is a well-established technology, which along with low temperature storage leads to maintenance of fruit and vegetable quality and to a net extension of the shelf life of these perishable products. However, the appropriate CO_2 and O_2 concentration for MAP storage in optimal conditions is different for each particular commodity, as explained in the following section.

9.4 Optimal CO_2 and O_2 concentration

Recommended gaseous concentration for equilibrium atmospheres and ranges of optimal temperatures for many whole and fresh-cut horticultural commodities stored under MAP conditions are reviewed by Beaudry (1999; 2000), Watkins (2000), Artés et al., (2006), and Sandhya (2010). For each particular fruit or vegetable, the recommendations for O_2 and CO_2 optimum concentrations generally represent the conditions that will result in maximum storage life of each commodity, being in an extremely wide range. However, if the level of O_2 drops below its critical value (extinction point), aerobic respiration finishes and anaerobic respiration becomes important, and when the level of CO_2 rises above a critical value, the produce develops physiological disorders.

The postharvest tolerances of most commercially important fruit and vegetables to high CO_2 concentrations have been established, the general goal being to identify the safe concentration that will result in maximum commodity storage without injury, since when a fruit or vegetable is subjected to atmospheres outside of the safe limits at any temperature/time combination, damage may be manifested as irregular ripening, initiation and/or aggravation of certain physiological disorders, development of off-flavor, and increased susceptibility to decay. Thus, whereas 1% CO_2 represents the upper levels for onion, cherimoya can tolerate 30% CO_2 concentration. In addition, tolerances of commodities to a particular CO_2 concentration increase with decreases in storage temperature and time of exposition, being also different among cultivars and higher in fresh-cut products than in whole fruits and vegetables (Watkins, 2000). Accordingly, the limit of O_2 concentration below which injury can occur varies widely depending on vegetable commodities, ranging from 0.5% for broccoli, lettuce, and spinach to 14% for orange sections (Beaudry, 2000). These O_2 limits not only refer to the fermentation threshold but may also relate to discoloration and other disorders.

9.5 *Importance of temperature stability*

As it has been addressed in Chapter 4, the most important factor in maintaining quality and extending the shelf life of fruit and vegetables after harvest is temperature, since most of the physical, biochemical, microbiological, and physiological reactions contributing to deterioration of produce quality are largely dependent on temperature. The creation and maintenance of an optimal atmosphere inside an MA package depends on the respiration rate of the product and the permeability of the films to O_2 and CO_2, both of which are affected by temperature (Beaudry et al., 1999). However, an increase in temperature has different effects on these two parameters: the increase in the respiration rate as a function of temperature, described by Q^R_{10}, is generally substantially greater than the increase in the permeability of packaging material (Q^P_{10}), which may favor the accumulation of CO_2 and depletion of O_2 inside the package.

In fact, metabolic processes including respiration, transpiration, and ripening are particularly temperature-dependent, the rates of biological reactions being generally increased two- to threefold for each 10°C increase in temperature. On the other hand, as temperature increases, the O_2 and CO_2 permeability of many packaging film increases markedly, although important differences exist depending on film type. Thus, for example, the permeation of O_2 and other gases through LPDE yields a 2.5-fold increase in permeability between 0 and 15°C. In contrast, the permeation of the gases through perforations has an extremely low temperature sensitivity factor, with only a 10% increase in the temperature range depicted (Beaudry, 2000).

A situation where respiratory demand for O_2 increases faster than O_2 permeation presents problems with maintaining adequate O_2 when the package undergoes a temperature increase. Then, maintenance of the desired atmosphere composition inside the packages depends on rigorous temperature control, since for a given temperature change, large differences between changes in produce respiration rate and in film permeability occur. Thus, for example, Tano et al. (2007) reported that the Q^R_{10} values for mushrooms, broccoli, and tomatoes were 3.0, 2.8, and 2.3 respectively while the Q^P_{10} of the package was lower than 1.2. This disparity resulted in an accumulation of CO_2 and a decrease in O_2 inside the packages subjected to temperature fluctuations, leading to anaerobic respiration (fermentation) in vegetable tissues. The exact O_2 concentration at which anaerobic respiration begins depends on the type of produce, on the storage temperature, and on the CO_2 concentration. However, once anaerobic respiration has been initiated, the O_2 concentration remains constant during subsequent fluctuation cycles, regardless of the temperature, presumably due to irreversible membrane damage and reduced mitochondrial activity. Thus, the damage caused by low O_2 and high CO_2 concentrations on fruit and vegetables is irreversible, its severity being dependent on the duration of storage under these conditions.

Moreover, proper control of RH in MAP containing fresh produce is a critical design consideration and is also affected by temperature. Most polymeric films used in MAP have lower WVTR relative to transpiration rates of fresh produce; therefore, excessive high RH may occur, causing moisture condensation, microbial growth, and decay of the produce. The condensation problem is aggravated by temperature abuse conditions, since the atmosphere in MAP maintained at constant temperature is saturated with moisture, while increasing the temperature decreases the RH inside the packages and increases the water vapor deficit and, consequently, the transpiration rate of fresh produce. This high rate of transpiration leads to accelerated produce weight loss and may explain the higher weight losses in packages subjected to temperature fluctuations than in those kept at constant temperature (Tano et al., 2007).

9.6 MAP and fruit quality maintenance

There are many similarities between the effects of low O_2 and high CO_2 on vegetable tissue metabolism, with most effects being suppression of various metabolic processes and even their effects are additives on maintaining quality of fruit and vegetables under MAP conditions. Vegetable tissue responses to modified CO_2 and O_2 levels include responses at the levels of primary and secondary metabolism, and these responses can be positive or negative. Then, the determination as to whether a particular plant organ can be favorably affected by reduced O_2 concentrations depends on positive and negative responses.

The use of MAP as a supplement to proper temperature maintenance in the effort of delayed fruit ripening and vegetable senescence, and associated physiological and biochemical changes, is generally beneficial for all commodities. Thus, successful applications of MAP on fruits include apples (Moodley et al., 2002), table grapes (Martínez-Romero et al., 2003b; Artés-Hernández et al., 2006), sweet cherries (Kappel et al., 2002; Serrano et al., 2005b), loquat (Amorós et al., 2008), litchi (Sivakumar and Korsten, 2006), papaya (González-Aguilar et al., 2003), and strawberries and raspberries (Nielsem and Leufvén, 2008; Lange, 2000), among others.

9.6.1 *Weight loss*

One of the main problems during postharvest storage of fruit and vegetables is weight loss, occurring mainly by transpiration rate, which affects its marketability, being responsible for important economic losses as commented in Chapter 3 (Section 3.3). In this sense, since films used in MAP have small water vapor diffusion, the internal atmosphere package becomes saturated with water vapor pressure and then transpiration of vegetable tissues decreases enormously, leading to low weight losses. For example, weight loss of control broccoli stored at 1°C in open air was 46% of their initial weight after 21 days, while broccoli stored in nonperforated and microperforated polypropylene bags lost less than 1.5% (Serrano et al., 2006). Similar results have been obtained in several fruits, such as loquat (Amorós et al., 2008), table grape (Martínez-Romero et al., 2003b), nectarines (Retamales et al., 2000), peaches (Akbudak and Eris, 2004), and cherries (Kappel et al., 2002; Serrano et al., 2005b), among others.

9.6.2 *Respiration rate*

Of the primary metabolic responses to low O_2, beneficial reaction includes a reduction in respiration, manifested as diminution in starch degradation and sugar consumption. The premise has been that reducing the respiration rate diminishes the rate of deterioration of the tissues, thereby extending storage life. A level of 50% reduction in respiration is suggested to be associated with sufficient enhancement of shelf life such that the cost of extra handling and materials resulting from MAP will be recovered (Beaudry, 2000). However, an important primary negative response to low O_2 is the induction of fermentation, as mentioned previously, leading to accumulation of acetaldehyde, ethanol, and lactate. Generally, the lower limit of O_2 content in the atmosphere is considered to be the O_2 level at which the fermentation is induced. In addition, in climacteric fruit, such as mango and papaya, apart from reduction of respiration rate, a delay on climacteric respiration peak has been reported (Yahia, 2006; Singh and Rao, 2005). Accordingly, high CO_2 was proposed to inhibit respiration rate by feedback inhibition or by controlling mitochondrial activity including an effect on Krebs cycle intermediates and enzymes. However, the influence of CO_2 on respiration rate is not clear, since there are examples in which respiration rate has been also increased or nonaffected by high CO_2 concentrations (Fonseca et al., 2002).

9.6.3 *Ethylene production*

Of the secondary metabolic responses to low O_2, important beneficial reactions include a reduction in ethylene biosynthesis and perception. In fact, low O_2 concentration is known to inhibit ACO activity, this effect being dependent of the ACC concentration, since as ACC increase the Km of the enzyme for O_2 decreases. Oxygen has also been reported to exert an effect on ethylene perception, which is reduced as O_2 concentration decreases. Therefore, in climacteric fruits, O_2 concentrations not low enough to reduce respiration rate still reduce the rate of ripening through an effect mediated by ethylene (Abeles et al., 1992). It has been known for several years that CO_2 is an antagonist of ethylene action and impedes its autocatalytic synthesis (Yang and Hoffman, 1984). In fact, CO_2 levels higher than 1% decrease or inhibit ethylene biosynthesis and consequently retard fruit ripening and deterioration, these effects being additive to those of reduced O_2 atmospheres (Artés et al., 2006).

This effect of MAP on inhibiting ethylene production is shown in Figure 9.3, in which it can be observed that ethylene production increased in Larry Ann and Black Amber plums during storage at 2°C, while in those plums stored under MAP conditions ethylene production was significantly lower. Accordingly, a clear inhibition of ethylene biosynthesis was observed in apricot stored in MAP, especially with films of low permeability in which concentration of 20% CO_2 were reached (Pretel et al., 1993).

9.6.4 *Color, ripening index, and firmness*

Color evolution associated with the postharvest ripening process is generally delayed in fruits stored under MAP conditions, as compared to those stored in open air, as has been shown in mango (Pesis et al., 2002), table grape (Martínez-Romero et al., 2003b), and loquat (Amorós et al., 2008). Accordingly, all individual color parameters (L*, a*, and b*)

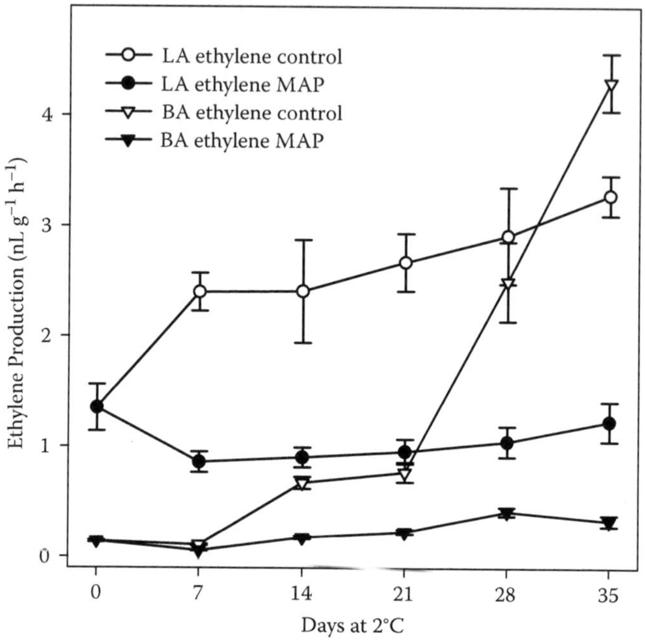

Figure 9.3 Ethylene production rate of Larry Ann (LA) and Black Amber (BA) plum cultivars during storage at 2°C in open air (control) or under MAP conditions using microperforated polyester/polypropylene (12/60 µm thickness) films. Ethylene production was measured at 2°C and 2 hours after plum fruits were taken out of MA packages.

significantly increased in unwrapped control broccoli during storage, which was related to both the yellowing process of broccoli inflorescences and the decrease in chlorophyll (a + b) concentration. However, broccoli under MAP conditions retained the green color characteristic of freshly harvested broccoli after 21 days of storage and chlorophyll concentration close to those found at harvest (Serrano et al., 2006). These effects could be attributed to the action of low O_2 on reducing chlorophyll degradation and browning mediated by the inhibition of pheophorbide oxigenase and PPO, responsible for chlorophyll loss and browning, respectively (Beaudry, 2000). In addition, color preservation by MAP storage has been related to the delay in anthocyanin and carotenoid biosynthesis, thus preserving alteration of color (Artés et al., 2006).

Ripening index generally increases during postharvest storage in a wide range of fruits as explained in Chapter 3 (Section 3.6), being mainly due to a decrease in TA and sometimes also to an increase in TSS. Thus, as shown in Figure 9.4, ripening index at harvest increased after 21 days of storage in four plum cultivars stored at 2°C in open air, while these increases were significantly lower in plum stored under MAP conditions, Accordingly, TSS increased and TA decreased in peaches and nectarines stored in air, while in MAP conditions no changes were observed (Akbudad and Eris, 2004). Moreover, in loquat fruit individual sugars and malic acid decreased over cold storage, these changes being delayed in MAP-stored fruits, showing a clear effect of MAP on decreasing fruit metabolism, especially loss of respiration substrates, and, in turn, on delaying the postharvest ripening process (Amorós et al., 2008).

MAP is also effective in delaying the softening process that usually occurs during postharvest storage, as displayed in Figure 9.4 for four plum cultivars. In general, MAP with 5–20% CO_2 and 5–10% O_2 are effective on retarding firmness losses during storage in a wide range of fruits, such as strawberries (García et al., 1998), apricot (Pretel et al., 1993), kiwifruit (Agar et al., 1999), loquat (Amorós et al., 2008), peaches, and nectarines (Akbudak and Eris, 2004). Accordingly, in table grapes packaged in nonperforated PP film, berry and skin firmness were almost double than in control fruits after 14 days of cold storage (Martínez-Romero et al., 2003b). This effect has been attributed to the reduction of cell-wall-degrading enzymes, such as PG, by high CO_2 and low O_2 (Femenia et al., 1998). Nevertheless, the effect of MAP on delaying softening could be also an ethylene-mediated effect, since in apricots decreased film permeability led to increased CO_2 concentration and decreased

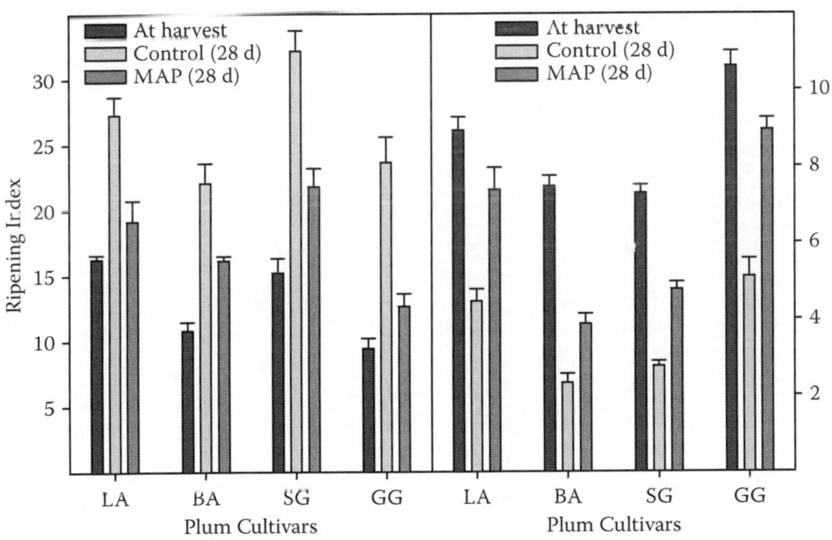

Figure 9.4 Fruit ripening index and firmness of four plum cultivars (LA, Larry Ann; BA, Black Amber; SG, Songold; and GG, Golden Globe) at harvest and after 28 days of storage at 2°C in open air (control) and under MAP conditions with microperforated polyester/polypropylene (12/60 µm thickness) films.

ethylene production and softening (Pretel et al., 1993). However, it has been also found that low O_2 concentration is more effective at inhibiting fruit softening than high CO_2 (Pretel et al., 1999).

9.6.5 Phytochemical compounds

MAP storage has been shown to have a beneficial effect on maintaining bioactive compounds of fruit and vegetables, although currently there are only a few reports about this issue. Thus, broccoli heads lost half of their initial H-TAA, phenolics, and ascorbic acid after 21 days of cold storage, while these losses were minimized in broccoli packaged with microperforated and nonperforated PP films (Figure 9.5). In addition, H-TAA has been correlated in broccoli with total phenolics and in less extension with ascorbic acid (Serrano et al., 2006). Accordingly, important losses in ascorbic acid occurred in loquat stored at 2°C, while levels at harvest were maintained in loquat stored under MAP conditions (Amorós et al., 2008). In papaya, MAP helped in maintenance of antioxidant potential of fruit by retaining acceptable levels of antioxidants, such as ascorbic acid and lycopene (Singh and Rao, 2005).

Anthocyanins tend to increase with ripening during postharvest storage in many fruits, such as apples, sweet cherries, strawberries, blueberries, and raspberries, as well as lycopene in tomato and watermelon (as

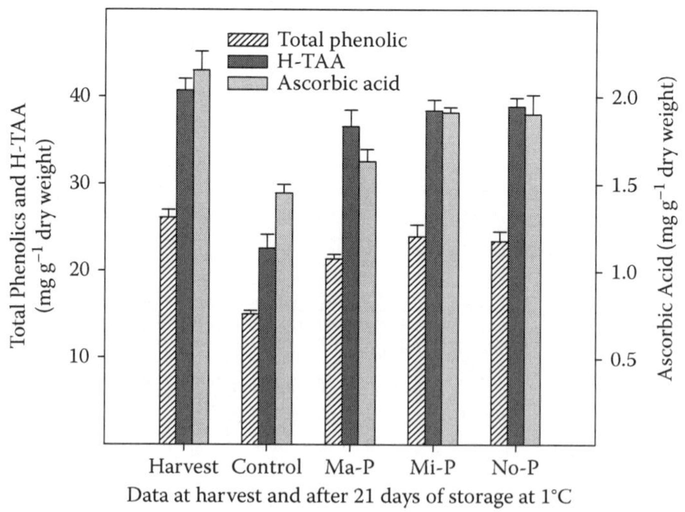

Figure 9.5 Total phenolic and ascorbic acid concentration and total antioxidant activity in the hydrophilic fraction (H-TAA) in broccoli at harvest and after 21 days of storage at 1°C in open air (control) and in MAP conditions, with macroperforated (Ma-P), microperforated (Mi-P), and nonperforated (No-P) polypropylene films.

explained in Chapter 3, Section 3.7). However, under MAP conditions, these increases have been reported to be lower than in control fruits stored at open air, due to the effect of MAP on delaying the evolution of the postharvest ripening process (Jones, 2007).

9.6.6 Decay and sensory quality

The effect of MAP on reducing postharvest spoilage is of particular importance in fresh-cut fruits and vegetables, as will be addressed in Section 9.7. However, some reports have also found an effect of MAP on reducing spoilage in storage of whole fruits. Thus, MAP decreased decay index in peaches and nectarines leading to high scores of overall appearance and taste in fruits stored under MAP conditions as compared with those stored on open air (Akbudad and Eris, 2004). Accordingly, MAP significantly reduced brown rot in sweet cherry as compared to air-stored fruits (Spotts et al., 2002).

Sensory properties are also maintained in fruit under MAP conditions with appropriate atmosphere composition. Thus, for example, scores for crunchiness and juiciness were higher in nonperforated and perforated polypropylene film packaged table grapes than in controls after 18 days of storage at 1°C, and even after 53 days no modifications were observed with respect to the scores at day 18 (Marínez-Romero et al., 2003a). However, negative secondary responses to low O_2 and high CO_2 may also occur, including reduced aroma biosynthesis and the possibility of off-flavor generation. The effect on aroma production is mediated by ethylene but also likely via action of O_2 on oxidative process, including respiration required for substrate production, although aroma generation is recovered when fruits are restored to normal air (Beaudry, 1999; Kader and Watkins, 2000; Artés et al., 2006).

Finally, atmospheres with very low O_2 content (<1%) and very high CO_2 levels (>50–80%) have also insecticidal effect when vegetable products are treated within a period of 2–4 days at room temperature or only 2–4 hours at higher temperatures. This technique has commercially been tried for grains and dry fruits and vegetables, but it is not yet well developed for fresh fruits, since the needed gas concentration induces fermentation and off flavors (Yahia, 2006).

9.6.7 Susceptibility to chilling injury

The beneficial effects of MAP on maintaining fruit quality during postharvest storage is even greater for tropical fruits than for temperate ones, due to the reduction of chilling sensitivity by atmospheres with high CO_2 and low O_2 concentrations (Yahia, 2006; Sandhya, 2010). Thus, the increase of electrolyte leakage on papaya fruit was coincident and correlated with the occurrence of CI symptoms, both process being decreased in MAP stored fruits (Singh and Rao, 2005). MAP also alleviated CI symptoms in pepper fruits (Serrano et al., 1997) and the red spots around lenticels occurred in mangos, although this effect was attributed to both the MA surrounding the fruits and maintenance of a high RH in the bags (Pesis et al., 2000). In peaches it has been also reported that MAP might prevent development of CI by maintaining high humidity inside the packages, since water loss causes excessive production of active oxygen species and then the high humidity in MAP could prevent chilling-induced oxidative stress (Hodges et al., 2004).

9.7 MAP benefits for storage of fresh-cut fruits and vegetables

A rapid expansion of MAP has occurred in the last 20 years for minimally processed fruits and vegetables, since MAP is especially important for these commodities, due to their greater susceptibility to water loss and surface browning, high respiration rate, enhanced ethylene biosynthesis and action with effect on the onset or progression of ripening in climacteric fruit, and microbial spoilage, all these process being increased by mechanical damage suffered during preparation, shipping, handling, and processing. Thus, extended shelf life has been observed in fresh-cut mangoes, pineapples, tomato apples, kiwifruit, melon, and fruit mixes using appropriate semi-rigid containers packaged in MAP, as well as in fresh-cut vegetables and prepared salads (Kader and Watkins, 2000; Soliva-Fortuny and Martin-Belloso, 2003; Artés et al., 2006; 2007; Singh et al., 2007; Rojas-Graü et al., 2009; Sandhya, 2010).

One important problem of fresh-cut fruits is the cut-edge browning due to the destruction of cellular compartmentalization by cutting, which allows the oxidation of phenolic compounds by PPO, originating colorless quinones that later on polymerize forming melanins, the O_2 being necessary for these browning reactions. Thus, at low O_2 concentration (0.25–5%) decreased PPO activity and also moderate level of CO_2 (10–20%) can inhibit the biosynthesis of phenolic compounds, substrates of PPO, that usually are induced in response to cutting damage, the combination of two gases leading to maintain visual appearance of several fresh-cut fruits, such as peach, kiwifruit, mango, and melon. However, MAP cannot effectively inhibit browning in apple, banana, pear, and artichoke, because of their high phenolic content, and the combination of MAP with antioxidant compounds, such as ascorbic acid, cysteine, or reduced glutathione, is necessary. Nevertheless, these and other antioxidants should be applied with caution, since they may alter the sensory quality and nutritional value of the products (Artés et al., 2007; Rojas-Graü et al., 2009).

Color of fresh-cut fruit is probably the main quality attribute considered by consumers, and research in the last few years has been focused on the prevention of discoloration, due to dehydration of the cut surface. Thus, avoiding desiccation of the cut surface by calcium or calcium plus ascorbate treatments is critical for maintaining acceptable visual appearance (Salcini and Massantini, 2005; Artés et al., 2007). On the other hand, pectin enzymes that are released during cutting operation can cause tissue softening, although their impact is mostly restricted to the parts of the fruit in contact with cut surface. However, in climacteric fruits, the ethylene produced by the physical action of cutting is sufficient to accelerate softening as it has been observed in banana and kiwifruit, and the use of MAP is not always effective enough to keep the firmness levels at harvest, unless that combination with calcium treatments are used (Artés et al., 2007).

Microbial decay is the major source of spoilage of fresh-cut produce, since the presence of damaged cells and the loss of cellular components during processing operations provide optimum conditions for the development of microorganisms. The type and species of microorganism varies with the fruit or vegetable, the cultivation practices, and the hygienic conditions during handling and processing. Chlorinated water is frequently used in the minimally fresh-cut processing factories for disinfection, but it is impossible to eliminate the entire microorganism present in the commodities. Consequently, the minimal processing industry wants safer alternatives. Several antimicrobial washing solutions such as O_3, and some physical treatments including UV-C radiation and super high O_2 (see Chapter 11), intense light pulses, N_2O, and noble gases, alone or in combination, are presently considered as promising treatments (Artés et al., 2009).

After cutting and handling processes, packaging under appropriate atmosphere conditions can effectively control the growth of microorganisms on the surface of fresh-cut fruits. The proliferation of aerobic microorganisms can be substantially delayed with reduced O_2 levels. High CO_2 concentrations are also generally effective in controlling the growth of most aerobic microorganisms, specifically Gram-negative bacteria and molds, but fail to inhibit most yeasts; the growth of fruit bacterial populations appeared to be at least as fast as under atmospheric conditions (Al-Ati and Hotchkiss, 2003; Soliva-Fortuny and Martín-Belloso, 2003; Rojas-Graü et al., 2009). On the contrary, too low O_2 concentrations inside packages of fresh-cut vegetables may pose a safety risk, as the growth of anaerobic foodborne pathogens such as *Yersinia enterocolitica, Aeromonas hydrophila, A. caviae, Clostridium botulinum,* and *Listeria monocytogenes* might be allowed or even stimulated. Therefore, an appropriate combination of gas composition, to ensure that O_2 levels inside the packages are high enough to avoid the triggering of anaerobic fermentative processes and package dimensions and permeability adapted to the respiration of the product, is critical to reach a sustainable equilibrium of gas concentrations (Martín-Belloso et al., 2007; Rojas-Graü et al., 2009). Appropriate combination of MAP with refrigeration may help to maintain vitamin C concentration by limiting ascorbic acid oxidation (Rojas-Graü et al., 2009).

Development of off-flavors and off-odors are some of the most common reasons for depleted quality of fresh-cut fruit. Nevertheless, the presence of off-odors and the persistent off-flavors should not be confused with the strong aromas detected just after opening the packages that quickly disappear, without affecting their sensory quality. MAP severely modifies the fruit volatiles profile if O_2 partial pressure decreases below the fermentation limit, since anaerobic respiration starts with the corresponding production of off-flavors and off-odors. In addition, some treatments applied before cutting, such as ethanol vapor, may induce off-flavor after shelf life (Plotto et al., 2006; Rojas-Graü et al., 2009).

9.8 Future research needs

The current trend of using MAP for extending the commercial life of many plant species and varieties, either whole or minimally processed, for transport, commercial distribution, and retail sale is expected to continue. Some improvements in MAP have been recently developed, including the fast achievement of the optimal atmosphere by injection of N_2 or a preprepared gaseous mixture into the package, or by including O_2 and CO_2 scavengers within packages. In addition, the use of intelligent or dynamic packages that suddenly increase their permeability to O_2 when increasing the temperature or polymers that incorporate in their manufacture antimicrobial substances, or ethylene scrubbers, like MnO_4K could also improve MAP results. In the same way the aroma could be improved in MAP systems with in-package additives or the use of a biosensor capable of measuring ethanol in the gas phase and to indirectly detect low O_2 levels.

chapter ten

Active packaging

10.1 *Introduction*

There are continuous changes in both current consumer demands and market trends toward mildly preserved convenience foods that have high fresh-like qualities and changes in retail and distribution practices (e.g., centralization of activities, internationalization of markets, and new trends such as Internet shopping) requiring increased distribution distances and longer storage times. In response to these demands, the concept of active packaging has been introduced in the last two decades as an innovative food packaging concept. In the case of fresh commodities, packaging that maintains fruits and vegetables in a fresh state for longer periods during transport and prevents contamination from foodborne pathogens is strictly required to meet these various challenges.

Traditionally, the basic functions of packaging have been classified into four categories: protection, communication, convenience, and containment. The package is used to protect the product against the deteriorative effects of the external environment, communicate with the consumer as a marketing tool, provide the consumer with greater ease of use and time-saving convenience, and contain products of various sizes and shapes. Although traditional packaging has contributed greatly to the early development of the food distribution systems, it is no longer sufficient because today's society has become increasingly complex. Innovative packaging with enhanced functions is constantly sought in response to the consumer demands for minimally processed foods with fewer preservatives, increased regulatory requirements, market globalization, and concern for food safety. Within the concept of innovative packaging, it is necessary to define and distinguish between *active packaging* and *intelligent packaging*.

Active packaging has been defined as a system in which the product, the package, and the environment interact in a positive way to extend shelf life or to achieve some characteristics that cannot be obtained otherwise. It has also been defined as a packaging system that actively changes the condition of the package to extend shelf life or improve food safety or sensory properties, and maintains the quality of the produce (Vermeiren et al., 1999). Active packaging systems have been developed to modify the environmental or physiological conditions within the food package. These systems usually involve the scavenging or absorption of undesirable compounds such as oxygen, carbon dioxide, ethylene, and excessive water. Other active packaging systems add or release compounds such as carbon dioxide, antioxidants, and preservatives into the headspace of the package; these compounds are generally administered by sachets, labels, or films.

Intelligent packaging has been defined as a packaging system that is capable of carrying out intelligent functions (such as detecting, sensing, recording, tracing, communicating, and applying scientific logic) to facilitate decision making to extend shelf life, enhance safety, improve quality, provide information, and warn about possible problems (Yam et al., 2005). Taking into account the four basic functions mentioned earlier, the uniqueness of intelligent packaging is in its ability to communicate: because the package and the food move constantly together throughout the supply chain cycle, the package is the food's best companion and is in the best position to communicate the conditions of the food. A variety of sensors have been developed based on chemical, enzymatic, immunochemical, or mechanical reactions. These sensors can be placed in or on the package. They can be used to detect and communicate such information as time/temperature conditions and history, oxygen and carbon dioxide levels, package leakage or spoilage, commodity ripeness and freshness, microbial growth, and specific foodborne human pathogen identification (Wilson, 2007).

This chapter will focus on active packaging with application in fruits and vegetables, in which MAP serves as a basis for active packaging, by using either films or edible coatings.

10.2 Active packaging technologies

The beneficial effects of MAP by reducing of oxygen levels and increasing the carbon dioxide on fruit quality maintenance with respect to air storage were studied in detail in Chapter 9. However, there are many situations in which the MA is not low or high enough with respect to oxygen and carbon dioxide, respectively, and in these cases active packaging can alter the physiology of harvested fruits and vegetables in a desirable manner, resulting in an improvement in the overall quality. Active packaging includes various aspects that may play a role in determining the shelf life of packaged fruits, such as physiological (respiration of fresh fruit and vegetables), chemical (lipid oxidation), and physical processes (dehydration), together with microbiological aspects (spoilage by microorganisms). The application of appropriate active packaging systems can be regulated in numerous ways, and depending on the requirements of the packaged produce, fruit deterioration can be significantly reduced.

The active packaging techniques for preservation and improving quality and safety of foods can be divided into two categories: absorbers (scavengers) and releasing systems (emitters). Absorbing or scavenging systems remove undesired compounds such as oxygen, carbon dioxide, ethylene, excessive water, and other specific compounds, while releasing systems actively add or emit compounds to the packaged food or into the headspace of the package, such as carbon dioxide, antioxidants, and preservatives. Depending on the physical form of active packaging systems, absorbers and releasers can be a sachet, label, or film type. Sachets are placed freely in the headspace of the package, and labels are attached into the lid of the package. Direct contact with food should be avoided because it impairs the function of the system and may cause migration problems.

10.3 Ethylene adsorbers

The development of packaging that absorbs or actively scavenges ethylene has been derived from research designed to remove it from storage atmospheres for a wide range of produce.

The active packaging that intends to remove undesirable ethylene from the headspace of a package through absorption, adsorption, or scavenging is the best known and most widely used for fruits. The achievement of this function can be gained by the incorporation of a physical or chemical absorbent or adsorbent in the packaging material, or added to the package by means of a sachet. In most research papers, the term *absorption* is used loosely to describe any system that removes a substance from the headspace, although there is a significant difference between absorption and adsorption. Adsorption is a two-dimensional phenomenon involving a substance being taken onto the bulk of a phase, while absorption is three-dimensional and involves a substance being taken into a surface. Both absorption and adsorption are physical phenomena while scavenging implies a chemical reaction. This section focuses mainly on ethylene adsorbers.

Some phenomena related to adsorption are known from ancient times, although the first scientific evidences were carried out by Scheele (1773) and Fontana (1777), who reported some experiments about the efficacy of charcoal and clays on gas adsorption (Dąbrowski, 2001), these early discoveries being the origin of current applications and possibly of future developments. Adsorption is a surface phenomenon in which particles (gas or solid in solution) are held on the surface of solid material. The particles are commonly named as adsorbates and the trapping solid material as the adsorbent. Adsorption is distinguished from absorption by the fact that with the later, the absorbate is accumulated throughout the absorber, not only on its surface. Two different patterns of adsorption can be described: physico-adsorption involving binding through van der Waals forces, or chemi-adsorption, in which chemical linkages occur (Martínez-Romero et al., 2007a). The amount of adsorbed material depends on temperature, pressure, and adsorbate concentration.

The main compounds used as ethylene adsorbers are activated carbon and zeolites. The commercial application of activated carbon in the adsorption of gases and vapor started in the 1930s, although the specific use for ethylene was in the late 1950s. Any carbonaceous material may be used to make activated carbon, but the selection of the raw material should have low inorganic matter content, be easily activated, be easily available, have low cost, and have low degradation during storage (Dąbrowski, 2001). Thus, lignocellulosic material such as wood, fruit shells, fruit stones, apple pulp, wheat, cotton stalks, viscose rayon, and coal, among others, are often used for activated carbon production. There are both physical and chemical methods for carbon activation. Chemical procedures have advantages over physical ones, in terms of greater yield, no previous carbonization being necessary, lower temperatures of activation, and good development of the porous structure (Puziy et al., 2002).

The ability of activated carbon to act as an adsorber is dependent on a wide range of properties (Aygün et al., 2003), such as magnitude and distribution of pore volume (pore structure), surface area, and type and quality of surface-bound functional groups (surface chemistry). The adsorption capacity is proportionally related to both large surface area and pore volume. For commercial food grade, activated carbons with surface areas ranging between 300 and 2000 $m^2\ g^{-1}$ are used, although some of them could achieve surface areas as high as 5000 $m^2\ g^{-1}$. Specific uses of activated carbon in foods are as decolorizing agents, taste-odor removing agents, and purification agents.

Activated carbon can be granular, powdered, or fibered (Ahmedna et al., 2000). However, the granular type is preferred due to its easier regeneration and versatility. The adsorption process of ethylene on these adsorbers fits a model proposed by Langmuir in 1916. Using this model, it is assumed that the rate of adsorption is directly related to ethylene pressure (temperature and RH) and the surface of the adsorber, reaching a dynamic equilibrium between adsorption and desorption.

A comparative study about the ethylene adsorption capacity of three forms of activated carbon revealed that the best results in terms of ethylene adsorption were obtained with granular (over 80%) followed by powered (over 70%), while fibered had the lower adsorption capacity for this gas (over 40%). Moreover, the exogenous application of ethylene at 2.5, 5.0, or 7.5 $\mu L\ L^{-1}$ concentrations, to a constant mass of activated carbon, led to the same percentage of adsorbed ethylene, independently of the concentration of the applied ethylene. In addition, the adsorption capacity of these activated carbons was not affected by temperature in the range of 2–20°C (Martínez-Romero et al., 2007a). This means that the double bond of ethylene makes it a very reactive compound that can be altered or degraded in many ways. The use of granular activated carbon impregnated with palladium as catalyst improved the ethylene adsorption compared with activated carbon alone (Bailén et al., 2007), the efficacy being enhanced when Pd was used at 10% instead of 1% (98% and 85%, respectively). The increase in ethylene removal when Pd was added to the activated carbon as a catalyst was attributed to the fact that not only an adsorption phenomenon occurred but also an oxidation process. However, the main disadvantage of Pd is its high cost, which would limit the practical application, and thus GAC-1% Pd could be considered as satisfactory in terms of ethylene adsorption. This adsorber/catalyst system was added as sachets to tomatoes under MAP conditions to create an active packaging. A reduction in color evolution (both internal and external) as well as a delay in the softening process was shown in tomatoes in MAP packages containing 1% Pd, which indicated a net delay of the tomato ripening process and an increase in shelf life. Interestingly, odor intensity was reduced by the use of activated carbon-1% Pd, which was associated with lower off-flavor and attributed to the capacity of the adsorber to trap volatiles (Figure 10.1). The active packaging was also effective in reducing the ethylene accumulation inside the packages, the weight loss, and decay incidence (Bailén et al., 2006). In addition, 23 compounds were identified in control tomatoes under MAP conditions, the main being aldehydes and alcohols, while in

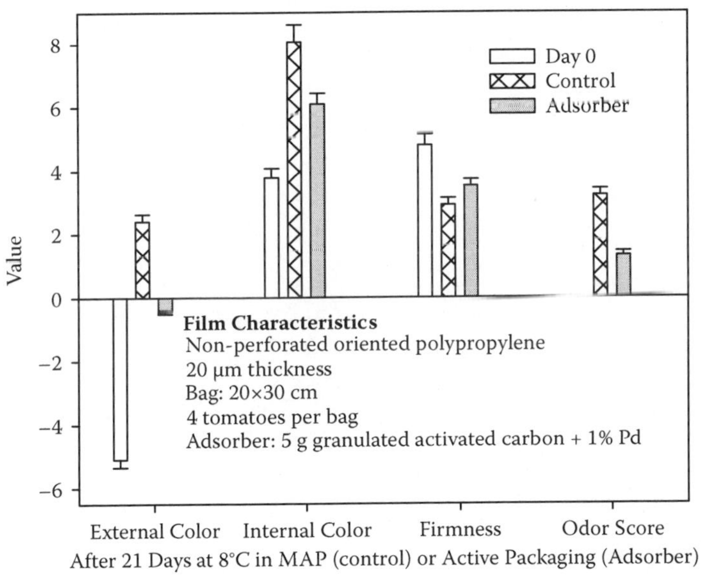

Figure 10.1 Changes in some tomato fruit ripening parameters from harvest (Day 0) and after 21 days of cold storage in control (MAP packages) and active packaged fruits with the system adsorber/catalyst. Color expressed as a* parameter, firmness as N mm^{-1}, and odor scores intensity on a ranked scale of 1 to 5, where 1 = absence, 2 = slight odor, 3 = moderate, 4 = severe off-flavor, and 5 = extremely off-flavor.

those packaged in MAP containing GAC-1% Pd the alcohols became the predominant while acids, ketones, and hydrocarbons disappeared. It is interesting to point out that this decrease of volatiles was not correlated to those results obtained from the sensorial panel, since panelists judged better the treated tomatoes than controls in terms of odor and flavor.

Other active packaging has been developed by using adsorbers and potassium permanganate as oxidizer. To be effective, $KMnO_4$ must be adsorbed on a suitable inert carrier with a large surface area (zeolite, vermiculite, silica gel, alumina pellets, or activated carbon) containing about 4–6% $KMnO_4$. The oxidation of ethylene with $KMnO_4$ can be thought of as a two-step process. Ethylene is initially oxidized to acetaldehyde, which in turn is oxidized to acetic acid and further oxidized to carbon dioxide and water. Following these reactions, potassium permanganate adsorbers change from purple to brown as the MnO_4^- is reduced to MnO_2, indicating the remaining adsorbing capacity. However, the adsorbent materials containing $KMnO_4$ cannot be integrated into fruit-contact packaging but are supplied only as sachets because of their toxicity and purple color.

To solve this problem, very recently a scrubber to remove ethylene continuously from stored environments has been developed (Martínez-Romero et al., 2009a). The scrubber is composed by a cartridge heater tightly joined to the activated carbon-1% Pd, and the application of heat pulses led to an increase in the ethylene oxidation and to auto-regeneration of the activated carbon; this fact is considered as very important due to low maintenance cost and the increased adsorbing capacity, which has been considered as one of the limiting factors of the classical ethylene adsorbers. Since the efficacy on ethylene removal was higher as was the number of heat pulses, several heater core temperatures were assayed (100–325°C), and it was concluded that temperatures ranging between 150–200°C eliminated 96–99% of ethylene, with low CO_2 accumulation (0.10–0.18 kPa), and in turn less activated carbon degraded without affecting the temperature of the storage environment. This hybrid was used in stored tomatoes in cold rooms, and the parameters related to ripening such as respiration rate, ethylene production, ACC (free and conjugated), color changes, softening, decrease in TA (mainly citric and ascorbic acids), and lycopene were significantly lower in stored tomato fruits with the adsorbent-catalyst system working continuously. Although this scrubber device could not be considered as an active packaging since it is applied to large storage cold rooms, a further step in the concept of a new tool to eliminate the ethylene surrounding fruit and vegetables in the storage areas, avoiding the detrimental effects of ethylene action and leading to maintenance of their postharvest quality, has been given. Other additional advantages are the auto-regeneration process, when heat pulses were applied to the adsorbent-catalyst system, and that is an environmentally friendly technology (Martínez-Romero et al., 2009b).

10.4 Antimicrobial fruit packaging

Antimicrobial packaging is one of the main applications of active packaging and can be defined as the packaging system that is able to kill or inhibit spoilage and pathogenic microorganisms that are present in contaminating foods by adding active ingredients in the packaging system and/or using actively functional polymers (Han, 2003). When the packaging system acquires antimicrobial activity, the packaging system (or material) limits or prevents microbial growth by extending the lag period and by reducing the growth rate or decreasing live counts of microorganisms. Some food products are not sensitive to microbial spoilage or contamination, and in these cases the antimicrobial packaging system is not necessary; however, most foods including fruits are perishable and susceptible to contamination, and therefore the use of an antimicrobial packaging will ensure safety, maintain quality, and increase shelf life.

Antimicrobial active packaging systems can be divided in four groups according to the localization of the antimicrobial compound: (1) the antimicrobial is released to the headspace of the package to interact with the produce surface, (2) the antimicrobial compound is included in the packaging material and is released to the product by a migration process, (3) the antimicrobial compound is immobilized in the surface of the package, and (4) the package material has inherent antimicrobial activity.

The first developments in antimicrobial packaging derived from antimicrobial substances being incorporated in or coated onto film materials (Vermeiren et al., 1999), although their applications mostly include meat, fish, bakery, and cheese products, and fewer results exist for fruits and vegetables. Initially, Ag-substituted zeolite was incorporated into plastic films due to the strong antimicrobial activity of Ag^+ ions, but the regulatory restriction of the addition of Ag to foods has discharged its commercial use. Several other compounds have been proposed and/or tested for antimicrobial activity in food packaging including organic acids (sorbate, propionate, and benzoate), bacteriocins (nisin), and enzymes (lysozyme), but many of the incorporated antimicrobials are not yet permitted for food use, and the election of the antimicrobial is often limited by the incompatibility of the component with the packaging material or by the heat lability of the component during extrusion process during film manufacture.

Other systems gradually release SO_2 to control mold growth in some fruits, such as table grapes. However, excessive release of SO_2 from pads of sodium metabisulphite incorporated to microporous material has been shown to cause partial bleaching problems in grapes. The accumulation or absorption of the excess SO_2 by foods could cause toxicological problems, compromising the safety in SO_2-releasing active packaging systems. Finally, ethanol has been used either by spraying onto foods prior to package or by using sachets that generate ethanol vapor. A major disadvantage of ethanol vapor is its absorption by the food product. In some cases the ethanol concentration in the product might have legislative problems, and the cost of the sachets limits their use to products with low profit margins (Ozdemir and Floros, 2004).

However, research has continued to find alternatives to these chemical substances, and the results have revealed that exploitation of some natural substances exhibiting antimicrobial and antifungal activities (Tripathi and Dubey, 2004) can be used as part of the active packaging. Among these natural compounds, the antimicrobial properties of essential oils derived from many plant organs have been empirically recognized for centuries, but only came to scientific attention recently (Appendini and Hotchkiss, 2002; Burt, 2004). In addition, these volatiles have been also exhibited antioxidant properties (Ruberto and Baratta, 2000).

Essential oils or the so-called volatile or ethereal oils (Guenther, 1948) are aromatic oily liquids obtained from plant organs: flower, bud, seed, leave, twig, bark, herb wood fruit, and root. The term *essential oil* is thought to derive from the word *Quinta essentia* with medical use attributed to Paracelsus. Essential oils are used as flavoring foods due to their flavor and fragrance, but nowadays essential oils and their pure components are gaining increasing interest from the point of view of their safe status, wide acceptance by consumers, and their exploitation for multi-purpose uses (Cowan, 1999). The most common essential oils as well as the major component used in the food industry with description of antioxidant or antimicrobial properties *in vitro* have been recently reviewed (Serrano et al., 2008a). These natural compounds belong to the genera *Thymus, Origanum, Syzygium, Mentha*, and *Eucalyptus*. Very recently, the essential oils from *Citrus* species have been postulated as potential antimicrobials. The components of *Citrus* essential oils contain 85–99% volatile and 1–15% nonvolatile components. The volatile constituents are a mixture of monoterpene (limonene) and sesquiterpene hydrocarbons and their oxygenated derivatives including aldehydes (citral), ketones, acids, alcohols (linalool), and esters (Fisher and Phillips, 2008). The whole essential oils show antioxidant activity, but their fractionation has indicated that the main components responsible for the antioxidant effect are carvacrol for oregano, thymol for thyme, eugenol for clove, menthol for mint, and eucalyptol for eucalyptus. The chemical structures of these natural essential oils are shown in Figure 10.2, in which eugenol, thymol, and carvacrol are phenols, while eucalyptol and menthol are terpenoids. For these compounds, the activity as antioxidants has been reported to be close to that of α-tocopherol (Ruberto and Baratta, 2000; Sacchetti et al., 2005) or vitamin C (Kim and Lee, 2004), and mainly due to the presence of hydroxyl groups in the benzene ring. However, the main biological activity and the possible use of the essential oils in the food industry are derived from their capacity to kill microorganisms. The *in vitro* antimicrobial activity of eugenol,

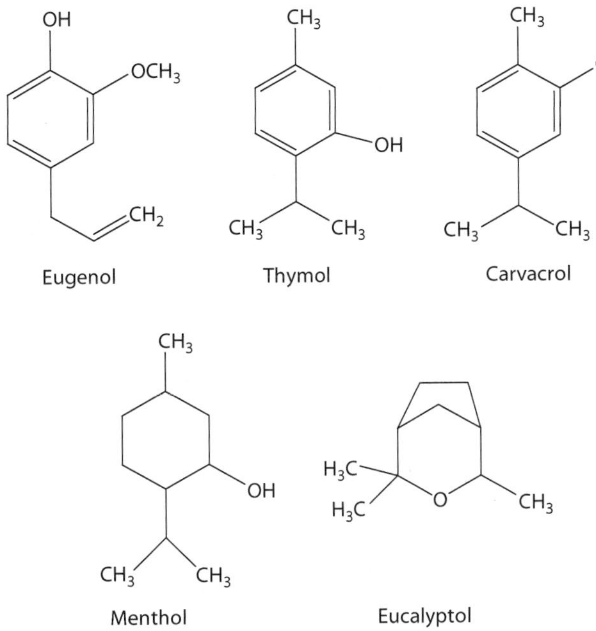

Figure 10.2 Chemical structures of the main essential oils exhibiting both antioxidant and antimicrobial activities.

thymol, and carvacrol has been reported against bacteria (Periago et al., 2004), yeasts (Arora and Kaur, 1999), and fungi (Vázquez et al., 2001). Among bacteria, essential oils are generally more inhibitory against Gram-positive than against Gram-negative (Holley and Patel, 2005). However, the *in vivo* efficacy and practical activity of only a few of the essential oils have been studied. The exact mechanism of action of the essential oils was not fully elucidated. Some authors have attributed it to their hydrophobicity, which enables them to partition in the lipids of the cell membrane disturbing its integrity and the inorganic ions equilibrium (Bagamboula et al., 2004), but others have postulated that the presence of the phenolic ring may be necessary for the antimicrobial activity of eugenol and thymol (Ultee et al., 2002). Moreover, the site(s) and number of hydroxyl groups on the phenol ring are thought to be related to their relative toxicity to microorganisms, with evidence that increased hydroxylation results in increased toxicity (Cowan, 1999). For those essential oils with an absence of phenolic groups like menthol, it has been speculated that the mechanism of action involves membrane disruption by the lipophilic compounds (Serrano et al., 2008a). Specifically, aromatic and phenolic compounds exert their antimicrobial effects at the cytoplasmic membrane by altering its structure and function. Efflux of K^+ is usually an early sign of damage and is often followed by efflux of cytoplasmic constituents (Cowan, 1999; Ultee et al., 2002). The loss of the differential permeability character of the cytoplasmic membrane is frequently identified as the cause of cell death. Other events that could lead to membrane dysfunction and subsequent disruption include dissipation of the two components of the proton motive force in cells (the pH gradient and the electrical potential) either by changes in ion transport or by depolarization through structural changes in the membrane; interference with the energy (ATP) generation system in the cell; or enzyme inhibition preventing substrate utilization for energy production (Holley and Patel, 2005).

The European Commission has registered a number of essential oils and their components to be applied in foodstuffs, including eugenol, menthol, and thymol (Commission Decision, 23 January 2002, CE). These compounds appear also in EAFUS (Everything Added to Food in the US) and GRAS (Generally Recognized as Safe) lists. In foods, the potential use of essential oils as natural preservatives has been reported in cheese, bakery products, and meat, among others (Burt, 2004), with the main disadvantages for the use of these natural compounds being related to persistence of strong aroma and the fact that they sometimes would change the organoleptic properties of food adversely. In fruits, the use of natural compounds such as hexanal, 2-(E)-hexenal, and hexyl acetate improved shelf life and safety of minimally processed fruits (Lanciotti et al., 2004). In this review, authors postulated that future trends in the use of natural compounds would be focused on the use of specific active packaging able to release the active molecules slowly over time in the headspace.

With these premises, the first active packaging by combination of MAP and pure essential oils was reported in sweet cherry (Serrano et al., 2005b) and several cultivars of table grapes such as Crimson, Autumn Royal, and Aledo (Valverde et al., 2005a; Valero, et al., 2006; Guillén et al., 2007b). With this active packaging, the overall quality of products can be improved in terms of maintenance of organoleptic and functional properties together with safety.

Table 10.1 shows the efficacy of the essential oils added to MAP in reducing the total mesophilic aerobic and yeast and mold counts in table grape and sweet cherry with respect to contamination in fruits stored in MAP. It is clear that the essential oils showed higher effectiveness in reducing the yeast and molds than mesophilic aerobics for both fruit types, which was related to the lower decay incidence reported in these fruits as compared to those stored in MAP. The microbial spoilage increased during fruit storage under MAP conditions only (control) because the concentration of CO_2 achieved inside the bags (below 3 kPa) was not high enough to act as antimicrobial. In these reports the pure volatiles (eugenol, thymol, carvacrol, or menthol) were used instead of the whole essential oils. Although the fungitoxic properties of the volatile constituents of higher plants have been reported, little attention has been paid to the fungitoxicity of

Table 10.1 Effect of the Addition of Essential Oils to MAP Packages on Microbial Spoilage in Table Grape and Sweet Cherry[1]

	Total mesophilic aerobics ($CFU\ g^{-1}$)		Yeasts and molds ($CFU\ g^{-1}$)	
	Table grape	Sweet cherry	Table grape	Sweet cherry
At harvest	4.77 a	4.20 a	4.61 a	2.10 a
Control	4.90 a	4.77 a	5.04 a	4.89 b
Eugenol	3.33 b	2.93 b	2.10 b	1.11 c
Thymol	3.41 b	2.84 b	2.46 b	0.95 c
Menthol	3.60 b	2.69 b	3.24 c	1.48 d

[1] Each package contains 500 μL of the corresponding essential oil, except in control, in which no essential oils were added. Data obtained after 16 and 35 days of cold storage in MAP packages for sweet cherry and table grape, respectively. For each column, different letters are significantly different at $P < 0.05$.

these substances when combined. It has been described that essential oils may induce fungitoxic potency, which may be due to synergism between their components. In fact, in Aledo table grape a mixture of essential oils (carvacrol, thymol, and eugenol) was used and lower concentration was needed to control microbial spoilage (Guillén et al., 2007b) with respect to these essential oils used alone (Valverde et al., 2005a; Valero et al., 2006). This information is highly valuable for future research since the fungitoxic potency of most of the fungicides has been reported to be enhanced when combined (Tripathi and Dubey, 2004) as well as the antimicrobial activity (Burt, 2004). The enhancement of fungitoxic potential of mixtures of the oils may be due to the joint action of two or more substances present in the oils. This synergism would be beneficial in postharvest protection because the pathogen would not easily produce resistance against the components. However, more work on the synergistic action of plant products under *in vitro* and *in vivo* conditions is required. The literature is also scarce on the mode of action of the essential oils as postharvest antifungal.

This active packaging was able to maintain color and to reduce softening in both sweet cherry and table grape (Figure 10.3) compared to those control fruits under MAP conditions. Similarly, the increase in ripening index or ratio TSS/TA was delayed in those fruits under active packaging as compared with those in MAP alone (Figure 10.4). Thus, the combination of MAP and essential oils delays the evolution of these parameters related to postharvest ripening more than MAP alone, the effects being attributed to the essential oils added, since gas composition was similar (11–12 O_2 and 2–3 kPa CO_2 for sweet cherry, and 10–14 O_2 and 1.3–2.0 kPa CO_2 for table grapes) in both control bags and active packages.

The responsible compounds for the human health beneficial properties associated with fruit and vegetable intake are those with antioxidant

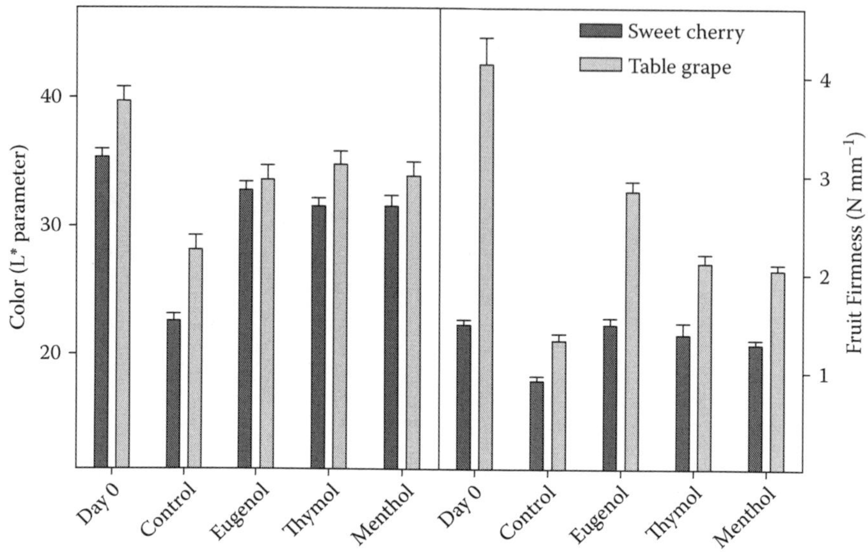

Figure 10.3 Values at harvest (Day 0) and after storage at 2°C in color luminosity (L* parameter) and fruit firmness in sweet cherry and table grapes under MAP packages (control) and in active packaging (500 µL of eugenol, thymol, or menthol). Storage times were 16 and 35 days for sweet cherry and table grapes, respectively.

activity, including carotenoids, ascorbic acid, flavonoids, anthocyanins, and other phenolic compounds (see Chapter 2, Section 2.3.5). However, little attention has been paid to the possible role of active packaging on the behavior of these bioactive compounds. In grape, the aforementioned loss of quality during storage was also accompanied by diminution of both total phenolics and anthocyanins in the skin (Figure 10.5) and in the flesh (Figure 10.6), which were responsible for the reduction of H-TAA found in both skin and flesh. Contrarily, the addition of eugenol or thymol inside the packages led to a delay in the loss of total phenolics and total anthocyanins in the skin and ascorbic acid in the flesh. In addition, total phenolics and TAA were increased with the use of the active packaging. Since eugenol and thymol have been described to exhibit a natural antioxidant activity (Sacchetti et al., 2005) close to that of vitamin C (Kim and Lee, 2004), and given their phenolic nature, the combined use of both compounds together with MAP storage as an active packaging would help maintain or increase the antioxidant capacity of fruits.

A strong impulse in the development of this technology is required for commercial application, since antimicrobial active packaging is an emerging and exciting concept in food technology that confers many benefits, fulfilling consumers' demand for safe products that avoid the use of

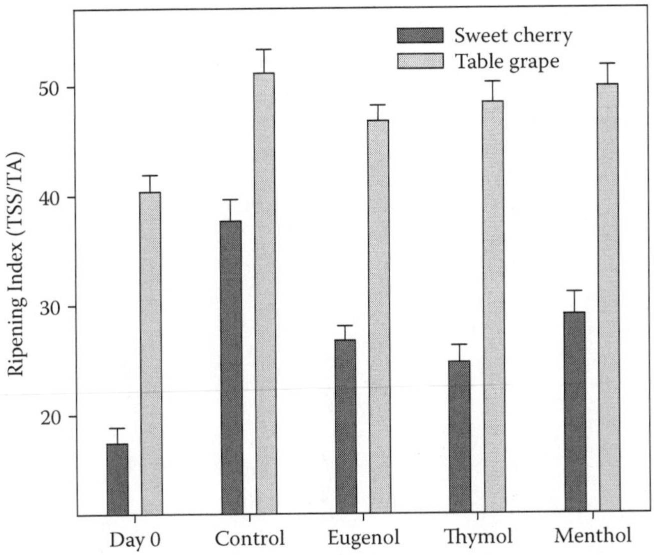

Figure 10.4 Values at harvest (Day 0) and after storage at 2°C in ripening index in sweet cherry and table grapes under MAP packages (control) and in active packaging (500 μL of eugenol, thymol, or menthol). Storage times were 16 and 35 days for sweet cherry and table grapes, respectively.

chemicals as a mean of preservation. Further studies are needed for a better understanding of the mechanism/s by which these essential oils affect the fruit physiology modulating the ripening process as well as their ability to kill microorganisms. In addition, the effectiveness of a combination of two or more of these compounds (with different functional groups) should be advisable.

10.5 *Edible coatings*

During the last two decades, both food and packaging industries have joined efforts to reduce the amount of food packaging materials mainly due to environmental and consumer concerns. In this sense, the concept of biobased materials for food packaging was introduced at the end of the last century (Petersen et al., 1999), although these materials are not necessarily biodegradable. Biobased packaging materials include both edible films and edible coatings along with primary and secondary packaging materials. Edible coatings may be defined as a thin layer of material that covers the surface of the food and can be eaten as part of the whole product. The election of a biobased packaging material will depend on the applicable food product: meat, fish, fruit and vegetable, seafood, egg, or dairy products, since deteriorative reactions (enzymatic, chemical, physical, or microbiological)

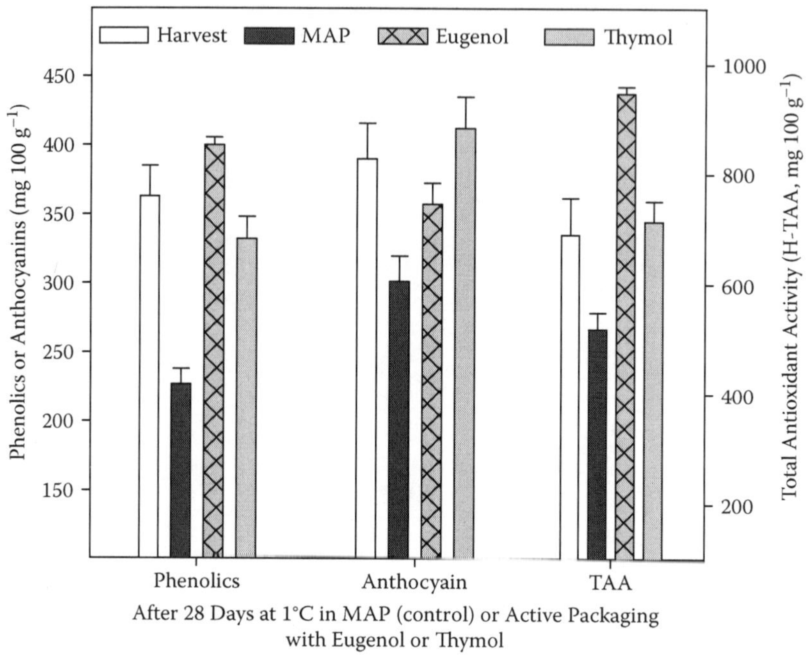

Figure 10.5 Bioactive compounds (total phenolics and anthocyanins) and hydrophilic antioxidant activity (H-TAA) in the table grape skin from control MAP packages and those with active packaging by adding eugenol or thymol after 28 days at 2°C. Each package contains 150 μL of the corresponding essential oil.

are quite specific. In this section, the edible films and coatings with possible use in fruits and vegetables will be provided.

The application of an edible coating onto the fruit surface modifies the internal atmosphere in the same way that plastic films do (see Chapter 9): by increasing the carbon dioxide and lowering the oxygen concentrations. Then, the effects of edible coatings on internal gas composition and their interactions on quality parameters must be determined for coated fresh produce. Success of edible coatings for fruits depends mainly on selecting films or coatings that can give a desirable internal gas composition that is appropriate for a specific product. Also, if a coating is too thick detrimental effects can result due to an internal oxygen concentration below a desirable beneficial level and an associated increase in carbon dioxide concentration above a critical tolerable level. On a general basis, oxygen permeability of most edible coatings is lower than that of the conventional plastic films (Park, 1999).

Biopolymer-based packaging is defined as packaging that contains raw materials from agricultural and marine sources. There are three such categories of biopolymers: (1) extracted directly from natural raw materials,

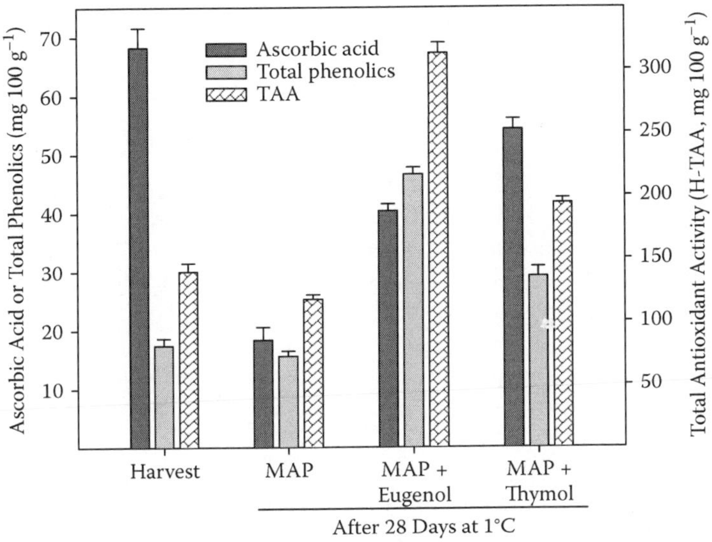

Figure 10.6 Bioactive compounds (total phenolics and ascorbic acid) and hydrophilic antioxidant activity (H-TAA) in table grape flesh from control MAP packages and those with active packaging by adding eugenol or thymol after 28 days at 2°C. Each package contains 150 μL of the corresponding essential oil.

such as starch, cellulose, protein, and marine prokaryotes; (2) produced by chemical synthesis from bioderived monomers; and (3) produced by microorganisms such as hydroxy-butyrate and hydroxy-valerate (Cha and Chinnan, 2004). Components of edible films and coatings can be divided into three categories: hydrocolloids, lipids, and composites. Hydrocolloids include proteins and polysaccharides, such as starch, alginate, cellulose derivatives, chitosan, and agar. Lipids include waxes, acylglycerols, and fatty acids. Composites contain both hydrocolloid components and lipids. The choice of materials for a film or coating is largely dependent on its desired function.

Among polysaccharides, starch is very biodegradable and cost effective but is also very hydrophilic. Films based on starch have moderate gas barrier properties and their mechanical properties are generally inferior to synthetic polymer films. Amylose is responsible for the film-forming capacity of starches. Amylose, the linear fraction of starch, is known to form a coherent and relatively strong, freestanding film, in contrast to amylopectin films, which are brittle and noncontinuous (Cha and Chinnan, 2004). Native granular starch is converted into a thermoplastic material by conventional methods in the presence of plasticizers, such as water and glycerol.

Another polysaccharide that is of high interest is chitosan, obtained from the deacetylation of chitin (poly-β-(1→4)-N-acetyl- D-glucosamine), which is mainly obtained from crab and shrimp shells. Films and coatings based on chitosan have selective permeability to gases (CO_2 and O_2) and good mechanical properties. However, their uses are limited mainly because of their high water vapor permeability. Moreover, chitosan shows antifungal and antibacterial properties, which are believed to originate from its polycationic nature, although the precise mechanism of its antimicrobial activity is still unknown (Srinivasa and Tharanathan, 2007). In addition, alginates, which are extracted from brown seaweeds of the *Phaephyceae* class, are the salts of alginic acid, a linear copolymer of D-mannuronic and L-glucuronic acid monomers. The ability of alginates to react with di-valent and trivalent cations is being utilized in alginate film formation. Calcium ions, which are more effective than magnesium, manganese, aluminum ferrous, and ferric ions, have been applied as gelling agents (Vargas et al., 2008).

Proteins that can be used in the formulation of edible coatings for fruits include those derived from animal sources, such as casein and whey protein, or obtained from plant sources like corn-zein, wheat gluten, soy protein, peanut protein, and cottonseed protein (Gennadios, 2002). Proteins exhibit a wide variety of different molecular characteristics depending on their biological origin and function that will determine the ability of particular proteins to form coatings and the characteristics of the coatings formed. Casein-based edible coatings are attractive for food applications due to their high nutritional quality, excellent sensory properties, and good potential for providing food products with adequate protection against their surrounding environment. Whey proteins have been the subject of intense investigation over the past decade or so. With the addition of plasticizer, heat-denatured whey proteins produce transparent and flexible water-based edible coatings with excellent oxygen, aroma, and oil barrier properties at low RH. However, the hydrophilic nature of whey protein coatings causes them to be less effective as moisture barriers.

Lipid-based edible coatings have a low affinity for water, which explains why they have low water vapor permeability, and thus the use of lipid coatings on fresh fruits and vegetables can help to control their desiccation and weight loss (Morillon et al., 2002).

According to the European Directives (ED, 1995; 1998) and the USA Code of Federal Regulations (FDA, 2006) edible coatings are those coatings that are formulated with food-grade additives, and for their application to fresh citrus fruits, the amount of edible coating ingredients used must be only that which is necessary to accomplish the intended effect, and the ingredients have to be GRAS and be listed in the aforementioned Code. Among the ingredients that can be incorporated into the formulation of edible coatings, the European Directive (1995) includes the following: arabic and karaya gum, pectins, shellac, beeswax, candelilla wax, and carnauba wax. This Directive was modified in 1998 by introducing new ingredients such as lecithin, polysorbates, fatty acids, and fatty acid salts. On the other hand, the Food and Drug Administration mentions other additives used as components of protective coatings applied to fresh fruits and vegetables like morpholine, polydextrose, sorbitan monostearate, sucrose fatty acid esters, cocoa butter, and castor oil.

Wax was the first edible coating used on fruits. The Chinese applied wax coatings to oranges and lemons in the 12th and 13th centuries. Although the Chinese did not realize that the full function of edible coatings was to slow down respiratory gas exchange, they found that wax-coated fruits could be stored longer than nonwaxed fruits. Park (1999) reviewed the development of systematic means of selecting edible coatings to maximize quality and shelf life of fresh fruits and vegetables. For these products, cellulose, casein, zein, soy protein, and chitosan were candidates to be used in fruits since they have the desirable characteristics of generally being odorless, tasteless, and transparent. In the past few years, research efforts have focused on the design of new eco-friendly coatings based on biodegradable polymers, which not only reduce the requirements of packaging but also lead to the conversion of by-products of the food industry into value-added film-forming components. Among these new materials for edible coatings *Aloe vera* gel was first used in table grape (Valverde et al., 2005b) and sweet cherry (Martínez-Romero et al., 2006) with satisfactory results in terms of reducing the weight loss and lowering the respiration rate during postharvest storage. In addition, *A. vera* gel delayed color changes, softening, and TA losses, maintaining fruit quality together with a reduction of both mesophilic aerobics and yeast and mold counts without affecting the sensory properties of the fruits.

Traditionally, edible coatings have been used as a barrier to minimize water loss and delay the natural senescence of coated fruits through selective permeability to gases. However, the new generation of edible coatings is being specifically designed to allow the incorporation and/or controlled release of antioxidants, vitamins, nutraceuticals, and natural antimicrobial agents by means of the application of promising technologies such as nano-encapsulation and the layer-by-layer assembly (Vargas et al., 2008).

In this sense, coated tomatoes with alginate or zein showed lower respiration rate and ethylene production than control ones, with a twofold lower concentration of the ethylene precursor. In addition, the evolution of parameters related to tomato quality losses, such as softening, color evolution, and weight loss, was significantly delayed (4–6 days on average) in coated tomatoes as compared to controls. Thereafter, sugars, organic acids (and especially ascorbic acid), and scores from sensory analysis remained at much higher levels at the end of storage in treated than in control tomatoes (Zapata et al., 2008). With the aim to reduce also the incidence

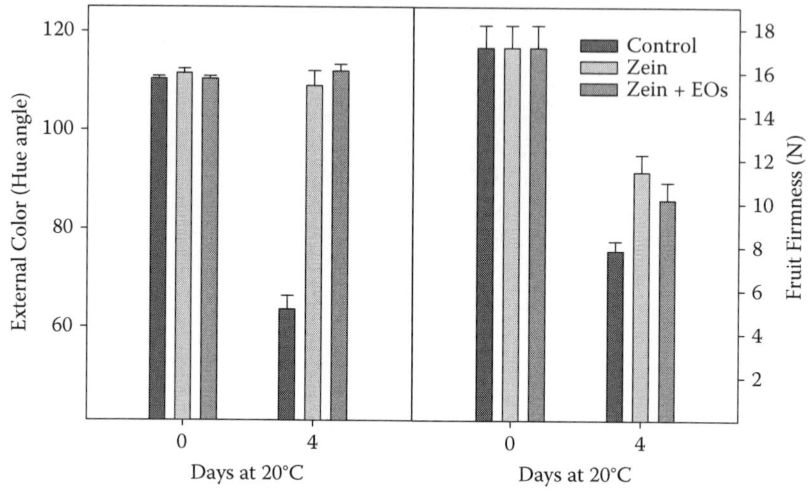

Figure 10.7 Values at harvest (Day 0) and after 4 days of storage at 20°C in external color and fruit firmness in control tomatoes and those coated with zein (5%) alone or with the addition of mixed essential oils (EOs). The coating solution contains 25 μL L^{-1} of each essential oil (eugenol, thymol, menthol, and carvacrol).

of decay, edible coatings based on zein (5%) alone or with the addition of mixed essential oils (thymol, carvacrol, eugenol, and menthol, 25 μL L^{-1} of each) as antimicrobials were assayed in tomato fruits, showing that these treatments were also effective in reducing the color changes and the softening process during postharvest storage at 20°C with respect to control fruits, although no differences were found between both treatments (Figure 10.7). However, the addition of essential oils to zein edible coating decreased fruit incidence decay, since 10% of decayed fruits were observed in zein coated fruits after 10 days of storage at 20°C, while no decayed fruits were found when essential oils were added to zein coating and a 30% of decay occurred in control fruits.

Accordingly, the softening process was delayed in Black Amber plums coated with 1% and 3% alginate, without or with the addition of essential oils (thymol, carvacrol, eugenol, and menthol, 25 μL L^{-1} of each), this effect being even higher when essential oils were added to the 3% alginate coating. These treatments also maintained higher levels of total acidity after storage with respect to control fruits, although in this parameter no differences were found among treatments (Figure 10.8). In addition, the decrease in color Chroma index of the flesh was also delayed in alginate coated plums (Figure 10.9). Thus, the effect of alginate on delaying the postharvest evolution of the ripening parameters on plum is clear, which could be attributed to its effect on inhibiting ethylene production, as observed in Figure 10.9.

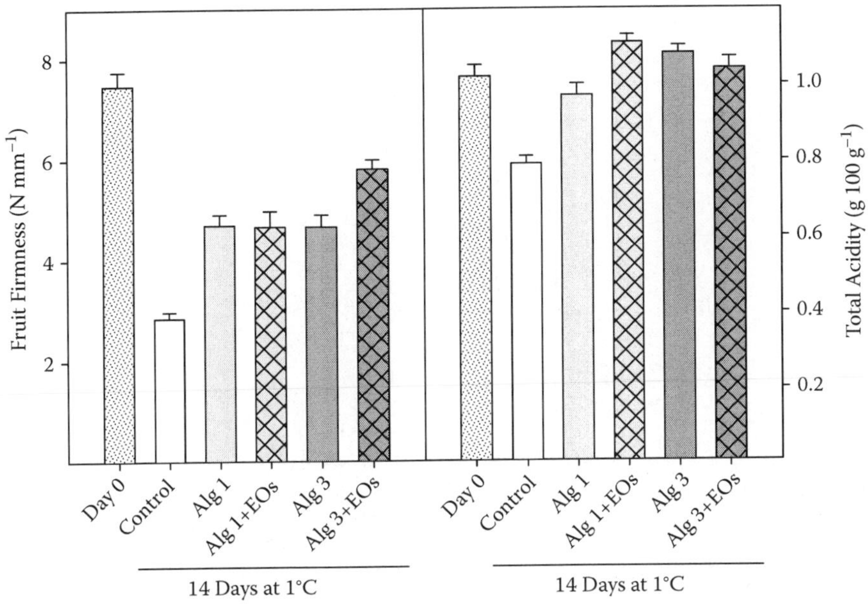

Figure 10.8 Firmness and total acidity in Black Amber plum at harvest (Day 0) and after 14 days of storage at 1°C, in control and 1% or 3% alginate coated fruits (Alg 1 and Alg 3, respectively) with or without the addition of essential oils (EOs, 25 μL L^{-1} of each: eugenol, thymol, menthol, and carvacrol)

10.6 Future trends

Although active packaging has been more successfully applied in the United States, Japan, and Australia than in Europe, this concept is still in its early stages and far from being applied on a large scale. The effectiveness of active packages has been deeply researched, but consumers are not always very keen on the use of sachets in food packaging, and precautions to minimize the risk of ingestion have been taken by clearly stating "Do not eat" on the label. On the contrary, active packaging will probably increase in developing countries in the near future due to consumer preferences for minimally processed and naturally preserved foods and the food industry's eagerness to invest in product quality and safety. The future trend in active packaging is to use absorbing or releasing compounds incorporated in the packaging film or in an adhesive label to get rid of separate objects in packaging, and thus to avoid consumer resistance toward new packaging techniques. The antimicrobial packaging materials are a potential way to decrease the amount of preservatives and focus the function of preservatives more precisely where microbial growth and spoilage mainly occur: on the surface of the food. The most significant challenges are to develop new antimicrobial packaging materials that are

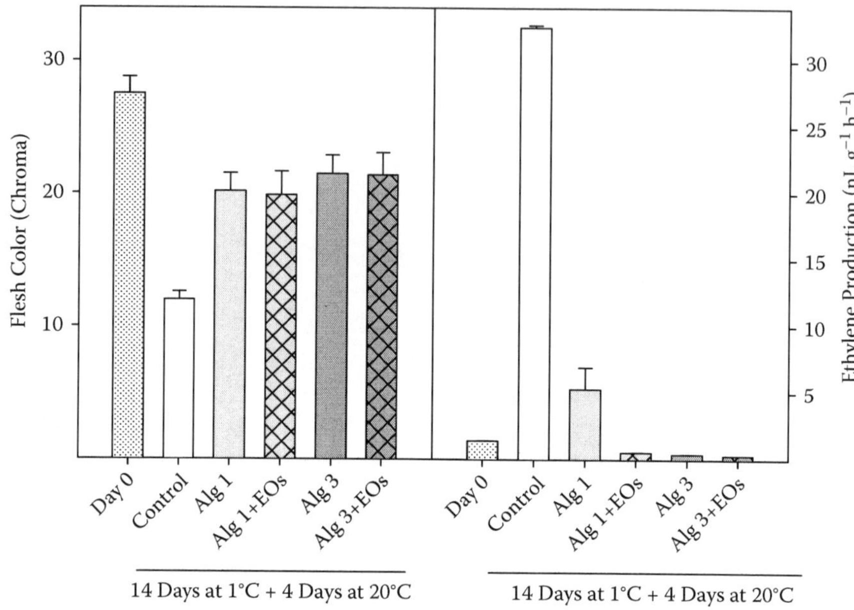

Figure 10.9 Flesh color (Chroma index) and ethylene production rate in Black Amber plum at harvest and after 14 days of storage at 1°C plus 4 days at 20°C, in control and 1% or 3% alginate coated fruits (Alg 1 and Alg 3, respectively) with or without the addition of essential oils (EOs, 25 μL L^{-1} of each: eugenol, thymol, menthol, and carvacrol).

effective against several spoilage and pathogenic microbes. This obviously means that more than one preservative should be incorporated into the same packaging material. It is self-evident that these novel materials should have proper permeability properties, good appearance, and good mechanical properties and must be reasonable in price, suitable for packaging machines already used in the food industry, and suitable for normal sealing procedures. In other words, they must have all those properties that traditional packaging materials have (Wilson, 2007).

chapter eleven

Emerging technologies

11.1 Introduction

In the previous chapters the most conventional postharvest technologies have been described, and most of them are being currently used in the horticultural industries. However, in recent years some new or emerging technologies are being investigated mainly with the aim to achieve an effective control on microbial spoilage of the fresh produce and thus to control the postharvest fungal decay. Among these emerging tools, in this chapter the use of atmospheres with high O_2, the biological control and the UV light will be provided. It is clear that there are other new technologies, but they are still in the initial steps of development or under investigations.

11.2 Atmospheres with high O_2

High O_2 MAP has a great impact in the fresh-cut fruit and vegetables industry. Packaging under appropriate atmosphere conditions can effectively control the growth of microorganisms on the surface of fresh-cut fruits. Recently, some researchers have claimed that super-atmospheric O_2 concentrations (>70 kPa) can be an alternative to low O_2-MA to prevent undesired anoxic respiration, inhibit the growth of naturally occurring spoilage microorganisms, and maintain fresh-like sensory quality of fresh-cut produce (Rojas-Graü et al., 2009).

High O_2 MAP could overcome the many disadvantages of low O_2 MAP. High O_2 MAP has been found to be particularly effective at inhibiting enzymatic discolorations, preventing anaerobic fermentation reactions, and inhibiting microbial growth. In addition, the high O_2 MAP of prepared produce items within inexpensive hermetically sealed plastic films is very effective at preventing undesirable moisture and odor losses. To gain these benefits, atmospheres about 80–95% O_2 and 5–20% N_2 are required, although to maximize the benefits of high O_2 MAP, it is desirable to maintain headspace levels of O_2 > 40% and CO_2 in the range of 10–25% during the cold storage of the produce (Hartley, 2000). With respect to PPO, the key enzyme primarily responsible for initiating discoloration on the cut surfaces of prepared produce and occurrence of colored melanine-type compounds, its activity can be inhibited by high O_2 through a feedback product inhibition (Day, 2002).

The experimental finding that high O_2 MAP is capable of inhibiting aerobic and anaerobic microbial growth can be explained by the growth profiles of aerobic and anaerobic microorganisms depending on the O_2 concentration in the surrounding atmosphere. Thus, at normal air atmosphere (21%), the growth rates of aerobic microorganisms are maxima and the enrichment of the atmosphere in O_2 leads to significant reduction. On the contrary, the growth rate of anaerobic microorganisms decreases as the percentage of O_2 increases in the atmosphere. It is hypothesized that ROS damage vital cellular macromolecules and thereby inhibit microbial growth when oxidative stresses overwhelm cellular protection systems. High levels of O_2, however, may lead to an enhanced formation of the superoxide anion (O^{2-}) inside cells, which is a highly reactive and destructive radical. The superoxide anion can be scavenged by SOD, an enzyme present in all aerobic organisms, which catalyses the conversion of superoxide into hydrogen peroxide and molecular oxygen.

Day (2002) studied a wide range of vegetables stored under high O_2 MAP, and for most prepared produce items, under defined storage and packaging conditions, high O_2 MAP was found to have beneficial effects on sensory quality in comparison with industry-standard air packing and low O_2 MAP. Thus, high O_2 MAP is effective for extending the shelf life of fresh cut iceberg lettuce, mushrooms, broccoli florets, baby-leaf spinach, parsley, raspberries, strawberries, grapes, and oranges, among others. Another important effect of high O_2 MAP was the inhibition of some spoilage and pathogenic microorganisms, such as *Aeromonas hydrophila*, *Salmonella enteritidis*, *Pseudomonas putida*, *R. stolonifer*, *B. cinerea*, *P. digitatum*, and *A. niger*, but failed in the control of *Pseudomonas fragi*, *B. cereus*, *Lactobacillus sake*, *Yersinia enterocolitica*, and *Listeria monocytogenes*. Accordingly, a combination of 80% oxygen and 20% carbon dioxide resulted in reduced growth of *R. stolonifer*, *B. cinerea*, and *P. discolor* compared with ambient atmosphere conditions when inoculated in Petri dishes (Hoogerwerf et al., 2002).

These authors state that novel high O_2 MAP has the potential to maintain the quality and ensure the microbial safety of fresh-cut products, although the commercial implementation and success of this new technology may encourage greater consumption of conveniently packed fresh prepared produce and help toward improving the health and well-being of consumers. In addition, further research on the effects of high O_2 MAP on the various spoilage and pathogenic microorganisms associated with fresh prepared produce items is necessary. Also, how high O_2 MAP affects the nutritive and bioactive compounds needs to be investigated, as well as how the potential synergy of high O_2 MAP and other active packaging devices will increase the availability of new packages to extend the shelf life of fresh commodities.

11.3 Biological control

As stated in Chapter 3 (Section 3.8), vegetable products are very sensitive to postharvest losses mainly due to decay incidence, which can be accelerated with the presence of wounds present on the plant organs during storage, often as a result of harvesting and transportation, which give microorganisms easy access. In recent years, great efforts have been made to find alternative tools to chemical fungicides since consumers are concerned about the safety of the fruits they eat, and they desire foods free from pesticide residues, toxins, and harmful microorganisms. The emerging technologies for the control of postharvest fungal diseases are essentially application of antagonistic microorganisms, application of natural antimicrobial substances, and application of sanitizing products. One of these alternatives has been the use of biological control or biocontrol. Biological control fits in well with the concept of sustainable agriculture because it mostly exploits natural microorganism cycles with reduced environmental impact. Among the biological strategies applicable to postharvest, the use of antagonistic microorganisms can be considered. Biocontrol using antagonists has proved to be one of the most promising alternatives, either alone or as part of an integrated pest management policy to reduce pesticide use (Spadaro and Gullino, 2004), through the exploitation of naturally occurring organisms, such as bacteria, viruses, and fungi, for the control of crop pests, weeds, and diseases.

Wilson and Pusey published a featured article in which they presented their ideas on the potential of postharvest biocontrol and discussed their use of a strain of *Bacillus subtilis* to control brown rot on peach, caused by *Monilinia fructicola* (Pusey and Wilson, 1984; Wilson and Pusey, 1985). After these first studies on biocontrol of postharvest disease appeared over 20 years ago, substantial progress has been achieved since then. Janisiewicz and Korsten (2002) presented an overview of biological control of postharvest diseases with antagonists describing the success and limitations of biocontrol agents under laboratory and semi-commercial conditions. Although commercial products have been registered by the early 2000s (Aspire™, *C. oleophila*, limited to the United States and Israel; BioSave™, *P. syringae*, limited to the United States) and many programs are currently under way worldwide to develop new antagonists biological control, this technology is not still routinely applied in the postharvest phase. In general, microbial antagonists are used as aqueous cell suspensions in postharvest spray, drench, or dip applications. The main reasons are based on the insufficient and inconsistent performance of biological control agents, the difficulty in obtaining an adequate formulation, and finally the difficulty in controlling rot caused by latent infections (Mari et al., 2007). More recently, attempts have been made to examine the field of postharvest biocontrol as it has developed over the past 20 years, define the reasons that have limited its commercialization, and identify areas of research that need to be addressed if the potential of postharvest biocontrol is to be achieved (Droby et al., 2009).

Spadaro and Gullino (2004) reviewed the main agents that are currently assayed as antagonist microorganisms including *Pseudomonas syringae* Van Hall, which are active against the genera *Botrytis, Penicillium, Mucor,* and *Geotrichum*. The yeast *Candida oleophila* Montrocher was found effective against *Botrytis* and *Penicillium* spp., while other yeasts such as *Aureobasidium pullulans, Candida saitoana, Candida sake,* and *Metschnikowia pulcherrima* are under development. It is important that evaluation of these microorganisms is carried out in a product formulation, since the formulation may improve or diminish antagonistic efficacy depending on the concentration of and the duration of exposure to the treatment.

The common mechanism of biocontrol among antagonists appears to be competition for nutrients and space, but other mechanisms may also be involved including production of antifungal metabolites, direct parasitism, and induced resistance sometimes associated with reduction of pathogen enzyme activity (Janisiewicz and Korsten, 2002). More than one mechanism was found to be implicated in biological control, but for each particular case a sole mechanism is involved. However, the exact mechanisms of action for most of the antagonists investigated are still incomplete because of the difficulties encountered during the study of the complex interactions between host, pathogen, antagonist, and other microorganisms present. This information is therefore necessary before developing appropriate formulations and methods of application and in order to obtain official approval.

Competition for nutrients and space seems to play a major role for controlling fungal pathogens, especially when yeasts are using as biocontrol agents. Yeasts act mainly competing for space or for the utilization of some nutrients with the pathogen and inhibiting its growth but leaving it alive (Spadaro and Gullino, 2004). In the competition for space, yeasts are helped by the formation of an extracellular polysaccharide capsule that can promote adhesion to the fruit surface. The biocontrol activity of microbial antagonists with most harvested commodities increased with the increasing concentrations of antagonists and decreasing concentrations of pathogen. This quantitative relationship, however, is highly dependent on the ability of the antagonists to multiply and grow at the wound site (Sharma et al., 2009).

There is little about the direct parasitism of the microbial antagonists in controlling postharvest diseases of fruits and vegetables. However, *Pichia guilliermondii* cells had the ability to attach to the hyphae of *B. cinerea* and *Penicillium* and induce partial degradation of the cell wall of *B. cinerea*. Thus, strong attachment of microbial antagonist with enhanced activity of cell wall degradation enzymes may be responsible for enhancing the efficacy of microbial agents in controlling the postharvest diseases of fruits and vegetables. In addition, attachment of the microbial antagonists to a site enhances their potential activity for the utilization of nutrients at the invasion site, avoiding the access of the pathogen to nutrients (El-Ghaouth et al., 2004).

With respect to antifungal production, some of the most active biocontrol agents are bacteria producing antibiotics, whose action, at least partially, determines their effectiveness. Thus, *B. subtilis* produces iturin, a powerful antifungal peptide, as well as gramicidin S (Edwards and Seddon, 2001). The main concern, related to the use of antibiotics in food products, is the development of human pathogens resistant to these compounds and the possible development of resistance in fruit pathogens. Even if antibiotic producers appear to be able to control wound infections established before antagonist application, at the moment, there are not such biological agents registered for use on fruit.

Related to induced resistance, peach inoculated with *Cryptococcus laurentii* as antagonist markedly induced activities of PPO, POX, and SOD during storage at 0 or 20°C, the increase in PPO being postulated as having a key role in the defense system at ambient temperature while during cold storage was related to CI (Wang et al., 2004).

The degree of control obtained by these microorganisms alone is often not satisfactory, so the addition of additives or chemical fungicides at low rates can enhance biocontrol activity and reduce the population of antagonist required to achieve effective control. Several methods have been reported to increase the antagonistic activity of yeasts and inhibit pathogenic infections, and thus enhancement of the biocontrol activity of antagonists could be obtained by many approaches. One example is the use of bicarbonate salts that have shown broad-spectrum antimicrobial properties for controlling postharvest pathogens. Accordingly, the addition of 2% (w/v) sodium bicarbonate in the suspensions of antagonistic yeasts *Cryptococcus laurentii* or *Trichosporon pullulans* against postharvest decay caused by *P. expansum* and *A. alternata* in pear fruits was significantly increased (Yao et al., 2004). The inhibitory effect of bicarbonate salts on postharvest pathogens is probably due to the reduction of fungal cell turgor pressure that results in collapse and shrinkage of hyphae and spores, and consequent inability of fungi to sporulate.

Taking into account the hurdle technology, the integrated heat treatment, biocontrol, and sodium bicarbonate were effective to reduce postharvest decay of apple caused by *Colletotrichum acutatum* and *P. expansum* (Conway et al., 2004). Thus, the need for finding suitable alternatives to fungicides to control postharvest decay has prompted research aimed at combining various alternatives into a control strategy that equals the effectiveness of synthetic chemicals. The ideal strategy would eradicate any pathogens present at the time of treatment and protect the commodity from further infection. In this sense, combinations of hot water dips, biological control, and controlled atmosphere storage decreased the gray mold growth on harvested strawberries (Wszelaki and Mitcham, 2003), although benefits were only obtained for a short period of time (2–20 days).

In some cases, pathogens attack fruits and vegetables in the field, and these latent infections become major factors for decay during transportation or storage of fruits and vegetables. Therefore, preharvest applications of microbial antagonistic culture are often effective to control postharvest decay of fruits and vegetables. Biological control has been also applied at preharvest to reduce the microbial spoilage on postharvest. Thus, the yeasts *Trichosporon pullulans*, *Cryptococcus laurentii*, and *Rhodotorula glutinis* were sprayed at a concentration of 1×10^8 CFU/mL onto sweet cherry fruit prior to harvest. Among the three yeasts, *C. laurentii* was the most effective antagonist for control of postharvest decay of sweet cherry, which could survive at high, relatively stable population levels on the surface of sweet cherry fruit under field conditions (Tian et al., 2004). The purpose of preharvest application is to precolonize the fruit surface with an antagonist immediately before harvest so that wounds inflicted during harvesting can be colonized by the antagonist before colonization by a pathogen, although this approach could not become commercially viable, because of poor survival of microbial antagonists in the field conditions (Sharma et al., 2009).

In conclusion, some significant progress has been made toward biological and integrated control of postharvest diseases on fruits. Some biological agents are already on the market in a few countries and will probably become more widely available as they are registered in more areas. However, biological control alone is not enough to gain a complete control of fungal diseases and is not as effective as pesticides. At the moment, biological control should be viewed as an important if not essential component of integrated disease management, although the use of microbial antagonists for the control of postharvest diseases of fruits and vegetables will be greatly expanded in the future and will definitely become an internationally adopted practice. In addition, registration is required by regulatory agencies (e.g., Environmental Protection Agency [EPA], and European agencies) before any biocontrol agent can be used commercially.

11.4 UV-irradiation

Ultraviolet (UV) light is used in the food industry for disinfecting surfaces, and apart from this use, there are relatively few applications of this technology in the food processing industry. The restricted range of commercially available equipment for disinfecting solids may contribute to its limited use. UV radiation is classified according to wavelength: UV-A, also known as near-ultraviolet radiation, ranges from 315 to 400 nm; UV-B, mid-range UV, from 280 to 315 nm; and UVC, far-UV, from 100 to 280 nm. In the following discussion, UV in general refers to UV-C, since most studies were performed with this range of radiation. Low doses of UV-C radiation (254 nm) elicit the resistance of fruits against pathogens and reduce decay of a wide array of fruits and vegetables when applied after harvest (Ben-Yehoshua, 2003).

Early studies of the ability of low doses of UV-C radiation to induce disease resistance in citrus fruits were reported (Rodov et al., 1992). They showed that the major effect of UV-C was not germicidal, since fruits inoculated after UV treatment were more resistant to pathogen invasion than those inoculated before the treatment, and the latter exhibited similar decay to that of the untreated fruits. Furthermore, these studies demonstrated that UV irradiation that inhibited decay of inoculated citrus fruits elicited the synthesis of the phytoalexins scoparone and scopoletin, and that UV irradiation induced the production of a new layer of lignin-like compounds on the fruit peel.

Some recent application of UV light has been in fresh-cut produce as sanitation procedure. The use of nonionizing, germicidal, and artificial ultraviolet light at a wavelength of 190–280 nm (UV-C) could be effective for surface decontamination of fresh-cut produce. The effectiveness of UV-C seems to be independent of the temperature in the range of 5–37°C but depends on the incident irradiation, as determined by the structure and surface of treated produce. Treatment with ultraviolet energy offers several advantages to food processors as it does not leave any residue, does not have legal restrictions, is easy to use and lethal to most types of microorganisms, and does not require extensive safety equipment to be implemented (Artés et al., 2009).

The use of UV as a postharvest treatment for fruits is permissible in the major fruit-producing countries, but further, commercial-scale studies of the effects of UV irradiation on each cultivar are still needed. This could indicate whether decay can be reduced without damage in large-scale operations. The crucial point is whether a safe dose can be found which would greatly impair pathogen growth without damaging the product (Ben-Yehoshua and Mercier, 2005). It must be borne in mind that UV radiation by itself, unlike the most effective chemical fungicides, does not prevent decay completely.

References

Abdi, N., Holford, P., McGlasson, W.B., and Mizrahi, Y. (1997). Ripening behaviour and responses to propylene in four cultivars of Japanese type plums. *Postharvest Biology and Technology*, 12, 21–34.

Abdi, N., McGlasson, W.B., Holford, P., Williams, M., and Mizrahi, Y. (1998). Responses of climacteric and suppressed-climacteric plums to treatment with propylene and 1-methylcyclopropene. *Postharvest Biology and Technology*, 14, 29–39.

Abeles, F.B., Morgan, P.W., and Saltveit, M.E. (1992). *Ethylene in Plant Biology*. San Diego: Academic Press.

Abu-Kpawoh, J.C., Xi, Y.E., Zhang, Y.Z., and Jin, Y.F. (2002). Polyamine accumulation following hot-water dips influences chilling injury and decay in "Friar" plum fruit. *Journal of Food Science*, 67, 2649–2653.

Acked, J. (2002). Maintaining the post-harvest quality of fruits and vegetables. In *Fruit and Vegetable* Processing, ed. W. Jongem, 121–149. Abington: Woodhead Publishing Limited.

Adams-Phillips, L., Barry, C., and Giovannoni, J. (2004). Signal transduction systems regulating fruit ripening. *Trends in Plant Science*, 9, 331–338.

Agar, I.T., Massantini, R., Hess-Pierce, B., and Kader, A.A. (1999). Postharvest CO_2 and ethylene production and quality maintenance of fresh-cut kiwifruit slices. *Journal of Food Science*, 64, 433–440.

Agriculture and Agri-Food Canada. (2000). *Produce Handler's Guide*, Dept. of Agriculture and marketing, Halifax, Nova Scotia.

Aguayo, E., Escalona, V.H., and Artés, F. (2008). Effect of hot water treatment and various calcium salts on quality of fresh-cut "Amarillo" melon. *Postharvest Biology and Technology*, 47, 397–406.

Agustí, M., Juan, M., Martínez-Fuentes, A., Mesejo, C., and Almela, V. (2004). Calcium nitrite delays climacteric of persimmon fruit. *Annals of Applied Biology*, 144, 65–69.

Ahmedna, M., Marshall, W.E., and Rao, R.M. (2000). Production of granular activated carbons from select agricultural by-products and evaluation of their physical, chemical and adsorption properties. *Bioresource Technology*, 71,113–123.

Akbudak, B., and Eris, A. (2004). Physical and chemical changes in peaches and nectarines during the modified atmosphere storage. *Food Control*, 15, 307–313.

Al-Ati T., and Hotchkiss J.H. (2003). The role of packaging film permselectivity in modified atmosphere packaging. *Journal of Agricultural and Food Chemistry*, 51, 4133–4138.

Alandes, L., Quiles, A., Pérez-Munuera, I., and Hernando, I. (2009). Improving the quality of fresh-cut apples, pears, and melons using natural additives. *Journal of Food Science*, 74, 590–596.

Albertini, M.E., Carcouet, E., Pailly, O., Gambotti, C., Luro, F., and Berti, L. (2006). Changes in organic acids and sugars during early stages of development of acidic and acidless Citrus fruits. *Journal of Agricultural and Food Chemistry*, 54, 8335–8339.

Alburquerque, N., Egea, J., Burgos, L., Martínez-Romero, D., Valero, D. and Serrano, M. (2006). The influence of polyamines on apricot ovary development and fruit set. *Annals of Applied Biology*, 149, 27–33.

Alcaraz-López, C., Botia, M., Alcaraz, F. and Riquelme, F. (2003). Effects of foliar sprays containing calcium, magnesium and titanium on plum (*Prunus domestica* L) fruit quality. *Journal of Plant Physiology*, 160, 1441–1446.

Alique, R., Zamorano, J.P., Martínez, A. and Alonso, J. (2005). Effect of heat and cold treatments on respiratory metabolism and shelf-life of sweet cherry, type picota cv "Ambrunés". *Postharvest Biology and Technology*, 35, 153–165.

Amorós, A., Pretel, M.T., Zapata, P.J., Botella, M.A., Romojaro, F., and Serrano, M. (2008). Use of modified atmosphere packaging with microperforated polypropylene films to maintain postharvest loquat quality. *Food Science and Technology International*, 14, 95–103.

Amorós, A., Zapata, P., Pretel, M.T., Botella, M.A. and Serrano, M. (2003). Physico-chemical and physiological changes during fruit development and ripening of five loquat (*Eriobotrya japonica* Lindl.) cultivars. *Food Science Technology International*, 9, 43–49.

Appendini, P., and Hotchkiss, J. H. (2002). Review of antimicrobial food packaging. *Innovative Food Science and Emerging Technology*, 3, 113–126.

Argenta, L.C., Fan, X.T., and Mattheis, J.P. (2003). Influence of 1-methylcyclopropene on ripening, storage life, and volatile production by d'Anjou cv. pear fruit. *Journal of Agricultural and Food Chemistry*, 51, 3858–3864.

Arias, M., Carbonell, J., and Agustí, M. (2005). Endogenous free polyamines and their role in fruit set of low and high parthenocarpic ability citrus cultivars. *Journal of Plant Physiology*, 162, 845–853.

Arora, D.S., and Kaur, J. (1999). Antimicrobial activity of spices. *International Journal of Antimicrobial Agents*, 12, 257–262.

Artés, F., Conesa, M.A., Hernández, S., and Gil, M.I. (1999). Keeping quality of fresh-cut tomato. *Postharvest Biology and Technology*, 17, 153–162.

Artés, F., Gómez, P.A., Aguayo, E., Escalona, V., and Artés-Hernández, F. (2009). Sustainable sanitation techniques for keeping quality and safety of fresh-cut plant commodities. *Postharvest Biology and Technology*, 51, 287–296.

Artés, F., Gómez, P.A., and Artés-Hernández, F. (2006). Modified atmosphere packaging of fruits and vegetables. *Stewart Postharvest Review*, 5:2.

Artés, F., Gómez, P.A., and Artés-Hernández, F. (2007). Physical, physiological and microbial deterioration of minimally fresh processed fruits and vegetables. *Food Science and Technology International*, 13, 177–188.

Artés, F., Sánchez, E., and Tijskens, L.M.M. (1998). Quality and shelf life of tomatoes improved by intermittent warming. *Lebensmittel Wissenschaft und-Technologie*, 31, 427–431.

Artés, F., Tudela, J.A., and Villaescusa, R. (2000). Thermal postharvest treatment for improving pomegranate quality and shelf life. *Postharvest Biology and Technology*, 18, 245–251.

Artés-Hernández, F., Tomas-Barberán, F.A., and Artés, F. (2006). Modified atmosphere packaging preserves quality of SO_2-free "Superior seedless" table grapes. *Postharvest Biology and Technology*, 39, 146–154.

Arvanitoyanni, I.S., and Mavromastis, A. (2009). Banana cultivars, cultivation practices, and physicochemical properties. *Critical Reviews in Food Science and Nutrition*, 49, 113–135.

Aubert, C., and Bourger, N. (2004). Investigation of volatiles in charentais cantaloupe melons (*Cucumis melo* Var. cantalupensis). Characterization of aroma constituents in some cultivars. *Journal of Agricultural and Food Chemistry*, 52, 4522–4528.

Aubert, C., and Chanforan, C. (2007). Postharvest changes in physicochemical properties and volatile constituents of apricot (*Prunus armeniaca* L.) characterization of 28 cultivars. *Journal of Agricultural and Food Chemistry*, 55, 3074–3082.

Aubert, C., Günata, Z., Ambid, C., and Baumes, R. (2003). Changes in physicochemical characteristics and volatile constituents of yellow- and white-fleshed nectarines during maturation and artificial ripening. *Journal of Agricultural and Food Chemistry*, 51, 3083–3091.

Aygün, A., Yenisoy-Karakaş, S., and Duman, I. (2003). Production of granular activated carbon from fruit stones and nutshells and evaluation of their physical, chemical and adsorption properties. *Microporous and Mesoporous Materials*, 66, 189–195.

Aziz, A., Brun, O., and Audran, J.C. (2001). Involvement of polyamines in the control of fruilet physiological abscission in grapevine (*Vitis vinifera*). *Physiologia Plantarum*, 113, 50–58.

Bagamboula, C. F., Uyttendaele, M., and Debevere, J. (2004). Inhibitory effect of thyme and basil essential oils, carvacrol, thymol, estragol, linalool and p-cymene towards *Shigella sonnei* and *S. flexneri*. *Food Microbiology*, 21, 33–42.

Bailén, G., Guillén, F., Castillo, S., Serrano, M., Valero, D., and Martínez-Romero, D. (2006). Use of activated carbon inside modified atmosphere packaging to maintain tomato fruit quality during cold storage. *Journal of Agricultural and Food Chemistry*, 54, 2229–2235.

Bailén, G., Guillén, F., Castillo, S., Zapata, P.J., Serrano, M., Valero, D., and Martínez-Romero, D. (2007). Use of a palladium catalyst to improve the capacity of activated carbon to absorb ethylene, and its effect on tomato ripening. *Spanish Journal of Agricultural Research*, 5, 579–586.

Bakshi, P., Masoodi, F.A., Chauhan, G.S., and Shah, T.A. (2005). Role of calcium in post-harvest life of temperate fruits: A review. *Journal of Food Science and Technology*, 42, 1–8.

Baldwin, E.A., Plotto, A., and Goodner, K. (2007). Shelf-life versus flavour-life for fruits and vegetables: How to evaluate this complex trait. *Stewart Postharvest Review*, 1, 1–10.

Bardocz, S., Duguid, T.J., Brown, D.S., Grant, G., Pusztai, A., White, A., and Ralph, A. (1995). The importance of dietary polyamines in cell regeneration and growth. *British Journal of Nutrition*, 73, 819–828.

Barkai-Golan, R. (2001). *Postharvest Diseases of Fruits and Vegetables. Development and Control*. Amsterdam: Elsevier Science.

Barry, C. and Giovannoni, J. (2007). Ethylene and fruit ripening. *Journal of Plant Growth Regulation*, 26, 143–159.

Basiouny, F.M. (1996). Blueberry fruit quality and storability influenced by postharvest application of polyamines and heat treatments. *Proceeding of the Florida State Horticultural Society*, 109, 269–272.

Beaudry, R.M. (1999). Effect of O_2 and CO_2 partial pressure on selected phenomena affecting fruit and vegetable quality. *Postharvest Biology and Technology*, 15, 293–303.

Beaudry, R.M. (2000). Responses of horticultural commodities to oxygen: Limits to the expended use of modified atmosphere packaging. *HortTechnology* 10, 491–500.

Becker, B.R., and Fricke, B.A. (2002). Hydrocooling time stimation methods. *International Communications in Heat and Mass Transfer*, 29, 165–174.

Beirão-da-Costa, S., Steiner, A., Correia, L., Empis, J., and Moldão-Martins, M. (2006). Effects of maturity stage and mild heat treatments on quality of minimally processed kiwifruit. *Journal of Food Engineering*. 76, 616–625.

Benedetti, S., Buratti, S., Spinardi, A., Mannino, S., and Mignani, I. (2008). Electronic nose as a non-destructive tool to characterise peach cultivars and to monitor their ripening stage during shelf-life. *Postharvest Biology and Technology*, 47, 181–188.

Bennett, A.B., and Labavitch, J.M. (2008). Ethylene and ripening-regulated expression and function of fruit cell wall modifying proteins. *Plant Science*, 175, 130–136.

Beno-Moualem, D., Gusev, L., Dvir, O., Pesis, E., Meir, S., and Lichter, A. (2004). The effects of ethylene, methyl jasmonate and 1-MCP on abscission of cherry tomatoes from the bunch and expression of endo-1,4-beta-glucanases. *Plant Science*, 167, 499–507.

Ben-Yehoshua, S. (1987). Transpiration, water stress and gas exchange. In *Postharvest Physiology of Vegetables*, ed. J. Weichmann, 113–170. New York: Marcel Dekker.

Ben-Yehoshua, S. (2003). Effects of postharvest heat and UV applications on decay, chilling injury and resistance against pathogens of citrus and other fruits and vegetables. *Acta Horticulturae*, 599, 159–173.

Ben-Yehoshua, S., and Mercier, J. (2005). UV irradiation, biological agents, and natural compounds for controlling postharvest decay in fresh fruits and vegetables. In *Environmentally Friendly Technologies for Agricultural Produce Quality*, ed. S. Ben-Yehoshua, 265–299. Boca Raton: Taylor and Francis.

Ben-Yehoshua, S., and Porat, R. (2005). Heat treatments to reduce decay. In *Environmentally Friendly Technologies for Agricultural Produce Quality*, ed. S. Ben-Yehoshua, 11–42. Boca Raton: Taylor and Francis.

Berüter, J. (2004). Carbohydrate metabolism in two apple genotypes that differ in malate accumulation. *Journal of Plant Physiology*, 161, 1011–1029.

Besada, C., Arnal, L., and Salvador, A. (2008). Improving storability of persimmon cv. Rojo Brillante by combined use of preharvest and postharvest treatments. *Postharvest Biology and Technology*, 50, 169–175.

Binder, B.M. (2008). The ethylene receptors: Complex perception for a simple gas. *Plant Science*, 175, 8–17.

Birtic, S., Ginies, C., Causse, M., Renard, C.M.G.C., and Page, D. (2009). Changes in volatiles and glycosides during fruit maturation of two contrasted tomato (*Solanum lycopersicum*) lines. *Journal of Agricultural and Food Chemistry*, 57, 591–598.

Blankenship, S.M., and Dole, J. M. (2003). 1-Methylcyclopropene: A review. *Postharvest Biology and Technology*, 28, 1–25.

Bleecker, A.B., and Kende, H. (2000). Ethylene: a gaseous signal molecule in plants. *Annual Review of Cell and Developmental Biology*, 16, 1–18.

Bollen, A.F., Woodhead, I.M., and Dela Rue, B.T. (1995). Compression forces and damage in the postharvest handling system, In *Harvest and Postharvest Technologies for Fresh Fruits and Vegetables*, ed. L. Kushwada, R. Serwatowski, and R. Brook, 168–175. Guanajuato: ASAE.

Bourne, M.C. (1980). Texture evaluation of horticultural crops. *HortScience*, 15, 51–56.

Brady, C.J. (1987). Fruit ripening. *Annual Review of Plant Physiology*, 38, 155–178.

Bregoli, A.M., Scaramagli, S., Costa, G., Sabatini, E., Ziosi, V., Biondi, S., and Torrigiani, P. (2002). Peach (*Prunus persica*) fruit ripening: Aminoetoxyvinilglycine (AVG) and exogenous polyamines affect ethylene emission and flesh firmness. *Physiologia Plantarum*, 114, 472–481.

Bregoli, A.M., Ziosi, V., Biondi, S., Rasori, A., Ciccioni, M., Costa, G., and Torrigiani, P. (2005). Postharvest 1-methylcyclopropene application in ripening control of "Stark Red Gold" nectarines: temperature-dependent effects on ethylene production and biosynthetic gene expression, fruit quality, and polyamine levels. *Postharvest Biology and Technology*, 37, 111–121.

Brody A.L. (2005). What's fresh about fresh-cut. *Food Technology*, 59, 74–77.

Brosnan, T., and Sun, D.W. (2001). Precooling techniques and applications for horticultural products: A review. *International Journal of Refrigeration*, 24, 154–170.

Brownleader, M.D., Lackson, P., Mobasheri, A., Pantelides, A.T., Sumar, S., Trevan, M., and Dey, P.M. (1999). Molecular aspects of cell wall modifications during fruit ripening. *Critical Reviews in Food Science and Nutrition*, 39, 149–164.

Brummell, D.A. (2006). Cell wall disassembly in ripening fruit. *Functional Plant Biology*, 33, 103–119.

Brummell, D.A., and Harpster, M.H. (2001). Cell wall metabolism in fruit softening and quality and its manipulation in transgenic plants. *Plant Molecular Biology*, 47, 311–340.

Burns, J.K. (2008). 1-Methylcyclopropene applications in preharvest systems: Focus on Citrus. *HortScience*, 43, 112–114.

Burns, J.K., Roka, F.M., Li, K.T., Pozo, L., and Buker, R.S. (2006). Late-season "Valencia" orange mechanical harvesting with an abscission agent and low-frequency harvesting. *HortScience*, 41, 660–663.

Burt, S. (2004). Essential oils: their antibacterial properties and potential applications in foods-a review. *International Journal of Food Microbiology*, 94, 223–253.

Burton, C.L., and Schulte-Paso, N.L. (1987). Carbon dioxide as an indicator of fruit impact damage. *HortScience* 22, 281–282.

Candan, A.P., Graell, J., and Larrigaudière, C. (2008). Roles of climacteric ethylene in the development of chilling injury in plums. *Postharvest Biology and Technology*, 47, 107–112.

Cantos, E., Espín, J.C., and Tomás-Barberán, F.A. (2002). Varietal differences among the polyphenol profiles of seven table grape cultivars studied by LC-DAD-MS-MS. *Journal of Agricultural and Food Chemistry*, 50, 5691–5696.

Cantu, D., Vicente, A.R., Greve, L.C., Dewey, F.M., Bennet, A.B., Labavitch, J.M., and Powell, A.L.T. (2009). The intersection between cell wall disassembly, ripening, and fruit susceptibility to *Botrytis cinerea*. *Proceedings of the National Academy of Sciences*, 105, 859–864.

Cara, B., and Giovannoni, J.J. (2008). Molecular biology of ethylene during tomato fruit development and maturation. *Plant Science*, 175, 106–113.

Carpita, N.C., and Gibeaut, D.M. (1993). Structural models of primary cell walls in flowering plants: Consistency of molecular structure with the physical properties of the walls during growth. *The Plant Journal*, 3, 1–30.

Carpita, N.C., and McCann, M. (2000). The cell wall. In *Biochemistry and Molecular Biology of Plants*, eds. B.B. Buchanan, W. Gruissem and R.L. Jones, 52–108. Rockville: American Society of Plant Biologist.

Carreño, J., Almela, L., Martínez, A., and Fernández-López, J.A. (1997). Chemotaxonomical classification of red table grapes based on anthocyanin profile and external colour. *Lebensmittel Wissenschaft und-Technologie*, 30, 256–265.

Cartea, M.E., and Velasco, P. (2008). Glucosinolates in *Brassica* foods: Bioavailability in food and significance for human health. *Phytochemistry Reviews*, 7, 213–229.

Cascales, A.I., Costell, E., and Romojaro, F. (2005). Effects of the degree of maturity on the chemical composition, physical characteristics and sensory attributes of peach (*Prunus persica*) cv. Caterin. *Food Science Technology International*, 11, 345–352.

Castañeda-Ovando, A., Pacheco-Hernández, M.L., Páez-Hernández, M.E., Rodríguez, J.A., and Galán-Vidal, A. (2009). Chemical studies of anthocyanins: A review. *Food Chemistry*, 113, 859–871.

Cevallos-Casals, B.A., Byrne, D., Okie, W.R., and Cisneros-Zevallos, L. (2006). Selecting new peach and plum genotypes rich in phenolic compounds and enhanced functional properties. *Food Chemistry*, 96, 273–280.

Cha, D.S., and Chinnan, M.S. (2004). Biopolymer-based antimicrobial packaging: A review. *Critical Review in Food Science and Nutrition*, 44, 223–237.

Chang, C., and Bleecker, A.B. (2004). Ethylene biology: More than a gas. *Plant Physiology*, 136, 2895–2899.

Chaovanalikit, A., and Wrolstad, R. E. (2004). Total anthocyanin and total phenolics of fresh and processed cherries and their antioxidant properties. *Journal of Food Science*, 69, FCT67-FCT72.

Chardonnet, C.O., Charron, C.S., Sam, C.E., and Conway, W.S. (2003). Chemical changes in the cortical tissue and cell wall of calcium-infiltrated "Golden Delicious" apples during cold storage. *Postharvest Biology and Technology*, 28, 97–111.

Chéour, F., Willemot, C., Arul, J., Desjardins, Y., Makhlouf, Y., Charrest, J., and Gosselin, A. (1990). Foliar application of calcium chloride delays postharvest ripening of strawberry. *Journal of the American Society for Horticultural Science*, 115, 789–792.

Cho, Y.S., Yeum, K.J., Chen, C.Y., Beretta, G., Tang, G., Krinsky, N.Y., Yoon, S., Lee-Kim, Y.C., Blumberg, J.B., and Russell, R.M. (2007). Phytonutrients affecting hydrophilic and lipophilic antioxidant activities in fruits, vegetables and legumes. *Journal of the Science of Food and Agriculture*, 87, 1096–1107.

Cipolla, B.G., Havouis, R., and Moulinoux, J.P. (2007). Polyamine contents in current foods: A basis for polyamine reduced diet and a study of its long term observance and tolerance in prostate carcinoma patients. *Amino Acids*, 33, 203–212.

Commission Decision of 23 January 2002 amending Commission Decision 1999/217/EC as regards the register of flavouring substances used in or on foodstuffs. 2002/113/EC: Official Journal L49 20/02/2002, pp. 1–160.

Cona, A., Rea, G., Angelini, R., Federico, R., and Tavladoraki, P. (2006). Functions of amino oxidases in plant development and defence. *Trends in Plant Science*, 11, 80–88.

Connor, A.M., Luby, J.J., Hancock, J.F., Berkheimer, S., and Hanson, E.J. (2002). *Journal of Agricultural and Food Chemistry*, 50, 893–898.

Conway, W.S., Janisiewiez, W.J., Klein, J.D., and Sams, C.E. (1999). Strategy of combining heat treatment, calcium infiltration, and biological control to reduce postharvest decay of "Gala" apples. *HortScience*, 34, 700–704.

Conway, W.S., Leverentz, B., Janisiewicz, W.J., Blodgett, A.B., Saftner, R.A., and Camp, M.J. (2004). Integrating heat treatment, biocontrol and sodium bicarbonate to reduce postharvest decay of apple caused by *Colletotrichum acutatum* and *Penicillium expansum*. *Postharvest Biology and Technology*, 34, 1–20.

Conway, W.S., Sams, C.E., Wang, C.Y., and Abbott, J.A. (1994). Additive effects of postharvest calcium and heat treatment on reducing decay and maintaining quality in apples. *Journal of the American Society for Horticultural Science*, 119, 49–53.

Cosgrove, D.J. (2001). Wall structure and wall loosening: A look backwards and forwards. *Plant Physiology*, 125, 131–134.

Cowan, M. M. (1999). Plant products as antimicrobial agents. *Clinical Microbiology Reviews*, 12, 564–582.

Crisosto, C.H., Crisosto, G.M., and Metheney, P. (2003). Consumer acceptance of "Brooks" and "Bing" cherries is mainly dependent on fruit SSC and visual skin color. *Postharvest Biology and Technology*, 28, 159–167.

Crisosto, C.H., Crisosto, G.M., and Ritenour, M.A. (2002). Testing the reliability of skin color as an indicator of quality for early season "Brooks" (*Prunus avium* L.) cherry. *Postharvest Biology and Technology*, 24, 147–154.

Crisosto, C.H., Day, K.R., Johnson, R.S., and Garner, D. (2000). Influence of in-season foliar calcium sprays on fruit quality and surface discoloration incidence of peaches and nectarines. *Fruits Varieties Journal*, 54, 118–122.

Crisosto, C.H., Mitchell, F.G., and Ju, Z. (1999). Susceptibility to chilling injury of peach, nectarine and plum cultivars grown in California. *HortScience*, 34, 1116–1118.

Crisosto, G.M., Crisosto, C.H., Echeverría, G., and Puy, J. (2007). Segregation of plum and pluot cultivars according to their organoleptic characteristics. *Postharvest Biology and Technology*, 44, 271–276.

Cristescu, S.M., De Martinis, D., Hekkert, S.L., Parker, D.H., and Harren, F.J.M. (2002). Ethylene production by *Botrytis cinerea in vitro* and in tomatoes. *Applied Environmental Microbiology*, 68, 5342–5350.

Cronje, R.B., Sivakumar, D., Mostert, P.G., and Korsten, L. (2009). Effect of different preharvest treatment regimes on fruit quality of litchi cultivar "Maritius". *Journal of Plant Nutrition*, 32, 19–29.

Daayf, F., and Lattancio, V. (2008). *Recent Advances in Polyphenol Research*. Chinchester: Blackwell Publishing Ltd.

Dąbrowski, A. (2001). Adsorption-from theory to practise. *Advances in Colloid Interface Science*, 93, 135–224.

Dang, K.T.H., Singh, Z., and Swinny, E.E. (2008). Impact of postharvest disease control methods and cold storage on volatiles, color development and fruit quality in ripe "Kensington Pride" mangoes. *Journal of Agricultural and Food Chemistry*, 56, 10667–10674.

D'Aquino, S., Palma, A., Fronteddu, F., and Tedde, M. (2005). Effect of preharvest and postharvest calcium treatments on chilling injury and decay of cold stored Fortune mandarins. *Acta Horticulturae*, 682, 631–637.

Davey, M.W., Montagu, M.V., Inzé, D., Sanmartin, M., Kanellis, A., Smirnoff, N., Benzie, I.J., Strain, J.J., and Favell, D. (2000). Plant L-ascorbic acid: Chemistry, function, metabolism, bioavailability and effects of processing. *Journal of the Science of Food and Agriculture*, 80, 825–860.

Day, B.P.F. (2002). New modified atmosphere packaging (MAP) techniques for fresh prepared fruit and vegetables. In *Fruit and Vegetable Processing*, ed. W. Jongem, 310–329. Abington: Woodhead Publishing Limited.

De Castro, L.R., Vigneault, C., and Cortez, L.A.B. (2005). Effect of container openings and airflow on energy required for forced air cooling of horticultural produce. *Canadian Biosystems Engineering*, 47, 1–9.

De Dios, P., Matilla, A.J., and Gallardo, M. (2006). Flower fertilization and fruit development prompt changes in free polyamines and ethylene in damson plum (*Prunus insititiu* L.). *Journal of Plant Physiology*, 163, 86–97.

DeEll, J. (2007). 1-MCP Applied preharvest or postharvest Improves the quality of "Bartlett" pears. *The Tender Fruit Grape Vine*, 11, 4–5.

Deepa, N., Kaur, C., George, B., Singh, B., and Kapoor, H.C. (2007). Antioxidant constituents in some red sweet pepper (*Capsicum annuum* L.) genotypes during maturity. *Lebensmittel Wissenschaft und-Technologie*, 40, 121–129.

Defilippi, B.G., Kader, A.A., and Dandekar, A.M. (2005). Apple aroma: Alcohol acyltransferase, a rate limiting step for ester biosynthesis, is regulated by ethylene. *Plant Science*, 168, 1199–1210.

Defilippi, B.G., San Juan, W., Valdés, H., Moya-León, M.A., Infante, R., and Campos-Vargas, R. (2009). The aroma development during storage of Castlebrite apricots as evaluated by gas chromatography, electronic nose, and sensory analysis. *Postharvest Biology and Technology*, 51, 212–219.

De Gara, L. (2004). Ascorbate and plant growth: from germination to cell death. In: *Vitamin C. Function and Biochemistry in Animals and Plants*, eds., H. Asard, J.M. May and N. Smirnoff, 92–105. New York: Garland Science/BIOS Scientific Publishers.

DellaPena, D., and Pogson, B.J. (2006). Vitamin synthesis in plants: Tocopherols and carotenoids. *Annual Review of Plant Biology*, 57, 711–718.

Del-Valle, V., Almenar, E., Lagarón, J.M., Catalá, R., and Gavara, R. (2003). Modelling permeation through porous polymeric films for modified atmosphere packaging. *Food Additives and Contaminants*, 20, 170–179.

De Paepe, A., and Van der Straeten, D. (2005). Ethylene biosynthesis and signaling: An overview. *Vitamins and Hormones*, 72, 399–430.

De Souza, M., Silva-Ferreira, K., Paes-Chaves, J.B., and Lopes-Texeira, S. (2008). L-ascorbic acid, ß-carotene and lycopene in papaya fruits (*Carica papaya*) with or without physiological skin freckles. *Scientia Agricola*, 65, 246–250.

Dias, M.G., Camões, M.F., and Oliveira, L. (2009). Carotenoids in traditional Portuguese fruits and vegetables. *Food Chemistry*, 113, 808–815.

Díaz-Mula, H.M., Castillo, S., Martínez-Romero, D., Valero, D., Zapata, P.J., Guillén, F., and Serrano, M. (2009a). Organoleptic, nutritive and functional properties of sweet cherry as affected by cultivar and ripening stage. *Food Science and Technology International*, In Press.

Díaz-Mula, H.M., Zapata, P.J., Guillén, F., Castillo, S., Martínez-Romero, D., Valero, D., and Serrano, M. (2008). Changes in physicochemical and nutritive parameters and bioactive compounds during development and on-tree ripening of eight plum cultivars: a comparative study. *Journal of the Science of Food and Agriculture*, 88, 2499–2507.

Díaz-Mula, H.M., Zapata, P.J., Guillén, F., Martínez-Romero, D., Castillo, S., Serrano, M., and Valero, D. (2009b). Changes in hydrophilic and lipophilic antioxidant activity and related bioactive compounds during postharvest storage of yellow and purple plum cultivars. *Postharvest Biology and Technology*, 51, 354–363.

Dibble, A.R.G., Davies, P.J., and Mutschler, M.A. (1988). Polyamine content of long-keeping Alcobaca tomato fruit. *Plant Physiology*, 86, 338–340.

Directive No 95/2/EC. (1995). European Parliament and Council of 20 February 1995 on food additives other than colours and sweeteners.

Directive No 98/72/CE (1998). European Parliament and Council of 15 October 1998 amending Directive 95/2/EC on food additives other than colours and sweeteners.

Dixon, J. and Hewett, E.W. (2000). Factors affecting apple aroma/flavour volatile concentration: A review. *New Zealand Journal of Crop Horticultural Science*, 28, 155–173.

Djioua, T., Charles, F., López-Lauri, F., Filgueiras, H., Coudret, A., Freire, M., Ducamp-Collin, M.N., and Sallanon, H. (2009). Improving the storage of minimally processed mangoes (*Mangifera indica L.*) by hot water treatments. *Postharvest Biology and Technology*, 52, 221–226.

Dong, C.X., Zhou, J.M., Fan, X.H., Wang, H.Y., Duan, Z.Q., and Tang, C. (2004). Application methods of calcium supplements affect nutrient levels and calcium forms in mature tomato fruits. *Journal of Plant Nutrition*, 27, 1443–1455.

Drake, S.R., Hansen, J.D., Elfving, D.C., Tang, J., and Wang, S. (2005). Hot water to control codling moth in sweet cherries: Efficacy and quality. *Journal of Food Quality*, 28, 361-376.

Droby, S., Wisniewski, M., Macarisin, D., and Wilson, C. (2009). Twenty years of postharvest biocontrol research: Is it time for a new paradigm? *Postharvest Biology and Technology*, 52, 137–145.

Druege, U. (2006). Ethylene and plant responses to abiotic stress. In *Ethylene Action in Plants*, eds. N.A. Khan, 81–118. Berlin: Springer-Verlag.

Ecker, W.L. (2002). The ethylene response pathway in Arabidopsis. *Annual Review of Plant Biology*, 48, 277–296.

Eden, M.A., Hill, R.A., Beresford, R., and Stewart, A. (1996). The influence of inoculum concentration, relative humidity, and temperature on infection of greenhouse tomatoes by *Botrytis cinerea*. *Plant Pathology*, 45, 798–806.

Edwards, S.G., and Seddon, B. (2001). Mode of antagonism of *Brevibacillus brevis* against *Botrytis cinerea in vitro*. *Journal of Applied Microbiology*, 91, 652–659.

Ekman, J.H., Clayton, M., Biasi, W.V., and Mitcham, E.J. (2004). Interactions between 1-MCP concentration, treatment interval and storage time for "Bartlett" pears. *Postharvest Biology and Technology*, 31, 127–136.

Elad, Y., and Eversen, K. (1995). Physiological aspects of resistance to *Botrytis cinerea*. *Phytopathology*, 8, 637–643.

El-Ghaouth, A., Wilson, C.L., and Wisniewski, M.E. (2004). Biologically based alternatives to synthetic fungicides for the postharvest diseases of fruit and vegetables. In *Diseases of Fruit and Vegetables*, ed. S.A.M.H. Naqvi, 511–535. Dordretch: Kluwer Academic Publishers.

Eliassen, K.A., Reistad, R., Risøen, U., and Rønning, H.F. (2002). Dietary polyamines. *Food Chemistry*, 78, 273–280.

Erkan, M., Pekmezci, M., and Wang, C.Y. (2005). Hot water and curing treatments reduce chilling injury and maintain post-harvest quality of "Valencia" oranges. *International Journal of Food Science and Technology*, 40, 91–96.

Eryani-Raqeeb, A.A., Mahmud, T.M.M., Omar, S.R.S., Mohamed, A.R., and Eryani, A.R.A. (2009). Effects of calcium and chitosan treatments on controlling Anthracnose and postharvest quality of papaya (*Carica papaya* L.). *International Journal of Agricultural Research*, 4, 53–68.

Escribano, M.I., and Merodio, C. (1994). The relevance of polyamine levels in cherimoya (*Annona cherimola* Mill.) fruit ripening. *Journal of Plant Physiology*, 143, 207–212.

Etienne, C., Moing, A., Dirlewanger, E., Raymond, P., Monet, R., and Rothan, C. (2002). Isolation and characterization of six peach cDNAs encoding key proteins in organic acid metabolism and solute accumulation: Involvement in regulating peach fruit acidity. *Physiologia Plantarum*, 114, 259–270.

Fallik, E. (2004). Prestorage hot water treatments (immersion, rinsing and brushing). *Postharvest Biology and Technology*, 32, 125–134.

Fallik, E., Aharoni, Y., Yekutieli, O., Wiseblum, A., Regev, R., Beres, H., and Bar-Lev, E. (1996). A method for simultaneously cleaning and disinfecting agricultural produce. Israel Patent Application No. 116965.

Fallik, E., Archbold, D.D., Hamilton-Kemp, T.R., Loughrin, J.H., and Collins, R.W. (1997). Heat treatment temporarily inhibits aroma volatile compound emission from Golden Delicious apples. *Journal of Agricultural and Food Chemistry*, 45, 4038–4041.

Fallik, E., Tuvia-Alkalai, S., Feng, X., and Lurie, S. (2001). Ripening characterisation and decay development of stored apples after short pre-storage hot water rinsing and brushing. *Innovative Food Science and Emerging Technologies*, 2, 127–132.

Fan, L., Forney, C.F., Song, J., Doucette, C., Jordan, M.A., McRae, K.B., and Walker, B.A. (2008). Effect of hot water treatments on quality of Highbush blueberries. *Journal of Food Science*, 70, M292–M296.

Fan, X., and Mattheis, J.P. (1999). Impact of 1-methylcyclopropene and methyl jasmonate on apple volatile production. *Journal of Agricultural and Food Chemistry*, 47, 2847–2853.

Fanasca, S., Colla, G., Maiani, G., Venneira, E., Rouphael, Y., Azzini, E., and Saccardo, F. (2006). Changes in antioxidant content of tomato fruits in response to cultivar and nutrient solution composition. *Journal of Agricultural and Food Chemistry*, 54, 4319–4325.

Fan-Chiang, H.J., and Wrolstad, R.E. (2005). Anthocyanin pigment composition of blackberries. *Journal of Food Science*, 70, C198–C202.

Fanciullino, A.L., Cercós, M., Dhuikue-Mayer, C., Froelicher, Y., Talón, M., Ollitrault, P., and Morillón, R. (2008). Changes in carotenoid content and biosynthetic gene expression in juice sacs of four orange varieties (*Citrus sinensis)* differing in flesh fruit color. *Journal of Agricultural and Food Chemistry*, 56, 3628–3638.

Fang, Y.Z., Yang, S., and Guoyao W. (2002). Free radicals, antioxidants, and nutrition. *Nutrition*, 18, 872–879.

Fawbush, F., Nock, J.F., and Watkins, C.B. (2009). Antioxidant contents and activity of 1-methylcyclopropene (1-MCP)-treated "Empire" apples in air and controlled atmosphere storage. *Postharvest Biology and Technology*, 52, 30–37.

Fawcett, H.S. (1936). *Citrus Diseases and Their Control*. New York: McGraw Hill.

FDA 21CFR172. (2006). Food additives permitted for direct addition to food for human consumption, Subpart C. Coatings, Films and Related Substances.

Femenia, A., Sánchez, E.S., Simal, S., and Roselló, C. (1998). Modification of cell wall composition of apricot (*Prunus armeniaca*) during drying and storage under modified atmospheres. *Journal of Agricultural and Food Chemistry*, 46, 5248–5253.

Feng, X., Hansen, J.D., Biasi, B., Tang, J., and Mitcham, E.J. (2004). Use of hot water treatment to control codling moths in harvested California "Bing" sweet cherries. *Postharvest Biology and Technology*, 31, 41–49.

Ferguson, I.B., Ben-Yehoshua, S., Mitcham, E.J., McDonald, R.E., and Lurie, S. (2000). Postharvest heat treatments: Introduction and workshop summary. *Postharvest Biology and Technology*, 21, 1–6.

Ferguson, I.B., and Boyd, L.M. (2001). Inorganic nutrients and fruit quality, In *Fruit Quality and Its Biological Basis*, ed. M. Knee, 17–45. Sheffield: Academic Press.

Fernández-López, J.A., Almela, L., Muñoz, J.A., Hidalgo, V., and Carreño, J. (1998). Dependence between colour and individual anthocyanin content in ripening grapes. *Food Research International*, 31, 667–672.

Fernández-Panchón, M.S., Villano, D., Troncoso, A.M., and García-Parrilla, M.C. (2008). Antioxidant activity of phenolic compounds: From *in vivo* results to *in vitro* evidence. *Critical Review in Food Science and Nutrition*, 24, 649–671.

Fisher, K., and Phillips, C. (2008). Potential antimicrobial uses of essential oils in food: is citrus the answer? *Trends in Food Science and Technology*, 19, 156–164.

Fonseca, S.C., Oliveira, F.A.R., and Brecht, J.K. (2002). Modelling respiration rate of fresh fruits and vegetables for modified atmosphere packages: A review. *Journal of Food Engineering*, 52, 99–119.

Francis, F.J. (1989). Food Colorants: Anthocyanins. *Critical Review in Food Science and Nutrition*, 28, 273–314.

Franco-Mora, O., Tanabe, K., Itai, A., Tamura, F., and Itamura, H. (2005a). Relationship between endogenous free polyamine content and ethylene evolution during fruit growth and ripening of Japanese pear (*Pyrus pyrifolia* Nakai). *Journal of the Japanese Society for Horticultural Science*, 74, 221–227.

Franco-Mora, O., Tanabe, K., Tamura, F., and Itai, A. (2005b). Effects of putrescine application on fruit set in "Housui" Japanese pear (*Pyrus pyrifolia* Nakai). *Scientia Horticulturae*, 104, 265–273.

Friedman, M. (1996). Food browning and its prevention: An overview. *Journal of Agricultural and Food Chemistry*, 44, 631–653.

Gane, R. (1934). Production of ethylene by some fruits. *Nature*, 134, 1008.

Gao, L., and Mazza, G. (1995). Characterization, quantification, and distribution of anthocyanins and colorless phenolic in sweet cherries. *Journal of Agricultural and Food Chemistry*, 43, 343–346.

García, J.M., Herrera, S., and Morilla, A. (1996). Effects of postharvest dips in calcium chloride on strawberry. *Journal of Agricultural and Food Chemistry*, 44, 30–33.

García, J.M., Medina, R.J., and Olías, J.M. (1998). Quality of strawberries automatically packed in different plastic films. *Journal of Food Science*, 63, 1037–1041.

García-Mariño, N., de la Torre, F., and Matilla, A.J. (2008). Organic acids and soluble sugars in edible and non edible parts of Damson plum (*Prunus domestica* L. subsp. *insititia* cv. Syriaca) fruits during development and ripening. *Food Science Technology International*, 14, 187–193.

Gebhardt, S.E., and Thomas, R.G. (2004). *Nutritive Value of Foods*. Beltsville: U.S. Department of Agriculture, Agricultural Research Service, Nutrient Data Laboratory.

Gennadios, A. (2002). *Protein-Based Edible Films and Coatings*. Boca Raton. CRC Press.

Gerasopoulos, D., and Richardson, D.G. (1999). Storage temperature and fruit calcium alter the sequence of ripening events of "d'Anjou" pears. *HortScience*, 34, 316–318.

Gil, M.I., Tomás-Barberán, F.A., Hess-Pierce, B., and Kader, S.A. (2002). Antioxidant capacities, phenolic compounds, carotenoids, and vitamin C contents of nectarine, peach, and plum cultivars from California. *Journal of Agricultural and Food Chemistry*, 50, 4976–4982.

Giovannoni, J. (2001). Molecular biology of fruit maturation and ripening. *Annual Review of Plant Physiology and Plant Molecular Biology*, 52, 725–749.

Giovannoni, J. (2004). Genetic regulation of fruit development and ripening. *Plant Cell*, 16, S170–S180.

Giovannoni, J. (2007). Fruit ripening mutants yields insights into ripening control. *Current Opinion in Plant Biology*, 10, 283–289.

Girardi, C.L., Corrent, A.R., Lucchetta, L., Zanuzo, M.R., Costa, T.S.D., Brackmann, A., Twyman, R.M., and Rombaldi, C.V. (2005). Effect of ethylene, intermittent warming and controlled atmosphere on postharvest quality and the occurrence of woolliness in peach (*Prunus persica* cv. Chiripá) during cold storage. *Postharvest Biology and Technology*, 38, 25–33.

Glew, R.H., Ayaz, F.A., Millson, M., Huang, H.S., Chuang, L.T., Sanz, C., and Golding, J.B. (2005). Changes in sugars, acids and fatty acids in naturally parthenocarpic date plum persimmon (*Diospyros lotus* L.) fruit during maturation and ripening. *European Food Research and Technology*, 221, 113–118.

Goff, S., and Klee, J. (2006). Plant volatile compounds: sensory cues for health and nutritional value. *Science*, 311, 815–819.

Golding, J.B., Shearer, D., McGlasson, W.B., and Wyllie, S.G. (1999). Relationships between respiration, ethylene, and aroma production in ripening banana. *Journal of Agricultural and Food Chemistry*, 47, 1646–1651.

Golding, J.B., Shearer, D., Wyllie, S.G., and McGlasson, W.B. (1998). Application of 1-MCP and propylene to identify ethylene-dependent ripening processes in mature banana fruit. *Postharvest Biology and Technology*, 14, 87–98.

Goldschmidt, E.E., Huberman, M., and Goren, R. (1993). Probing the role of endogenous ethylene in the degreening of citrus fruit with ethylene antagonists. *Plant Growth Regulation*, 12, 325–329.

Gómez-Galindo, F., Herppich, W., Gekas, V., and Sjöholm, I. (2004). Factors affecting quality and postharvest properties of vegetables: Integration of water relations and metabolism. *Critical Review in Food Science and Nutrition*, 44, 139–154.

Gómez-Galindo, F., Sjöholm, I., Rasnusson, A.G., Widell, S., and Kaack, K. (2007). Plant stress physiology: opportunities and challenges for the food industry. *Critical Review in Food Science and Nutrition*, 46, 749–763.

Gonçalves, B., Landbo, A.K., Knudse, D., Silva, A.P., Moutinho-Pereia, J., Rosa, E., and Meyer, A.S. (2004). Effect of ripeness and postharvest storage on the phenolic profiles of cherries (*Prunus avium* L.). *Journal of Agricultural and Food Chemistry*, 52, 523–530.

Gonçalves, B., Silva, A.P., Moutinho-Pereia, J., Bacelar, E., Rosa, E., and Meyer, A.S. (2007). Effect of ripeness and postharvest storage on the evolution of color and anthocyanins in cherries (*Prunus avium* L.). *Food Chemistry*, 103, 976–984.

Gong, Y., Fan, X., and Mattheis, J.P. (2002). Responses of "Bing" and "Rainier" sweet cherries to ethylene and 1-methylcyclopropene. *Journal of the American Society for Horticultural Science*, 127, 831–835.

González-Aguilar, G.A., Buta, J.G., and Wang, C.Y. (2003). Methyl jasmonate and modified atmosphere packaging (MAP) reduce decay and maintain postharvest quality of papaya "Sunrise." *Postharvest Biology and Technology*, 28, 361–370.

González-Aguilar, G.A., Gayoso, L., Cruz, R., Fortiz, J., Báez, R., and Wang, C.Y. (2000a). Polyamines induced by hot water treatments reduce chilling injury and decay in pepper fruit. *Postharvest Biology and Technology*, 18, 19–26.

González-Aguilar, G.A., Zacarías, L., Perez-Amador, M.A., Carbonell, J., and Lafuente, M.T. (2000b). Polyamine content and chilling susceptibility are affected by seasonal changes in temperature and by conditioning temperature in cold-stored "Fortune" mandarin fruit. *Physiologia Plantarum*, 108, 140–146.

González-Buesa, J., Ferrer-Mairal, A., Oria, R., and Salvador, M.L. (2009). A mathematical model for packaging with microperforated films of fresh-cut fruits and vegetables. *Journal of Food Engineering*, 95, 158–165.

González-Neves, G., Charamelo, D., Balado, J., Barreiro, L., Bochicchio, R., Gatto, G., Gil, G., Tessore, A., Carbonneau, A., and Moutounet, M. (2004). Phenolic potential of Tannat, Cabernet-Sauvignon and Merlot grapes and their correspondence with wine composition. *Analytica Chimica Acta*, 513, 191–196.

Gonzali, S., Mazzucati, A., and Perata, P. (2009). Purple as a tomato: Towards high anthocyanin tomatoes. *Trends in Plant Science*, 14, 237–241.

Goulao, L.F., and Oliveira, C.M. (2008). Cell wall modifications during fruit ripening: When a fruit is not the fruit. *Trends in Food Science and Technology*, 19, 4–25.

Goyette, B., Hui, C.K.P., and Vigneault, C. (2000). An improved continuous liquid-ice system based on submerged mixing of water and ice. *Applied Engineering in Agriculture*, 16, 259–263.

Gras, M.L., Vidal, D., Betoret, N., Chirat, A., and Fito, P. (2003). Calcium fortification of vegetables by vacuum impregnation interactions with cellular matrix. *Journal of Food Engineering*, 56, 279–284.

Guenther, E. (1948). *The Essential Oils*. D. New York: Van Nostrand.

Guillén, F. (2009). 1-MCP como estrategia de conservación. *Horticultura Extra 2009 Poscosecha*, 69, 18–24.

Guillén, F., Castillo, S., Zapata, P.J., Martínez-Romero, D., Serrano, M., and Valero, D. (2007a). Efficacy of 1-MCP treatment in tomato fruit. 1. Duration and concentration of 1-MCP treatment to gain an effective delay of postharvest ripening. *Postharvest Biology and Technology*, 43, 23–27.

Guillén, F., Castillo, S., Zapata, P.J., Martínez-Romero, D., Valero, D., and Serrano, M. (2006). Efficacy of 1-MCP treatment in tomato fruit. 2. Effect of cultivar and ripening stage at harvest. *Postharvest Biology and Technology*, 42, 235–242.

Guillén, F., Zapata, P. J., Martínez-Romero, D., Castillo, S., Serrano, M., and Valero, D. (2007b). Improvement of the overall quality of table grapes stored under modified atmosphere packaging in combination with natural antimicrobial compounds. *Journal of Food Science*, 72, S185–S190.

Guillot, S., Peytavi, L., Bureau, S., Boulanger, R., Lepoutre, J.P., Crouzet, J., and Scorr-Galindo, S. (2006). Aroma characterization of various apricot varieties using headspace-solid phase microextraction combined with gas chromatography-mass spectrometry and gas chromatography-olfactometry. *Food Chemistry*, 96, 147–155.

Guo, H., and Ecker, J.R. (2004). The ethylene signalling pathway: New insights. *Current Opinion in Plant Biology*, 7, 40–49.

Halliwell, B. (2007). Dietary polyphenols: Good, bad, or indifferent for your health? *Cardiovascular Research*, 73, 341–347.

Han, J.H. (2003). Antimicrobial food packaging. In *Novel Food Packaging Techniques*, ed. R. Ahvenainen, 66–68. Abington: Woodhead Publishing Limited.

Hanson, E.J., Beggs, J.L., and Beaudry, R.M. (1993). Applying calcium chloride postharvest to improve higbush blueberry firmness. *HortScience*, 28, 1033–1034.

Hardfenburg, R.E., Watada, A. E., and Wang, C.Y. (1986). The Commercial Storage of Fruits, Vegetable, and Florist and Nursery Stock. USDA Agric. Hdbk No. 66, Washington, D.C.

Hartley, D.R. (2000). The product design perspective on fresh produce packaging. *Postharvest News and Information*, 11, 35N–38N.

Hernández-Muñoz, P., Almenar, E., Del Valle, V., Velez, D., and Gavara, R. (2008). Effect of chitosan coating combined with postharvest calcium treatment on strawberry (*Fragaria x ananassa*) quality during refrigerated storage. *Food Chemistry*, 110, 428–435.

Hernández-Muñoz, P., Almenar, E., Ocio, M.J., and Gavara, R. (2006). Effect of calcium dips and chitosan coatings on postharvest life of strawberries (*Fragaria x ananassa*). *Postharvest Biology and Technology*, 39, 247–253.

Hewajulige, I.G.N., Wilson Wijeratnam, R.S., Wijesundera, R.L.C., and Abeysekere, M. (2003). Fruit calcium concentration and chilling injury during low temperature storage of pineapple. *Journal of the Science of Food and Agriculture*, 83, 1451–1454.

Hoa, T.T., Clark, C.J., Waddell, B.C., and Woolf, A.B. (2006). Postharvest quality of Gragon fruit (*Hylocereus undatus*) following disinfesting hot air treatment. *Postharvest Biology and Technology*, 41, 62–69.

Hodges, D.M., Lester, G.E., Munro, K.D., and Toivonen, P.M.A. (2004). Oxidative stress: importance for postharvest quality. *HortScience*, 39, 924–929.

Hoeberichts, F.A., Van der Plas, L.H.W., and Woltering, E.J. (2002). Ethylene perception is required for the expression of tomato ripening related genes and associated physiological changes even at advanced stages of ripening. *Postharvest Biology and Technology*, 26, 125–133.

Holland, N., Menezes, H.C., and Lafuente, M.T. (2002). Carbohydrates as related to the heat-induced chilling tolerance and respiratory rate of "Fortune" mandarin fruit harvested at different maturity stages. *Postharvest Biology and Technology*, 25, 181–191.

Holley, R.A., and Patel, D. (2005). Improvement in shelf-life and safety of perishable foods by plant essential oils and smoke antimicrobials. *Food Microbiology*, 22, 273–292.

Hoogerwerf, S.W., Kets, E.P.W., and Dijksterhuis, J. (2002). High-oxygen and high carbon dioxide containing atmospheres inhibit growth of food associated moulds. *Letters in Applied Microbiology*, 35, 419–22.

Hopkirk, G., Harker, F.R., and Harman, J.E. (1990). Calcium and the firmness of kiwifruit. *New Zealand Journal of Crop and Horticultural Science*, 18, 227–230.

Ishikawa, T., Dowdle, J., and Smirnoff, N. (2006). Progress in manipulating ascorbic acid biosynthesis and accumulation in plants. *Physiologia Plantarum*, 126, 343–355.

Izumi, H., and Watada, A.E. (1995). Calcium treatment to maintain quality of zucchini squash slices. *Journal of Food Science*, 60, 789–793.

Jaime, P., Salvador, M.L., and Oria, R. (2001). Respiration rate of sweet cherries: "Burlat", "Sunburst" and "Sweetheart" cultivars. *Journal of Food Science*, 66, 43–47.

Janisiewicz, W.J., and Korsten, L. (2002). Biological control of postharvest diseases of fruits. *Annual Review of Phytopathology*, 40, 411–441.

Jarvis, M.C., Briggs, S.P.H., and Knox, J.P. (2003). Intercellular adhesion and cell separation in plants. *Plant, Cell and Environment*, 26, 977–989.

Javeri, H., Toledo, R., and Wicker, L. (1991). Vacuum infusion of citrus pectinmethylesterase and calcium effects on firmness of peaches. *Journal of Food Science*, 56, 739–742.

Jeong, S.K., Kim, S.Y., Kim, D.R., Jo, S.C., Nam, K.C., Ahn, D.U., and Lee, S.C. (2004). Effect of heat treatment on the antioxidant activity of extracts from Citrus peels. *Journal of Agricultural and Food Chemistry*, 52, 3389–3393.

Jiang, Y., Joyce, D.C., and Terry, L.A. (2001). 1-Methylcyclopropene treatment affects strawberry fruit decay. *Postharvest Biology and Technology*, 23, 227–232.

Jin, P., Zheng, Y., Tang, S., Rui, H., and Wang, C.Y. (2009). A combination of hot air and methyl jasmonate vapour treatment alleviates chilling injury of peach fruit. *Postharvest Biology and Technology*, 52, 24–29.

Johnson, I.T. (2002). Glucosinolates in the human diet: Bioavailability and implications for health. *Phytochemistry Reviews*, 1, 183–188.

Johnstone, P.R., Hartz, T.K., and May, D.M. (2008). Calcium fertigation ineffective at increasing fruit yield and quality of muskmelon and honeydew melons in California. *HortTechnology*, 18, 685–689.

Jomori, M.L.L., Kluge, R.A., and Jacomino, A.P. (2003). Cold storage of "Tahiti" lime treated with 1-methylcyclopropene. *Scientia Agricola*, 60, 785–788.

Jones, R.B. (2007). The effects of postharvest handling conditions and cooking on anthocyanin, lycopene and glucosinolate content and bioavailability in fruits and vegetables. *New Zealand Journal of Crop and Horticultural Science*, 35, 219–227.

Kader, A.A. (2002). *Postharvest Technology of Horticultural Crops*. Regents of the University of California, Division of Agricultural and Natural Resources, Oakland, CA, USA.

Kader, A.A., and Watkins, C.B. 2000. Modified atmosphere packaging—Towards 2000 and beyond. *HortTechnology*, 10, 483–486.

Kader, A.A., Zagory, D., and Kerbel, E.L. (1989). Modified atmosphere packaging of fruits and vegetables. *Critical Review on Food Science and Nutrition*, 28, 1–30.

Kadir, S.A. (2004). Fruit quality at harvest of "Jonathan" apple treated with foliarly-applied calcium chloride. *Journal of Plant Nutrition*, 27, 1991–2006.

Kafkas, E., Koşar, M., Paydaş, S., Kafkas, S., and Başer, K.H.C. (2007). Quality characteristics of strawberry genotypes at different maturation stages. *Food Chemistry*, 100, 1229–1236.

Kalač, P., and Krausová, P. (2005). A review of dietary polyamines: Formation, implications for growth and health and occurrence in foods. *Food Chemistry*, 90, 219–230.

Kalač, P., Křížek, M., Pelikánová, T., Langová, M., and Veškrna, O. (2005). Content of polyamines in selected foods. *Food Chemistry*, 90, 561–564.

Kalač, P., Švecová, S., and Pelikánová, T. (2002). Levels of biogenic amines in typical vegetable products. *Food Chemistry*, 77, 349–351.

Kappel, E., Toivonen, P., Mckenzie, K.L., and Stan, S. (2002). Storage characteristics of new sweet cherry cultivars. *HortScience*, 37, 139–143.

Kato, M., Hayakawa, Y., Hyodo, H., Ikoma, Y., and Yano, M. (2000). Wound-induced ethylene synthesis and expression of 1-aminocyclopropane-1-carboxylate (ACC) synthase, ACC oxidase, phenylalanine ammonia-lyase, and peroxidase in wounded mesocarp tissue of *Cucurbita maxima*. *Plant Cell Physiology*, 41, 440–447.

Kaur, D., Sharma, R., Wani, A.A., Gill, B.S., and Sogi, D.S. (2006). Physicochemical changes in seven tomato (*Lycopersicon esculentum*) cultivars during ripening. *International Journal of Food Properties*, 9, 747–757.

Kende, H. (1993). Ethylene biosynthesis. *Annual Review of Plant Physiology and Plant Molecular Biology*, 44, 283–307.

Ketsa, S., and Atantee, S. (1998). Phenolics, lignin, peroxidase activity and increased firmness of damaged pericarp of mangosteen fruit after impact. *Postharvest Biology and Technology*, 14, 117–124.

Khan, A.S., Singh, Z., Abbasi, N.A., and Swinny, E.E. (2008). Pre- or post-harvest applications of putrescine at low temperature storage affect fruit ripening and quality of "Angelino" plum. *Journal of the Science of Food and Agriculture*, 88, 1686–1695.

Khan, A.S., Singh, Z., and Swinny, E.E. (2009). Postharvest application of 1-methylcyclopropene modulates fruit ripening, storage life and quality of "Tegan Blue" Japanese plum kept in ambient and cold storage. *International Journal of Food Science and Technology*, 44, 1272–1280.

Kim, D.O., and Lee, C.Y. (2004). Comprehensive study on vitamin C equivalent antioxidant capacity (VCEAC) of various polyphenolics in scavenging a free radical and its structural relationship. *Critical Review in Food Science and Nutrition*, 44, 153–273.

Kim, H.S., and Jin, C.D. (2006). Polyamines as antioxidant protectors against paraquat damage in radish (*Raphanus sativus* L.) cotyledons. *Journal of Plant Biology*, 49, 237–246.

Kim, Y., Lounds-Singleton, A.J., and Talcott, S.T. (2009). Antioxidant phytochemical and quality changes associated with hot water immersion treatments with mangoes (*Mangifera indica* L.). *Food Chemistry*, 115, 989–993.

King, R.E., Bomser, J.A., and Min, D.B. (2006). Bioactivity of resveratrol. *Comprehensive Reviews in Food Science and Food Safety*, 5, 65–70.

Klee, H., and Tieman, D. (2002). The tomato ethylene receptor gene family: Form and function. *Physiologia Plantarum*, 115, 336–341.

Kondo, S., Ponrod, W., and Sutthiwal, S. (2003). Polyamines in developing mangosteens and their relationship to postharvest chilling injury. *Journal of the Japanese Society for Horticultural Science*, 72, 318–320.

Kortstee, A.J., Appeldoorn, N.J.G., Oortwijn, M.E.P., and Visser, R.G.F. (2007). Differences in regulation of carbohydrate metabolism during early fruit development between domesticated tomato and two wild relatives. *Planta*, 226, 929–939.

Koukounaras, A., Diamantidis, G., and Sfakiotakis, E. (2008). The effect of heat treatment on quality retention of fresh-cut peach. *Postharvest Biology and Technology*, 48, 30–36.

Kramer, G. F., Wang, C. Y., and Conway, W. S. (1991). Inhibition of softening by polyamine application in "Golden Delicious" and "McIntosh" apples. *Journal of the American Society for Horticultural Science*, 116, 813–817.

Kratsch, H.A., and Wise, R.R. (2000). The ultrastructure of chilling stress. *Plant, Cell and Environment*, 23, 337–350.

Krinsky, N.I., and Johnson, E.J. (2005). Carotenoid actions and their relation to health and disease. *Molecular Aspects of Medicine*, 26, 459–516.

Kris-Etherton, P.M., Hecker, K.D., Bonanome, A., Koval, S.M., Binkoski, A.M., Hilpert, K.F., Griel, A.E., and Etherton, T.D. (2002). Bioactive compounds in foods: Their role in the prevention of cardiovascular disease and cancer. *Excerpta Medica*, 71S–88S.

Krumbein, A., Peters, P., and Brückner, B. (2004). Flavour compounds and a quantitative descriptive analysis of tomatoes (*Lycopersicon esculentum* Mill.) of different cultivars in short-term storage. *Postharvest Biology and Technology*, 32, 15–28.

Kukura, J.L., Beelman, R.B., Peiffer, V., and Walsh, R. (1998). Calcium chloride added to irrigation water of mushrooms (*Agaricus bisporus*) reduces postharvest browning. *Journal of Food Science*, 63, 454–457.

Kumar, A., Altabella, T., Taylor, M.A., and Tiburcio, A.F. (1997). Recent advances in polyamine research. *Trends in Plant Sciences*, 2, 124–130.

Kurz, C., Carle, R., and Schieber, A. (2008). HPLC-DAD-MS characterization of carotenoids from apricots and pumpkins for the evaluation of fruit product authenticity. *Food Chemistry*, 110, 522–530.

Kusano, T., Yamaguchi, K., Berberich, T., and Takahashi, Y. (2007). Advances in polyamine research in 2007. *Journal of Plant Research*, 120, 345–350.

Kushad, M.M. (1998). Changes in polyamine levels in relationship to the double-sigmoidal growth curve of peaches. *Journal of the American Society for Horticultural Science*, 123, 950–955.

Kushad, M.M., Yelenosky, G., and Knight, R. (1988). Interrelationship of polyamine and ethylene biosynthesis during avocado fruit development and ripening. *Plant Physiology*, 87, 463–467.

Lafuente, M.T., and Sala, J.M. (2002). Abscisic acid levels and the influence of ethylene, humidity and storage temperature on the incidence of postharvest rind staning of "Navelina" orange (*Citrus sinensis* L. Osbeck) fruit. *Postharvest Biology and Technology*, 25, 49–57.

Lamikanra, O., Bett-Garber, K.L., Ingram, D.A., and Watson, M.A. (2005). Use of mild heat pre-treatment for quality retention of fresh-cut cantaloupe melon. *Journal of Food Science*, 70, C53–C57.

Lamikanra, O., and Watson, M.A. (2007). Mild heat and calcium treatment effects on fresh-cut cantaloupe melon during storage. *Food Chemistry*, 102, 1383–1388.

Lanciotti, R., Gianotti, A., Patrignani, F., Belletti, N., Guerzoni, M. E., and Gardini, F. (2004). Use of natural aroma compounds to improve shelf-life and safety of minimally processed fruits. *Trends in Food Science and Technology*, 15, 201–208.

Lange, D.L. (2000). New film technologies for horticultural products. *HortTechnology*, 10, 487–490.

Lara, I., García, P., and Vendrell, M. (2004). Modifications in cell wall composition after cold storage of calcium-treated strawberry (*Fragaria ananassa* Duch.). *Postharvest Biology and Technology*, 34, 331–339.

Lara, I., García, P., and Vendrell, M. (2006). Post-harvest heat treatments modify cell wall composition of strawberry (*Fragaria x ananassa* Duch.) fruit. *Scientia Horticulturae*, 109, 48–53.

Larqué, E., Sabater-Molina, M., and Zamora, S. (2007). Biological significance of dietary polyamines. *Nutrition*, 23, 87–95.

Lasbrook, C.C. (2005). New insights into cell disassembly during fruit ripening. *Stewart Postharvest Review*, 3:2.

Law, D. M., Davies, P. J., and Mutschler, M. A. (4957757). Method of extending shelf life and enhancing keeping quality of fruits. US patent, 1988.

Lederman, I.E., Zauberman, G., Weksler, A., and Fuchs, Y. (1997). Ethylene-forming capacity during cold storage and chilling injury development in "Keitt" mango fruit. *Postharvest Biology and Technology*, 10, 107–112.

Lee, S.K., and Kader, A.A. (2000). Preharvest and postharvest factors influencing vitamin C content of horticultural crops. *Postharvest Biology and Technology*, 20, 207–220.

Lelièvre, J.M., Latché, A., Jones, B., Bouzayen, M., and Pech, J.C. (1997). Ethylene and fruit ripening. *Physiologia Plantarum*, 101, 727–739.

Lenucci, M.S., Cadinu, D., Taurino, M., Piro, G., and Dalessandro, G. (2006). Antioxidant composition in cherry and high-pigment tomato cultivars. *Journal of Agricultural and Food Chemistry*, 54, 2606–2613.

Lester, G.E. (2000). Polyamines and their cellular anti-senescence properties in honeydew muskmelon fruit. *Plant Science*, 160, 105–112.

Lester, G.E., and Grusak, M.A. (1999). Postharvest application of calcium and magnesium to honeydew and netted muskmelon: Effects on tissue ion concentrations, quality and senescence. *Journal of the American Society for Horticultural Science*, 124, 545–552.

Lester, G.E., and Grusak, M.A. (2004). Field application of chelated calcium: Postharvest effects on cantaloupe and honeydew fruit quality. *HortTechnology*, 14, 29–38.

Lila, M.A., and Raskin, I. (2005). Health-related interactions of phytochemicals. *Journal of Food Science*, 70, R20–R27.

Lister, C.E., Skinner, M.A., and Hunter, D.C. (2007). Fruits, vegetables, and their phytochemicals for bone and joint health. *Current Topics in Nutraceutical Research*, 5, 67–82.

Liu, J., Nada, K., Pang, X., Honda, C., Kitashiba, H., and Moriguchi, T. (2006b). Role of polyamines in peach fruit development and storage. *Tree Physiology*, 26, 791–798.

Liu, J.H., Honda, C., and Moriguchi, T. (2006a). Review: Involvement of polyamines in floral and fruit development. *Japan Agricultural Research Quarterly*, 40, 51–58.

Liu, R.H. (2003). Health benefits of fruit and vegetables are from additive and synergistic combinations of phytochemicals. *American Journal of Clinical Nutrition*, 78, 517S–520S.

Lobit, P., Génard, M., Wu, B.H., Soing, P., and Habib, R. (2003). Modelling citrate metabolism in fruits: Responses to growth and temperature. *Journal of Experimental Botany*, 54, 2489–2501.

Lohani, S., Trivedi, P.K., and Nath, P. (2004). Changes in activities of cell wall hydrolases during ethylene-induced ripening in banana: Effect of 1-MCP, ABA and IAA. , 31, 119–126.

Longo, L., and Vasapollo, G. (2006). Extraction and identification of anthocyanins from *Smilax aspera* L. berries. *Food Chemistry*, 94, 226–231.

Lopes-da-Silva, F., De Pascual-Teresa, S., Rivas-Gonzalo, J., and Santos-Buelga, C. (2002). Identification of anthocyanin pigments in strawberry (cv Camarosa) by LC using DAD and ESI-MS detection. *European Food Research and Technology*, 214, 248–253.

Lopes-da-Silva, F., Escribano-Bailón, M.T., and Santos-Buelga, C. (2007). Stability of pelargonidin 3-glucoside in model solutions in the presence and absence of flavanols. *American Journal of Food Technology*, 2, 602–617.

Löser, C. (2000). Polyamines in human and animal milk. *British Journal of Nutrition*, 84, Suppl. 1, S55–S58.

Lozano, M., Vidal-Aragón, M.C., Hernández, M.T., Ayuso, M.C., Bernalte, M.J. García, J., and Velardo, B. (2009). Physicochemical and nutritional properties and volatile constituents of six plum (*Prunus salicina* Lindl.) cultivars. *European Food Research and Technology*, 228, 403–410.

Lu, J., Vigneault, C., Charles, M.T., and Raghavan, G.S.V. (2007). Heat treatment application to increase fruit and vegetable quality. *Stewart Postharvest Review*, 3:4.

Luna-Guzmán, I., and Barret, D.M. (2000). Comparison of calcium chloride and calcium lactate effectiveness in maintaining shelf stability and quality of fresh-cut cantaloupes. *Postharvest Biology and Technology*, 19, 61–72.

Luna-Guzmán, I., Cantwell, M., and Barret, D.M. (1999). Fresh-cut cantaloupe: Effects of $CaCl_2$ dips and heat treatments on firmness and metabolic activity. *Postharvest Biology and Technology*, 17, 201–213.

Lurie, S. (1998). Postharvest heat treatments. *Postharvest Biology and Technology*, 14, 257–269.

Lurie, S., and Crisosto, C. (2005). Chilling injury in peach and nectarine. *Postharvest Biology and Technology*, 37, 199–208.

Madrid, R., Valverde, M., Alcolea, V., and Romojaro, F. (2004). Influence of calcium nutrition on water soaking disorder during ripening of cantaloupe melon. *Scientia Horticulturae*, 101, 69–79.

MAFF (1996). EC Quality Standards for Horticultural Produce: Fresh Fruit.

Mahmud, T.M.M., Eryani-Raqeeb, A.A., Omar, S.S.R., Mohamed, Z.A.R., and Eryani, A.A.R. (2008). Effects of different concentrations and applications of calcium on storage life and physicochemical characteristics of papaya (*Carica papaya* L.). *American Journal of Agricultural and Biological Sciences*, 3, 526–533.

Malik, A.U., and Singh, Z. (2005). Pre-storage application of polyamines improves shelf-life and fruit quality of mango. *Journal of Horticultural Science and Biotechnology*, 80, 363–369.

Malik, A.U., and Singh, Z. (2006). Improved fruit retention, yield and fruit quality in mango with exogenous application of polyamines. *Scientia Horticulturae*, 110, 167–174.

Malik, A.U., Singh, Z., and Dhaliwal, S.S. (2003). Exogenous application of putrescine affects mango fruit quality and shelf life. *Acta Horticulturae*, 628, 121–127.

Manganaris, G.A., Crisosto, C.H., Bremer, V., and Holcroft, D. (2008). Novel 1-methylcyclopropene immersion formulation extends shelf life of advanced maturity "Joanna Red" plums (*Prunus salicina* Lindell). *Postharvest Biology and Technology*, 47, 429–433.

Manganaris, G.A., Vasilakakis, M., Diamantidis, G., and Mignani, I. (2005a). Effects of post-harvest calcium treatments on the physicochemical properties of cell wall pectin in nectarine fruit during ripening after harvest or cold storage. *Journal of Horticultural Science and Biotechnology*, 80, 611–617.

Manganaris, G.A., Vasilakakis, M., Diamantidis, G., and Mignani, I. (2006). Effect of in-season calcium applications on cell wall physicochemical properties of nectarine fruit (*Prunus persica* var. *nectarina* Ait. Maxim) after harvest or cold storage. *Journal of the Science of Food and Agriculture*, 86, 2597–2602.

Manganaris, G.A., Vasilakakis, M., Diamantidis, G., and Mignani, I. (2007). The effect of postharvest calcium application on tissue calcium concentration, quality attributes incidence of flesh browning and cell wall physicochemical aspects of peach fruits. *Food Chemistry*, 100, 1385–1392.

Manganaris, G.A., Vasilakakis, M., Mignani, I., Diamantidis, G., and Tzavella-Klonari, K. (2005b). The effect of preharvest calcium sprays on quality attributes, physicochemical aspects of cell wall components and susceptibility to brown rot of peach fruits (*Prunus persica* L. cv. Andross). *Scientia Horticulturae*, 107, 43–50.

Mao, L.C., Que, F., and Donald, H.J. (2004). 1-Methylcyclopropene and CaCl2 treatments affect lipolytic enzymes in fresh-cut watermelon fruit. *Acta Botanica Sinica*, 46, 1402–1407.

Marcos, J.F., González-Candelas, L., and Zacarías, L. (2005). Involvement of ethylene biosynthesis and perception in the susceptibility of citrus fruits to *Penicillium digitatum* infection and the accumulation of defence-related mRNAs. *Journal of Experimental Botany*, 56, 2183–2193.

Mari, M., Neri, F., and Bertolini, P. (2007). Novel approaches to prevent and control postharvest diseases of fruit. *Stewart Postharvest Review*, 3:6.

Marín, A., Ferreres, F., Tomás-Barberán, F. A., and Gil, M. I. (2004). Characterization and quantitation of antioxidant constituents of sweet pepper (*Capsicum annuum* L.). *Journal of Agricultural and Food Chemistry*, 52, 3861–3869.

Marín, A., Rubio, J.S., Martínez, V., and Gil, M.I. (2009). Antioxidant compounds in green and red peppers as affected by irrigation frequency, salinity and nutrient solution composition. *Journal of the Science of Food and Agriculture*, 89, 1352–1359.

Martí, N., Pérez-Vicente, A., and García-Viguera, C. (2001). Influence of storage temperature and ascorbic acid addition on pomegranate juice. *Journal of the Science of Food and Agriculture*, 82, 217–221.

Martín-Belloso, O., Soliva-Fortuny, R., and Oms-Oliu, G. (2007). Fresh Cut Fruits. In *Handbook of Food Products Manufacturing*, ed. Y.H. Hui, 879–899. New Jersey: John Wiley and Sons, Inc.

Martín-Diana, A.B., Rico, D., Frías, J.M., Barat, J.M., Henehan, G.T.M., and Barry-Ryan, C. (2007). Calcium for extending the shelf life of fresh whole and minimally processed fruits and vegetables: A review. *Trends in Food Science and Technology*, 18, 210–218.

Martínez, G.A., and Civello, P.M. (2008). Effect of heat treatments on gene expression and enzyme activities associated to cell wall degradation in strawberry fruit. *Postharvest Biology and Technology*, 49, 38–45.

Martínez-Madrid, M.C., Serrano, M., Pretel, M.T., Martínez-Reina, G., and Romojaro, F. (2000). Note: The ripening of *Prunus persica* fruits with a dominant flat allele. *Food Science and Technology International*, 6, 399–405.

Martínez-Madrid, M.C., Serrano, M., Riquelme, F., and Romojaro, F. (1996). Polyamines, abscisic acid and ethylene production in tomato fruit. *Phytochemistry*, 43, 323–326.

Martínez-Romero, D., Alburquerque, N., Valverde, J.M., Guillén, F., Castillo, S., Valero, D., and Serrano, M. (2006). Postharvest sweet cherry quality and safety maintenance by *Aloe vera* treatment: a new edible coating. *Postharvest Biology and Technology*, 39, 93–100.

Martínez-Romero, D., Bailén, G., Serrano, M., Guillén, F., Valverde, J. M., Zapata, P., Castillo, S., and Valero, D. (2007a). Tools to maintain postharvest fruit and vegetable quality through the inhibition of the ethylene action. *Critical Review in Food Science and Nutrition*, 47, 543–560.

Martínez-Romero, D., Dupille, E., Guillen, F., Valverde, J.M., Serrano, M., and Valero D. (2003a). 1-Methylcyclopropene increases storability and shelf life in climacteric and nonclimacteric plums. *Journal of Agricultural and Food Chemistry*, 51, 4680–4686.

Martínez-Romero, D., Guillén, F. Castillo, S. Valero, D., and Serrano, M. (2003b). Modified atmosphere packaging maintains quality of table grape. *Journal of Food Science* 68, 1838–1843.

Martínez-Romero, D., Guillén, F., Castillo, S., Zapata, P.J., Serrano, M., and Valero, D. (2009a). Development of a carbon-heat hybrid ethylene scrubber for fresh horticultural produce storage purposes. *Postharvest Biology and Technology*, 51, 200–205.

Martínez-Romero, D., Guillén, F., Castillo, S., Zapata, P.J., Valero, D., and Serrano, M. (2009b). Effect of ethylene concentration on quality parameters of fresh tomatoes stored using a carbon-heat hybrid ethylene scrubber. *Postharvest Biology and Technology*, 51, 206–211.

Martínez-Romero, D., Guillén, F., Valverde, J. M., Bailén, G., Zapata, P. J., Serrano, M., Castillo, S., and Valero, D. (2007b). Influence of carvacrol on survival of *Botrytis cinerea* inoculated in table grapes. *International Journal of Food Microbiology*, 115, 144–148.

Martínez-Romero, D., Serrano, M., Carbonell, A., Burgos, L., Riquelme, F., and Valero, D. (2002). Effects of postharvest putrescine treatment on extending shelf life and reducing mechanical damage in apricot. *Journal of the Science of Food and Agriculture*, 67, 1706–1712.

Martínez-Romero, D., Serrano, M., Carbonell, A., Castillo, S., Riquelme, F., and Valero, D. (2004). Mechanical damage during fruit post-harvest handling: Technical and physiological implications. In *Production Practices and Quality Assessment of Food Crops. Vol. 3. Quality Handling and Evaluation*, eds. R. Dris, and S.M. Jain, 233–252. Dordrecht: Kluwer Academic Publishers.

Martínez-Romero, D., Serrano, M., and Valero, D. (2003c). Physiological changes in pepino (*Solanum muricatum* Ait) fruit stored at chilling and non-chilling temperatures. *Postharvest Biology and Technology*, 30, 177–186.

Martínez-Romero, D., Valero, D., Serrano, M., Burló, F., Carbonell, A., Burgos, L., and Riquelme, F. (2000). Exogenous polyamines and gibberellic acid effects on peach (*Prunus persica* L.) storability improvement. *Journal of Food Science*, 65, 288–294.

Martínez-Romero, D., Valero, D., Serrano, M., Martínez-Sánchez, F., and Riquelme, F. (1999). Effects of post-harvest putrescine and calcium treatments on reducing mechanical damage and polyamines and abscisic acid levels during lemon storage. *Journal of the Science of Food and Agriculture*, 79, 1589–1595.

Martínez-Téllez, M.A., Ramos-Clamont, M.G., Gardena, A.A., and Vargas-Arispuro, I. (2002). Effect of infiltrated polyamines on polygalacturonase activity and chilling injury responses in zucchini squash (*Cucurbita pepo* L). *Biochemical and Biophysical Research Communications*, 295, 98–101.

Martin-Tanguy, J. (1997). Conjugated polyamines and reproductive development: Biochemical, molecular and physiological approaches. *Physiologia Plantarum*, 100, 675–688.

Mathooko, F.M., Tsunashima, Y., Owino, W.Z.O., Kubo, Y., and Inaba, A. (2001). Regulation of genes encoding ethylene biosynthetic enzymes in peach (*Prunus persica* L.) fruit by carbon dioxide and 1-methylcyclopropene. *Postharvest Biology and Technology*, 21, 265–281.

Mato, I., Suárez-Luque, S., and Huidobro, J.F. (2005). A review of the analytical methods to determine organic acids in grape juices and wines. *Food Research International*, 38, 1175–1188.

Mattoo, A.K., and Handa, A.K. (2008). Higher polyamines restore and enhance metabolic memory in ripening fruit. *Plant Science*, 174, 386–393.

May, J.M. (1999). Is ascorbic acid an antioxidant for the plasma membrane? *The FASEB Journal*, 13, 995–1006.

McDonald, K., and Sun, D.W. (2000). Vacuum cooling technology for the food processing industry: A review. *Journal of Food Engineering*, 45, 55–65.

McDonald, R.E., McCollum, T.G., and Baldwin, E.A. (1999). Temperature of water heat treatments influences tomato fruit quality following low-temperature storage. *Postharvest Biology and Technology*, 16, 147–155.

Mehta, R.A., Cassol, T., Li, N., Ali, N., Handa, A.K., and Mattoo, A.K. (2002). Engineered polyamine accumulation in tomato enhances phytonutrient content, juice quality, and vine life. *Nature Biotechnology*, 20, 613–618.

Mencarelli, F., Massantini, R., and Botondi, R. (1996). Influence of impact surface and temperature on the ripening response of kiwifruit. *Postharvest Biology and Technology*, 8, 165–177.

Mercadente, A.Z., Steck, A., and Pfander, H. (1999). Carotenoids from guava (*Psidium guajava* L.): Isolation and structure elucidation. *Journal of Agricultural and Food Chemistry*, 47, 145–151.

Michailides, T.J., and Manganaris, G. (2009). Harvesting and handling effects on postharvest decay. *Stewart Postharvest Review*, 2009, 2:2.

Mignani, I., Greve, L.C., Ben-Arie, R., Stotz, H.U., Li, C., Shackel, K., and Lavabitch, J.M. (1995). The effects of GA_3 and divalent cations on aspects of pectin metabolism and tissue softening in ripening tomato pericarp. *Physiologia Plantarum*, 93, 108–115.

Miller, A.R. (1992). Physiology, biochemistry and detection of bruising (mechanical stress) in fruits and vegetables. *Postharvest News and Information*, 3, 53–58.

Miller, N.J., Sampson, J., Candeias, L.P., Bramley, P.M., and Rice-Evans, C.A. (1996). Antioxidant activities of carotenes and xantophylls. *FEBS Letters*, 384, 240–242.

Mirdehghan, S.H., Rahemi, M., Castillo, S., Martínez-Romero, D., Serrano, M., and Valero, D. (2007a). Pre-storage application of polyamines by pressure or immersion improves shelf-life of pomegranate stored at chilling temperature by increasing endogenous polyamine levels. *Postharvest Biology and Technology*, 44, 26–33.

Mirdehghan, S.H., Rahemi, M., Martínez-Romero, D., Guillén, F., Valverde, J.M., Zapata, P., Serrano, M., and Valero, D. (2007b). Reduction of pomegranate chilling injury during storage after heat treatments: Role of polyamines. *Postharvest Biology and Technology*, 44, 19–25.

Mirdehghan, S.H., Rahemi, M., Serrano, M., Guillén, F., Martínez-Romero, D., and Valero, D. (2006). Prestorage heat treatment to maintain nutritive and functional properties during postharvest cold storage of pomegranate. *Journal of Agricultural and Food Chemistry*, 54, 8495–8500.

Mirdehghan, S.H., Rahemi, M., Serrano, M., Guillén, F., Martínez-Romero, D., and Valero, D. (2007c). The application of polyamines by pressure or immersion as a tool to maintain functional properties in stored pomegranates arils. *Journal of Agricultural and Food Chemistry*, 55, 755–760.

Moinard, C., Cynober, L., and de Bandt, J.P. (2005). Polyamines: Metabolism and implications in human diseases. *Clinical Nutrition*, 24, 184–197.

Monselise, S.P. (1986). *CRC Handbook of Fruit Set and Development*. Boca Raton: CRC Press Inc.

Moodley, R.S., Govinden, R., and Odhav, B. (2002). The effect of modified atmosphere and packaging on patulin production in apples. *Journal of Food Protection*, 65, 867–871.

Morandi, B., Grappadelli, L.G., Rieger, M., and Lo Bianco, R. (2008). Carbohydrate availability affects growth and metabolism in peach fruit. *Physiologia Plantarum*, 133, 229–241.

Moreno, D.A., Carvajal, M., López-Berenguer, C., and García-Viguera, C. (2007). Chemical and biological characterisation of nutraceutical compounds of broccoli. *Food*, 1, 297–312.

Moret, S., Smela, D., Populin, T., and Conte, L.S. (2005). A survey on free biogenic content of fresh and preserved vegetables. *Food Chemistry*, 89, 355–361.

Morillon, V., Debeafort, F., Blond, G., Capelle, M., and Voilley, A. (2002). Factors affecting the moisture permeability of lipid-based edible films: A review. *Critical Review in Food Science and Nutrition*, 42, 67–89.

Moss, M.O. (2008). Fungi, quality, and safety issues in fresh fruits and vegetables. *Journal of Applied Microbiology*, 104, 1239–1243.

Mozetiĉ, B., Simcĩč, M., and Trebsě, P. (2006). Anthocyanins and hydroxycinnamic acids of Lambert Compact cherries (*Prunus avium* L.) after cold storage and 1-methylcyclopropene treatment. *Food Chemistry*, 97, 302–309.

Mozetiĉ, B., Trebŝe, P., and Hribar, J. (2002). Determination and quantisation of anthocyanins and hydroxycinnamic acids in different cultivars of sweet cherries (*Prunus avium* L.) from Nova Gorica Region (Slovenia). *Food Technology and Biotechnology*, 40, 207–212.

Mwaniki, M.W., Mathooko, F.M., Matsuzaki, M., Hiwasa, K., Tateishi, A., and Ushijima, K. (2005). Expression characteristics of seven members of the beta-galactosidase gene family in "La France" pear (*Pyrus communis* L.) fruit during growth and their regulation by 1-methylcyclopropene during postharvest ripening. *Postharvest Biology and Technology*, 36, 253–263.

Nagy, S. (1980). Vitamin C contents of citrus fruit and their products: a review. *Journal of Agricultural and Food Chemistry*, 28, 8–18.

Nair, S., and Singh, Z. (2004). Chilling injury in mango fruit in relation to biosynthesis of free polyamines. *Journal of Horticultural Science and Biotechnology*, 79, 515–522.

Neljubow, D.N. (1901). Uber die horizontale nutation der stengel von Pisium sativum und einiger anderer pflanzen. *Beitrage und Botanik Zentralblatt*, 10, 128–139.

Nguyen, M.L., and Schwartz, S.J. (1999). Lycopene: Chemical and biological properties. *Food Technology*, 53, 38–45.

Nichenametla, S.N., Taruscio, T.G., Barney, D.L., and Exon, J.H. (2006). A review of the effects and mechanisms of polyphenolics in cancer. *Critical Review in Food Science and Nutrition*, 46, 161–183.

Nielsem, T., and Leufvén, A. (2008). The effect of modified atmosphere packaging on the quality of Honeoye and Korona strawberries. *Food Chemistry*, 107, 1053–1063.

Nishibori, N., Fujihara, S., and Akatuki, T. (2007). Amounts of polyamines in foods in Japan and intake by Japanese. *Food Chemistry*, 100, 491–497.

Obenland, D.M., Arpaia, M.L., Austin, R.K., and MacKey, B.E. (1999). High-temperature forced-air treatment alters the quantity of flavor-related, volatile constituents present in Navel and Valencia oranges. *Journal of Agricultural and Food Chemistry*, 47, 5184–5188.

Omoni, A.O., and Aluko, R.E. (2005). The anti-carcinogenic and anti-atherogenic effects of lycopene: a review. *Trends in Food Science and Technology*, 16, 344–350.

Oms-Oliu, G., Hertog, M.L.A.T.M, Soliva-Fortuny, R., Martín-Belloso, O., and Nicolaï, B.M. (2009). Recent developments in the use of modified atmosphere packaging for fresh-cut fruits and vegetables. *Stewart Postharvest Review*, 4:3.

Orak, H.H. (2007). Total antioxidant activities, phenolics, anthocyanins, polyphenoloxidase activities of selected red grape cultivars and their correlation. *Scientia Horticulturae*, 111, 235–241.

Ortiz, A., Echeverria, G., Graell, J., and Lara, I. (2009). Calcium dips enhance volatile emission of cold-stored 'Fuji Kiku-8' apples. *Journal of Agricultural and Food Chemistry*, 57, 4931–4938.

Ozdemir, M., and Floros, J.D. (2004). Active food packaging technologies. *Critical Review in Food Science and Nutrition*, 44, 185–193.

Paksasorn, A., Hayasaka, T., Matsui, H., Ohara, H., and Hirata, N. (1995). Relationship of polyamine content to ACC content and ethylene evolution in Japanese apricot fruit. *Journal of the Japanese Society for Horticultural Science*, 63, 761–766.

Pandey, S., Ranade, S.A., Nagar, P.K., and Kumar, N. (2000). Role of polyamines and ethylene as modulators of plant senescence. *Journal of Bioscience*, 25, 291–299.

Pandit, S.S., Chiley, H.G., Kulkarni, R.S., Pujari, K.H., Giri, A.P., and Gupta, V.S. (2009). Cultivar relationships in mango based on fruit volatile profile. *Food Chemistry*, 114: 363–372.

Park, H.J. (1999). Development of advanced edible coatings for fruits. *Trends in Food Science and Technology*, 10, 254–260.

Park, S., Zhao, Y., Leonard, S.W., and Traber, M.G. (2005). Vitamin E and mineral fortification in fresh-cut apples (*Fuji*) using vacuum impregnation. *Nutrition and Food Science*, 35, 393–402.

Park, Y.S., Jung, S.T., Kang, S.G., Drzewiecki, J., Namiesnik, J., Haruenkit, R., Barasch, D., Trakhtenberg, S., and Gorinstein, S. (2006). *In vitro* studies of polyphenols, antioxidants and other dietary indices in kiwifruit *(Actinidia deliciosa). International Journal of Food Sciences and Nutrition* 57, 107–122.

Paull, R.E., and Chen, N.J. (2000). Heat treatment and fruit ripening. *Postharvest Biology and Technology*, 21, 21–37.

Pech, J.C., Bouzayen, M., and Latché, A. (2008). Climacteric fruit ripening: Ethylene-dependent and independent regulation of ripening pathways in melon fruit. *Plant Science*, 175, 114–120.

Pech, J.C., Latché, A., and Balagué, C. (1992). *Cellular and Molecular Aspects of the Plant Hormone Ethylene*. The Netherlands: Kluwer Academic Publishers.

Pennington, J.A.T. (2002). Food composition databases for bioactive food components. *Journal of Food Composition and Analysis*, 15, 419–434.

Pérez-Vicente, A., Martínez-Romero, D., Carbonell, A., Serrano, M., Riquelme, F., Guillén, F., and Valero, D. (2002). Role of polyamines in extending shelf life and the reduction of mechanical damage during plum (*Prunus salicina* Lindl) storage. *Postharvest Biology and Technology*, 25, 25–32.

Periago, P. M., Delgado, B., Fernández, P. S. and Palop, A. (2004). Use of carvacrol and cymene to control growth and viability of *Listeria monocytogenes* cells and predictions of survivors using frequency distribution functions. *Journal of Food Protection*, 67, 1408–1416.

Perkins-Veazie, P., Collins, J.K., Pair, S.D., and Roberts, W. (2001). Lycopene content differs among red-fleshed watermelon cultivars. *Journal of the Science of Food and Agriculture*, 81, 983–987.

Pesis, E., Ackerman, M., Ben-Arie, R., Feygenberg, O., Feng, X., Apelbaum, A., Goren, R., and Prusky, D. (2002). Ethylene involvement in chilling injury symptoms of avocado during cold storage. *Postharvest Biology and Technology*, 24, 171–181.

Pesis, E., Aharoni, D., Aharon, Z., Ben-Arie, R., Aharoni, N., and Fuchs, Y. (2000). Modified atmosphere and modified humidity packaging alleviates chilling injury symptoms in mango fruit. *Postharvest Biology and Technology*, 19, 93–101.

Petersen, K., Nielsen, P.G., Bertelsen, G., Lawther, M., Olsen, M.B., Nilsson, N.H., and Mortensen, G. (1999). Potential of biobased materials for food packaging. *Trends in Food Science and Technology*, 10, 52–28.

Peterson, D.L. (2005). Harvest mechanization progress and prospects for fresh market quality deciduous tree fruits. *HortTechnology*, 15, 72–75.

Petkou, I.T., Pritsa, T.S., and Sfakiotakis, E.M. (2004). Effects of polyamines on ethylene production, respiration and ripening of kiwifruit. *Journal of Horticultural Science and Biotechnology*, 79, 977–980.

Phakawatmongkol, W., Ketsa, S., and Van Doorn, W.G. (2004). Variation in fruit chilling injury among mango cultivars. *Postharvest Biology and Technology*, 32, 115–118.

Picchioni, G.A., Watada, A.E., Conway, W.S., Whitaker, B.D., and Sams, C.E. (1998). Postharvest calcium infiltration delays membrane lipid catabolism in apple fruit. *Journal of Agricultural and Food Chemistry*, 46, 2452–2457.

Pinheiro, S.C.F., and Almeida, D.P.F. (2008). Modulation of tomato pericarp firmness through pH and calcium: Implications for the texture of fresh-cut fruit. *Postharvest Biology and Technology*, 47, 119–125.

Pino, J.A., Mesa, J., Muñoz, Y., Martí, M.P., and Marbot, R.J. (2005). Volatile components from mango (*Mangifera indica* L.) cultivars. *Journal of Agricultural and Food Chemistry*, 53, 2213–2223.

Plotto, A, Bai, J, Narciso, J.A., Brecht, J.K., and Baldwin, E.A. (2006). Ethanol vapour prior to processing extends fresh-cut mango storage by decreasing spoilage, but does not always delay ripening. *Postharvest Biology and Technology*, 39, 134–145.

Polenta, G., Lucanngeli, C.D., Budde, C.O., González, C.B., and Murray, R.E. (2006). Heat and anaerobic treatments affected physiological and biochemical parameters in tomato fruits. *LWT-Food Science and Technology*, 39, 37–34.

Ponappa, T., and Miller, A.R. (1996). Polyamines in normal and auxin-induced strawberry fruit development. *Physiologia Plantarum*, 98, 447–454.

Porat, R., Weiss, B., Cohen, L., Daus, A., Goren, R., and Droby, S. (1999). Effects of ethylene and 1-methylcyclopropene on the postharvest qualities of "Shamouti" oranges. *Postharvest Biology and Technology*, 15, 155–163.

Prasanna, V., Prabha, T.N., and Tharanathan, R.N. (2007). Fruit ripening phenomena: An overview. *Critical Reviews in Food Science and Nutrition*, 47, 1–19.

Pretel, M.T., Serrano, M., Amorós, A., Riquelme, F., and Romojaro, F. (1995). Non-involvement of ACC and ACC oxidase activity in pepper fruit ripening. *Postharvest Biology and Technology*, 5, 295–302.

Pretel, M.T., Serrano, M., Amorós, A., and Romojaro, F. (1999). Ripening and ethylene biosynthesis in controlled atmosphere stored apricots. *European Food Research and Technology*, 209, 130–134.

Pretel, M.T., Serrano, M., Martínez, G., Riquelme, F., and Romojaro, F. (1993). Influence of films of different permeability on ethylene synthesis and ripening of MA-Packaged apricots. *Lebensmittel-Wissenschaft und Technologie*, 26, 8–13.

Promyou, S., Ketsa, S., and van Doorn, W.G. (2008). Hot water treatments delay cold-induced banana peel blackening. *Postharvest Biology and Technology*, 48, 132–138.

Prusky, D., and Lichter, A. (2008). Mechanisms modulating fungal attack in post-harvest pathogen interactions and their control. *European Journal of Plant Pathology*, 121, 281–289.

Pusey, P.L., and Wilson, C.L. (1984). Postharvest biological control of stone fruit brown rot by *Bacillus subtilis*. *Plant Disease*, 68, 753–756

Puziy, A.M., Poddubnaya, O.I., Martínez-Alonso, A., Suárez-García, F., and Tascón, J.M.D. (2002). Synthetic carbons activated with phosphoric acid. I. Surface chemistry and ion binding properties. *Carbon*, 40, 1493–1505.

Quiles, A., Hernando, I., Pérez-Munuera, I., and Lluch, M.A. (2007). Effect of calcium propionate on the microstructure and pectin methylesterase activity in the parenchyma of fresh-cut Fuji apples. *Journal of the Science of Food and Agriculture*, 87, 511–519.

Raffo, A., La Malfa, G., Fogliano, V., Maiani, G., and Quaglia, G. (2006). Seasonal variations in antioxidant components of cherry tomatoes (*Lycopersicon esculentum* cv. Naomi F1). *Journal of Food Composition and Analysis*, 19, 11–19.

Rai, D.R., and Paul, S. (2007). Packaging requirements of highly respiring produce under modified atmosphere: A review. *Journal of Science and Technology*, 44, 10–15.

Ramezanian, A., Rahemi, M., and Vazifehshenas, M.R. (2009). Effects of foliar application of calcium chloride and urea on quantitative and qualitative characteristics of pomegranate fruits. *Scientia Horticulturae*, 121, 171–175.

Randhawa, J.S., Jawandha, S.K., Mahajan, B.V.C., and Gill, P.P.S. (2009). Effect of different pre-harvest treatments on quality of ber fruit during cold storage. *Journal of Food Science and Technology*, 46, 174–176.

Rasori, A., Ruperti, B., Bonghi, C., Tonutti, P., and Ramina, A. (2002). Characterization of two putative ethylene receptor genes expressed during peach fruit development and abscission. *Journal of Experimental Botany*, 53, 2333–2339.

Recasens, I., Benavides, A., Puy, J., and Casero, T. (2004). Pre-harvest calcium treatments in relation to the respiration rate and ethylene production of "Golden Smoothee" apples. *Journal of the Science of Food and Agriculture*, 84, 765–771.

Rennie, T.J., Raghavan, G.S.V., Vigneault, C., and Gariépy, Y. (2001). Vacuum cooling of lettuce with various rates of pressure reduction. *Transaction of the ASAE*, 44, 89–93.

Retamales, J., Deffilippi, B., and Campos, R. (2000). Alleviation of cold storage disorders in nectarines by modified atmosphere packaging. *Fruits*, 55, 213–219.

Rhodes, M.J.C. (1980). The maturation and ripening of fruits. In *Senescence in Plants*, ed. K.V. Thimann, 157–205. Boca Raton: CRC Press.

Rodov, V., Ben-Yehoshua, S., Kim, J.J., Shapiro, B., and Ittah, Y. (1992). Ultraviolet illumination induces scoparone production in kumquat and orange fruit and improves decay resistance. *Journal of the American Society for Horticultural Science*, 117, 788–792.

Rodrigo, M.J., and Zacarías, L. (2006). Horticultural and quality aspects of citrus fruits. In *Handbook of Fruits and Fruit Processing*, ed. Y.H. Hui, 293–307. Oxford. Blackwell Publishing.

Rodriguez, S.C., López, B., and Chaves, A.R. (2001). Effect of different treatments on the evolution of polyamines during refrigerated storage of eggplants. *Journal of Agricultural and Food Chemistry*, 49, 4700–4705.

Rodriguez-Amaya, D.B., and Kimura, M. (2004). *Harvestplus Handbook for Carotenoid Analysis. HarvestPlus Technical Monograph 2*. Brasil: Harvestplus.

Rojas-Graü, M.A., Oms-Oliu, G., Soliva-Fortuny, R., and Martín-Belloso, O. (2009). The use of packaging techniques to maintain freshness in fresh-cut fruits and vegetables: A review. *International Journal of Food Science and Technology*, 44, 875–889.

Rose, J.C., and Bennett, A.B. (1999). Cooperative disassembly of the cellulose-xyloglucan network of plant cell walls: Parallels between cell expansion and fruit ripening. *Trends in Plant Science*, 4, 176–183.

Ruberto, G., and Baratta, M. T. (2000). Antioxidant activity of selected essential oil components in two lipid model systems. *Food Chemistry*, 69, 167–174.

Sacchetti, G., Maietti, S., Muzzoli, M., Scaglianti, M., Manfredini, S., Radice, M., and Bruni, R. (2005). Comparative evaluation of 11 essential oils of different origin as functional antioxidants, antiradicals and antimicrobials in foods. *Food Chemistry*, 91, 621–632.

Safizadeh, M.R., Rahemi, M., Tafazoli, E., and Eman, Y. (2007). Influence of postharvest vacuum infiltration with calcium on chilling injury, firmness and quality of Lisbon lemon fruit. *American Journal of Food Technology*, 2, 388–396.

Saftner, R.A., Bai, J., Abbott, J.A., and Lee, Y.S. (2003). Saltveit, M.E. and Morris, L.L. (1990). Overview of chilling injury of horticultural crops, In *Chilling Injury of Horticultural Crops*, ed. C.Y. Wang, 3–15. Boca Raton: CRC Press.

Salcini, M., and Massantini, R. (2005). Minimally processed fruits: An update on browning control. *Stewart Postharvest Review* 3:7.

Salftner, R.A., Bai, J., Abbott, J.A., and Lee, Y.S. (2003). Sanitary dips with calcium propionate, calcium chloride, or a calcium amino acid chelate maintain quality and shelf stability of fresh-cut honeydew chunks. *Postharvest Biology and Technology*, 29, 257–269.

Saltvert, M.E., and Morris, L.L. (1990). Overview of chilling injury of horticultural crops. In *Chilling Injury of Horticultural Crops*, ed. C.Y. Wang, 3–15. Boca Raton: CRC Press.

Sandhya. (2010). Modified atmosphere packaging of fresh produce: Current status and future needs. *Lebensmmittel Wissenschaft und Technologie*, 43, 381–392.

Saura-Calixto, F., and Goñi, I. (2006). Antioxidant capacity of the Spanish Mediterranean diet. *Food Chemistry*, 94, 442–447.

Saura-Calixto, F., and Goñi, I. (2009). Definition of the Mediterranean diet based on bioactive compounds. *Critical Review in Food Science and Nutrition*, 49, 145–152.

Scalbert, A., Manach, C., Morand, C., Rémésy, C., and Jiménez, L. (2005). Dietary polyphenols and the prevention of diseases. *Critical Review in Food Science and Nutrition*, 45, 287–306.

Schirra, M., Barbera, G., D'hallewin, G., Inglese, P., and La Mantia, T. (1997). Storage response of cactus pear fruit to $CaCl_2$ preharvest spray and postharvest heat treatment. *Journal of Horticultural Science*, 72, 371–377.

Schirra, M., and D'hallewin, (1997). Storage performance of Fortune mandarins following hot water dips. *Postharvest Biology and Technology*, 10, 229–238.

Schirra, M., D'hallewin, G.S., Ben-Yehoshua, S., and Fallik, E. (2000). Host-pathogen interactions modulated by heat treatment. *Postharvest Biology and Technology*, 21, 71–85.

Schirra, M., Palma, A., D'aquino, S., Angioni, A., Minello, E.V., Melis, M., and Cabras, P. (2008). Influence of postharvest hot water treatment on nutritional and functional properties of kumquat (*Fortunella japonica* Lour. Swingle Cv. Ovale) fruit. *Journal of Agricultural and Food Chemistry*, 56, 455–560.

Schreiner, M., and Huyskens-Keil, S. (2006). Phytochemicals in fruit and vegetables: health promotion and postharvest elicitors. *Critical Review in Plant Sciences*, 25, 267–278.

Seeram, N.P. (2008). Berry fruits for cancer prevention: current status and future prospects. *Journal of Agricultural and Food Chemistry*, 56, 630–635.

Seifried, H.E., Anderson, D.E., Fisher, E.I., and Milner, J.A. (2007). A review of the interactions among dietary antioxidants and reactive oxygen species. *Journal of Nutritional Biochemistry*, 18, 567–579.

Sen, C.K., Khanna, S., and Roy, S. (2007). Tocotrienols in health and disease: The other half of the natural vitamin E family. *Molecular Aspects of Medicine*, 28, 692–728.

Serrano, M., Amorós, A., Pretel, M.T., Martínez-Madrid, M.C., and Romojaro, F. (2002). Effect of calcium deficiency on melon (*Cucumis melo* L.) texture and glassiness incidence during ripening. *Food Science and Technology International*, 8, 147–154.

Serrano, M., Díaz-Mula, H.M., Zapata, P.J., Castillo, S., Guillén, F., Martínez-Romero, D., Valverde, J.M., and Valero, D. (2009). Maturity stage at harvest determines the fruit quality and antioxidant potential after storage of sweet cherry cultivars. *Journal of Agricultural and Food Chemistry*, 57, 3240–3246.

Serrano, M., Guillén, F., Martínez-Romero, D., Castillo, S., and Valero, D. (2005a). Chemical constituents and antioxidant activity of sweet cherry at different ripening stages. *Journal of Agricultural and Food Chemistry*, 53, 2741–2745.

Serrano, M., Martínez-Madrid, M.C., Martínez, G., Riquelme, F., Pretel, M.T., and Romojaro, F. (1996). Review: Role of polyamines in chilling injury of fruit and vegetables. *Food Science and Technology International*, 2, 195–199.

Serrano, M., Martínez-Madrid, M.C., Pretel, M.T., Riquelme, F., and Romojaro, F. (1997). Modified atmosphere packaging minimizes increases in putrescine and abscisic acid levels caused by chilling injury in pepper fruit. *Journal of Agricultural and Food Chemistry*, 45, 1668–1672.

Serrano, M., Martínez-Romero, D., Castillo, S., Guillén, F., and Valero, D. (2004a). Role of calcium and heat treatments in alleviating physiological changes induced by mechanical damage in plum. *Postharvest Biology and Technology*, 34, 155–157.

Serrano, M., Martínez-Romero, D., Castillo, S., Guillén, F., and Valero, D. (2004b). Effect of preharvest sprays containing calcium, magnesium and titanium on the quality of peaches and nectarines at harvest and during postharvest storage. *Journal of the Science of Food and Agriculture*, 84, 1270–1276.

Serrano, M., Martínez-Romero, D., Castillo, S., Guillén, F., and Valero, D. (2005b). The use of natural antifungal compounds improves the beneficial effect of MAP in sweet cherry storage. *Innovative Food Science and Emerging Technologies*, 6, 115–123.

Serrano, M., Martínez-Romero, D., Guillén, F., Castillo, S., and Valero, D. (2006). Maintenance of broccoli quality and functional properties during cold storage as affected by modified atmosphere packaging. *Postharvest Biology and Technology*, 39, 61–68.

Serrano M., Martínez-Romero D., Guillén F., and Valero D. (2003). Effects of exogenous putrescine on improving shelf life of four plum cultivars. *Postharvest Biology and Technology*, 30, 259–271.

Serrano, M., Martínez-Romero, D., Guillén, F., Valverde, J.M., Zapata, P.J., Castillo, S., and Valero, D. (2008a). The addition of essential oils to MAP as a tool to maintain the overall quality of fruits. *Trends in Food Science and Technology*, 19, 464–471.

Serrano, M., Martínez-Romero, D., Zuzunaga, M., Riquelme, F., and Valero, D. (2004c). Calcium, polyamine and gibberellin treatments to improve postharvest fruit quality. In *Production Practices and Quality Assessment of Food Crops. Vol. 4. Postharvest Treatment and Technology*, eds. R. Dris and S.M. Jain, 55–68. Dordrecht: Kluwer Academic Publishers.

Serrano, M., Pretel, M.T., Martínez-Madrid, M.C., Romojaro, F., and Riquelme, F. (1998). CO_2 treatment of zucchini squash reduces chilling-injured physiological changes. *Journal of Agricultural and Food Chemistry*, 46, 2465–2468.

Serrano, M., Zapata, P.J., Castillo, S., Guillén, F., Martínez-Romero, D., and Valero, D. (2010). Antioxidant and nutritive constituents during sweet pepper development and ripening are enhanced by nitrophenolate treatments. *Food Chemistry* 118, 497–503.

Serrano, M., Zapata, P.J., Guillén, F., Martínez-Romero, D., Castillo, S., and Valero, D. (2008b). Post-harvest ripening of tomato. In *Tomatoes and Tomato Products*, eds. V.R. Preedy and R.R. Watson, 67–84. Enfield: Science Publishers.

Sevillano, L., Sánchez-Ballesta, M.T., Romojaro, F., and Flores, F.B. (2009). Physiological, hormonal and molecular mechanisms regulating chilling injury in horticultural species: Postharvest technologies applied to reduce its impact. *Journal of the Science of Food and Agriculture*, 89, 555–573.

Sharma, R.R., Singh, D., and Singh, R. (2009). Biological control of postharvest diseases of fruits and vegetables by microbial antagonists: A review. *Biological Control*. 50, 205–221.

Sharon-Asa, L., Shalit, M., Frydman, A., Bar, E., Holland, D., Or, E., Lavi, U., Lewinsohn, E., and Eyal, Y. (2003). Citrus fruit flavor and aroma biosynthesis: isolation, functional characterization, and development regulation of Cstps1, a key gene in the production of the sesquiterpene aroma compound valencene. *The Plant Journal*, 36, 664–674.

Shewfelt, R.L. (1999). What is quality? *Postharvest Biology and Technology*, 15, 197–200.

Shiozaki, S., Ogata, T., and Horiuchi, S. (2000). Endogenous polyamines in the pericarp and seed of the grape berry during development and ripening. *Scientia Horticulturae*, 83, 33–41.

Shiratake, K., and Martinola, E. (2007). Transporters in fruit vacuoles. *Plant Biotechnology*, 24, 127–133.

Silva, F., Goyette, B., Bourgeois, G., and Vigneault, C. (2006). Comparing forced air cooling and water cooling for apples. *International Journal of Food, Agriculture and Environment*, 4, 33–36.

Simão, R.A., Silva, A.P., Gonçalves, F.H., Oliveira, J.R., Pereira, R., Lajolo, F.M., and Cordenunsi, B.R. (2008). Mango starch degradation. I. A microscopic view of the granule during ripening. *Journal of Agricultural and Food Chemistry*, 56, 7410–7415.

Singh, R., Singh, P., Pathak, N., Singh, V.K., and Dwivedi, U.N. (2007). Modulation of mango ripening by chemicals: physiological and biochemical aspects. *Plant Growth Regulation*, 53, 137–145.

Singh, S.P., and Rao, D.V.S. (2005). Effect of modified atmosphere packaging (MAP) on the alleviation of chilling injury and dietary antioxidants levels in "Solo" papaya during low temperature storage. *European Journal of Horticultural Science*, 70, 246–252.

Sisler, E.C. (2006). The discovery and development of compounds counteracting ethylene at the receptor level. *Biotechnology Advances*, 24, 357–367.

Sisler, E.C., and Pian, A. (1973). Effect of ethylene and cyclic olefins on tobacco leaves. *Tobacco Science*, 17, 68–72.

Sisler, E.C., and Serek, M. (1997). Inhibitors of ethylene responses in plants at the receptor level: Recent developments. *Physiologia Plantarum*, 100, 577–582.

Sivakumar, D., and Korsten, S. (2006). Influence of modified atmosphere packaging and postharvest treatments on quality retention of litchi cv. Mauritius. *Postharvest Biology and Technology*, 41, 135–142.

Smilanick, J.L., Mansour, M.F., and Sorenson, D. (2006). Pre- and postharvest treatments to control green mold of Citrus fruits during ethylene degreening. *Plant Disease*, 90, 89–96.

Soliva-Fortuny, R.C., and Martín-Belloso, O. (2003). New advances in extending the shelf-life of fresh-cut fruits: A review. *Trends in Food Science and Technology*, 14, 341–353.

Song, J., and Forney, C.F. (2008). Flavour volatile production and regulation in fruit. *Canadian Journal of Plant Science*, 88, 537–550.

Soto-Zamora, G., Yahia, E.M., Brecht, J.K., and Gadea, A. (2005). Effects of postharvest hot air treatments on the quality and antioxidant levels in tomato fruit. *Lebensmmittel Wissenschaft und Technologie*, 38, 657–663.

Sozzi, G.O., and Beaudry, R.M. (2007). Current perspectives on the use of 1-methylcyclopropene in tree fruit crops: An international survey. *Stewart Postharvest Review*, 2:8.

Spadaro, D., and Gullino, M.L. (2004). State of the art and future prospects of the biological control of postharvest fruit diseases. *International Journal of Food Microbiology*, 91, 185–194.

Spotts, R.A., Cervantes, L.A., and Facteau, T.J. (2002). Integrated control of brown rot of sweet cherry fruit with a preharvest fungicide, a postharvest yeast, modified atmosphere packaging, and cold storage temperature. *Postharvest Biology and Technology*, 24, 251–257.

Spotts, R.A., Cervantes, L.A., and Mielke, E.A. (1999). Variability in postharvest decay among apple cultivars. *Plant Disease*, 83, 1051–1054.

Srinivasa, P.C., and Tharanathan, R.N. (2007). Chitin/Chitosan–Safe, ecofriendly packaging materials with multiple potential uses. *Food Reviews International*, 23, 53–72.

Stearns, J.C., and Glick, B.R. (2003). Transgenic plants with altered ethylene biosynthesis or perception. *Biotechnology Advances*, 21, 193–210.

Stintzing, F.C., and Carle, R. (2004). Functional properties of anthocyanins and betalains in plants, food, and in human nutrition. *Trends in Food Science and Technology*, 15, 19–38.

Stückrath, R., Quevedo, R., De La Fuente, L., Hernández, A., and Sepúlveda, V. (2008). Effect of calcium foliar application on the characteristics of blueberry fruit during storage. *Journal of Plant Nutrition*, 31, 849–866.

Suntharalingam, S., (1996). Postharvest treatment of mangoes with calcium. *Tropical Science*, 36, 14–17.

Tang, J., Mitcham, E., Wang, S., and Lurie, S. (2007). *Heat treatments for Postharvest Pest Control: Theory and Practice*. Oxon: CAB International.

Tano, K., Oulé, K., Doyon, G., Lencki, R.W., and Arul, J. (2007). Comparative evaluation of the effect of storage temperature fluctuation on modified atmosphere packages of selected fruit and vegetables. *Postharvest Biology and Technology*, 46, 212–221.

Taylor, M., and Ramsay, G. (2005). Carotenoid biosynthesis in plant storage organs: recent advances and prospects for improving plant food quality. *Physiologia Plantarum*, 124, 143–151.

Teruel, B., Kieckbusch, T., and Cortez, L. (2004). Cooling parameters for fruits and vegetables of different sizes in a hydrocooling system. *Science of Agriculture*, 61, 655–658.

Thanaraj, T., Terry, L.A., and Bessant, C. (2009). Chemometric profiling of pre-climacteric Sri Lankan mango fruit (*Mangifera indica* L.). *Food Chemistry*, 112, 786–794.

Tian, S.P., Qin, G.Z., and Xu, Y. (2004). Survival of antagonistic yeasts under field conditions and their biocontrol ability against postharvest diseases of sweet cherry. *Postharvest Biology and Technology*, 33, 327–331.

Toivonen, P.M.A. (2007). Fruit maturation and ripening and their relationship to quality. *Stewart Postharvest Review*, 2:7.

Tomás-Barberán, F.A., Gil, M.I., Cremin, P., Waterhouse, A.L., Hess-Pierce, B., and Kader, A.A. (2001). HPLD-DAD-ESIMS analysis of phenolic compounds in nectarines, peaches, and plums. *Journal of Agricultural and Food Chemistry*, 49, 4748–4760.

Topuz, A., and Ozdemir, F. (2007). Assessment of carotenoids, capsaicinoids and ascorbic acid composition of some selected pepper cultivars (*Capsicum annuum* L.) grown in Turkey. *Journal of Food Composition and Analysis*, 20, 596–602.

Torrigiani, P., Bregoli, A.M., Ziosi, V., and Costa, G. (2008). Molecular and biochemical aspects underlying polyamine modulation of fruit development and ripening. *Stewart Postharvest Review*, 2:10.

Torrigiani, P., Bregoli, A.M., Ziosi, V., Scaramagli, S., Ciriaci, T., Rasori, A., Biondi, S., and Costa, G. (2004). Pre-harvest polyamine and aminoethoxyvinylglycine (AVG) applications modulate fruit ripening in Stark Red Gold nectarines (*Prunus persica* L. Batsch). *Postharvest Biology and Technology*, 33, 293–308.

Traka, M., and Mithen, R. (2009). Glucosinolates, isothiocyanates and human health. *Phytochemistry Reviews*, 8, 269–282.

Tripathi, P., and Dubey, N.K. (2004). Exploitation of natural products as alternative strategy to control postharvest fungal rotting of fruit and vegetables. *Postharvest Biology and Technology*, 32, 235–245.

Tsao, R., and Akhtar, M.H. (2005). Nutraceuticals and functional foods: I. Current trend in phytochemical antioxidant research. *Journal of Food Agriculture and Environment*, 3, 10–17.

Tucker, G., and Robards, K. (2008). Bioactivity and structure of biophenols as mediators of chronic diseases. *Critical Review in Food Science and Nutrition*, 48, 929–966.

Tucker, G.A., and Grierson, D. (1987). Fruit ripening. In *The Biochemistry of Plants* Vol. 12, ed. D. Davies, 265–319. New York: Academic Press, Inc.

Ultee, A., Bennik, M. H. J., and Moezelaar, R. (2002). The phenolic hydroxyl group of carvacrol is essential for action against the food-borne pathogen: *Bacillus cereus*. *Applied Environmental Microbiology*, 68, 1561–1568.

Usenik V., Fabčič J., and Štampar F. (2008). Sugars, organic acids, phenolic composition and antioxidant activity of sweet cherry (*Prunus avium* L.). *Food Chemistry*, 107, 185–192.

Valero, D., Martínez, D., Riquelme, F., and Serrano, M. (1998a). Polyamine response to external mechanical bruising in two mandarin cultivars. *HortScience*, 33, 1220–1223.

Valero, D., Martínez-Romero, D., and Serrano, M., (2002a). The role of polyamines in the improvement of the shelf life of fruit. *Trends in Food Science and Technology*, 13, 228–234.

Valero, D., Martínez-Romero, D., Serrano, M., and Riquelme F. (1998b). Postharvest gibberellin and heat treatment effects on polyamines, abscisic acid and firmness in lemons. *Journal of Food Science*, 63, 611–615.

Valero, D., Martínez-Romero, D., Serrano, M., and Riquelme F. (1998c). Influence of postharvest putrescine and calcium on endogenous polyamines, firmness, and abscisic acid in lemon (*Citrus lemon* L. Burn Cv Verna). *Journal of Agricultural and Food Chemistry*, 46, 2102–2109.

Valero, D., Martínez-Romero, D., Serrano, M., and Riquelme F. (1999). Polyamine roles on the post-harvest of fruits: A review. In *Recent Research Developments in Agricultural and Food Chemistry*, ed. S. Pandalai, 39–55. Trivandrum: Research Signpost.

Valero, D., Martínez-Romero, D., Valverde, J.M., Guillén, F., Castillo, S., and Serrano, M. (2004). Could the 1-MCP treatment effectiveness on plum be affected by packaging? *Postharvest Biology and Technology*, 34, 295–303.

Valero, D., Martínez-Romero, D., Valverde, J.M., Guillén, F., and Serrano, M. (2003). Quality improvement and extension of shelf life by 1-methylcyclopropene in plum as affected by ripening stage at harvest. *Innovative Food Science and Emerging Technologies*, 4, 339–348.

Valero, D., Pérez-Vicente, A., Martínez-Romero, D., Castillo, S., Guillén, F., and Serrano, M. (2002b). Plum storability improved after calcium and heat treatments: role of polyamines. *Journal of Food Science*, 67, 2571–2575.

Valero, D., Serrano, M., Martínez-Madrid, M.C., and Riquelme, F. (1997). Polyamines, ethylene, and physicochemical changes in low-temperature-stored peach (*Prunus persica* L. Cv. Maycrest). *Journal of Agricultural and Food Chemistry*, 45, 3406–3410.

Valero, D., Valverde, J.M., Martínez-Romero, D., Guillén, F., Castillo, S., and Serrano, M. (2006). The combination of modified atmosphere packaging with eugenol or thymol to maintain quality, safety and functional properties of table grapes. *Postharvest Biology and Technology*, 41, 317–327.

Valpuesta, V., and Botella, M.A. (2004). Biosynthesis of L-ascorbic acid in plants: New pathways for an old antioxidant. *Trends in Plant Science*, 9, 573–577.

Valverde, J.M., Guillén, F., Martínez-Romero, D., Castillo, S., Serrano, M., and Valero, D. (2005a). Improvement of table grapes quality and safety by the combination of modified atmosphere packaging (MAP) and eugenol, menthol or thymol. *Journal of Agricultural and Food Chemistry*, 53, 7458–7464.

Valverde, J.M., Valero, D., Martínez-Romero, D., Guillén, F., Castillo, S., and Serrano, M. (2005b). Novel edible coating based on *Aloe vera* gel to maintain table grape quality and safety. *Journal of Agricultural and Food Chemistry*, 53, 7807–7813.

Van Rooyen, Z., and Bower, J.P. (2005). The role of fruit mineral composition on fruit softness and mesocarp discolouration in "Pinkerton" avocado (*Persea americana* Mill.). *Journal of Horticultural Science and Biotechnology*, 80, 793–799.

Vargas, M., Pastor, C., Chiralt, A., McClements, J., and González-Martínez, C. (2008). Recent advances in edible coatings for fresh and minimally processed fruits. *Critical Review in Food Science and Nutrition*, 48, 496–511.

Vázquez, B. I., Gente, C., Franco, C. M., Vázquez, M.J., and Cepeda, A. (2001). Inhibitory effects of eugenol and thymol on *Penicillium citrinum* strains in culture media and cheese. *International Journal of Food Microbiology*, 67, 157–163.

Vermeiren, L., Devlieghere, F., van Beest, M., de Kruijf, N., and Debevere, J. (1999). Developments in the active packaging of foods. *Trends in Food Science and Technology*, 10, 77–86.

Vicente, A.R., Costa, M.L., Martínez, G.A., Chaves, A., and Civello, P.M. (2005). Effect of heat treatments on cell wall degradation and softening in strawberry. *Postharvest Biology and Technology*, 38, 213–222.

Vicente, A.R., Martínez, G.A., Chaves, A.R., and Civello, P.M. (2006). Effect of heat treatment on strawberry fruit damage and oxidative metabolism during storage. *Postharvest Biology and Technology*, 40, 116–122.

Vigneault, C., and Goyette, B. (2001). Loss of ice through container openings during liquid-ice cooling of horticultural crops. *Canadian Agricultural Engineering*, 43, 45–48.

Vigneault, C., Goyette, B., and De Castro, L.R. (2006). Maximum slat width for cooling efficiency of horticultural produce in wooden crates. *Postharvest Biology and Technology*, 40, 308–313.

Vigneault, C., Goyette, B., Markarian, N.H., Hui, C.K.P., Côté, S., Charles, M.T., and Émond, J.P. (2004). Plastic container opening area for optimum hydrocooling. *Canadian Biosystems Engineering*, 46, 41–44.

Vigneault, C., Rennie, T.J., and Toussaint, V. (2008). Cooling of freshly harvested fruits and vegetables. *Stewart Postharvest Review*, 3:4.

Vigneault, C., Sargent, S.A., and Bartz, J.A. (2000). Postharvest decay risk associated with hydrocooling tomatoes. *Plant Disease*, 84, 1314–1318.

Vilaplana, R., Valentines, M.C., Toivonen, P., and Larrigaudiere, C. (2006). Antioxidant potential and peroxidative state of "Golden Smoothee" apples treated with 1-methylcyclopropene. *Journal of the American Society for Horticultural Science*, 131, 104–109.

Villatoro, C., Altisent, R., Echeverría, G., Graell, J., López, M.T., and Lara, I. (2008). Changes in biosynthesis of aroma volatile compounds during on-tree maturation of "Pink Lady" apples. *Postharvest Biology and Technology*, 47, 286–295.

Vincken, J.P., Schols, H.A., Oomen, R.J.F.J., McCann, M.C., Ulvskov, K.P., Voragen, A.G.J., and Visser, R.G.F. (2003). If homogalacturonan were a side chain of rhamnogalacturonan I. Implications for cell wall architecture. *Plant Physiology*, 132, 1781–1798.

Vizzotto, M., Cisneros-Zevallos, L., Byrne, D.H., Ramming, D.W., and Okie, W.R. (2007). Large variation found in the phytochemical and antioxidant activity of peach and plum germplasm. *Journal of the American Society for Horticultural Science*, 132, 334–340.

Voutilainen, S., Nurmi, T., Mursu, J., and Rissanen, T.H. (2006). Carotenoids and cardiovascular health. *American Journal of Clinical Nutrition*, 83, 1265–1271.

Wang, B., Wang, J., Feng, X., Lin, L., Zhao, Y., and Jiang, W. (2009). Effects of 1-MCP and exogenous ethylene on fruit ripening and antioxidants in stored mango. *Plant Growth Regulation*, 57, 185–192.

Wang, C.Y., Conway, W.S., Abbott, J.A., Kramer, G.F., and Sams, C.E. (1993). Postharvest infiltration of polyamines and calcium influences ethylene production and texture changes in "Golden Delicious" apples. *Journal of the American Society for Horticultural Science*, 118, 801–806.

Wang, C.Y., and Qi, L. (1997). Modified atmosphere packaging alleviates chilling injury in cucumbers. *Postharvest Biology and Technology*, 10, 195–200.

Wang, J.Y. (1994). Combined treatment of heat shock and low-temperature conditioning reduces chilling injury in zucchini squash. *Postharvest Biology and Technology*, 4, 65–73.

Wang, J.Y., and Casero, R.A. (2006). *Polyamine cell signaling*. New Jersey: Humana Press Inc.

Wang, K.L.C., Li, H., and Ecker, J.R. (2002). Ethylene biosynthesis and signalling networks. *Plant Cell*, Supplement 2002, S131–S151.

Wang, S.Y., Chen, C.T., Sciarappa, W., Wang, C.Y., and Camp, M.J. (2008). Fruit quality, antioxidant capacity, and flavonoid content of organically and conventionally grown blueberries. *Journal of Agricultural and Food Chemistry*, 56, 5788–5794.

Wang, S.Y., and Lin, H.S. (2000). Antioxidant activity in fruits and leaves of blackberry, raspberry, and strawberry varies with cultivar and developmental stage. *Journal of Agricultural and Food Chemistry*, 48, 140–146.

Wang, Y., Lu, W., Jiang, Y., Luo, Y., Jiang, W., and Joyce, D. (2006a). Expression of ethylene-related expansin genes in cool-stored ripening banana fruit. *Plant Science*, 170, 962–967.

Wang, Y.S., Tian, S.P., Xu, Y., Qin, G.Z., and Yao, H. (2004). Changes in the activities of pro- and anti-oxidant enzymes in peach fruit inoculated with *Cryptococcus laurentii* or *Penicillium expansum* at 0 or 20°C. *Postharvest Biology and Technology*, 34, 21–28.

Wang, W.Y., Zhu, B.Z., Lü, J., and Luo, Y.B. (2006b). No difference in the regulation pattern of calcium on ethylene biosynthesis between wild-type and *Never-Ripe* tomato fruit at mature green stage. *Russian Journal of Plant Physiology*, 53, 54–61.

Watkins, C.B. (2000). Responses to horticultural commodities to high carbon dioxide as related to modified atmosphere packaging. *HortTechnology*, 10, 501–506.

Watkins, C.B. (2006). The use of 1-methylcyclopropene (1-MCP) on fruits and vegetables. *Biotechnology Advances*, 24, 389–409.

Watkins, C.B. (2007). The effect of 1-MCP on the development of physiological storage disorders in horticultural crops. *Stewart Postharvest Review*, 2:11.

Watkins, C.B. (2008). Overview of 1-methylcyclopropene trials and uses for edible horticultural crops. *HortScience*, 43, 86–94.

Watkins, C.B., and Miller, W.B. (2005). A summary of physiological processes or disorders in fruits, vegetables and ornamental plants that are delayed or decreased, increased, or unaffected by application of 1-MCP. Accessed August 2009. http://www.hort.cornell.edu/mcp.

Watkins, C.B., Nock, J.F., and Whitaker, B.D. (2000). Responses of early, mid and late season apple cultivars to postharvest application of 1-methylcyclopropene (1-MCP) under air and controlled atmosphere storage conditions. *Postharvest Biology and Technology*, 19, 17–32.

Welch, C.R., Wu, Q., and Simon, J.E, (2008). Recent advances in anthocyanin analysis and characterization. *Current Analytical Chemistry*, 4, 75–101.

White, P.J., and Broadley, M.R. (2003). Calcium in plants. *Annals of Botany*, 92, 487–511.

Willcox, J.K., Ash, S.L., and Catignani, G.L. (2004). Antioxidants and prevention of chronic disease. *Critical Review in Food Science and Nutrition*, 44, 275–295.

Wills, R.B.H., and Ku, V.V.V. (2002). Use of 1-MCP to extend the time to ripen of green tomatoes and postharvest life of ripe tomatoes. *Postharvest Biology and Technology*, 26, 85–90.

Wills, R.B.H., Tirmazi, S.I.H., and Scott, K. (1977). Use of calcium to delay ripening of tomatoes. *HortScience*, 12, 551–552.

Wilson, C., and Pusey, P.L. (1985). Potential for biological control of postharvest plant diseases. *Plant Disease*, 69, 375–378.

Wilson, C.L. (2007). *Intelligent and Active Packaging for Fruit and Vegetables*. Boca Raton: CRC Press.

Woods, J.L. (1990). Moisture loss from fruits and vegetables. *Postharvest News and Information*, 1, 195–199.

Woolf, A.B., and Ferguson, I.B. (2000). Postharvest responses to high fruit temperatures in the field. *Postharvest Biology and Technology*, 21, 7–20.

Woolf, A.B., Requejo-Tapia, C., Cox, K.A., Jackman, R.C., Gunson, A., Arpaia, M.L., and White, A. (2005). 1-MCP reduces physiological storage disorders of "Hass" avocados. *Postharvest Biology and Technology*, 35, 43–60.

Wrolstad, R.E., Dursta, R.W., and Lee, J. (2005). Tracking color and pigment changes in anthocyanin products. *Trends in Food Science and Technology*, 16, 423–428.

Wszelaki, A.L., and Mitcham, E.J. (2003). Effect of combinations of hot water dips, biological control and controlled atmospheres for control of gray mold on harvested strawberries. *Postharvest Biology and Technology*, 27, 255–264.

Wu, X., Beecher, G.R., Holden, J.M., Haytowitz, D.B., Gebhardt, S.E., and Prior, R.L. (2004). Lipophilic and hydrophilic antioxidant capacities of common foods in the United States. *Journal of Agricultural and Food Chemistry*, 53, 4026–4037.

Xu, C., Jin, Z., and Yang, S. (2005). Polyamines induced by heat treatment before cold-storage reduce mealiness and decay in peach fruit. *Journal of Horticultural Science and Biotechnology*, 80, 557–560.

Yahia, E.M. (2006). Modified atmosphere for atmospheres for tropical fruits. *Stewart Postharvest Review*, 5:6.

Yahia, E. M., Contreras-Padilla, M., and González-Aguilar, G. (2001). Ascorbic acid content in relation to ascorbic acid oxidase and polyamine content in tomato and bell pepper fruits during development, maturation and senescence. *Lebensmmittel Wissenschaft und Technologie*, 34, 452–457.

Yahia, E.M., Soto-Zamora, G., Brecht, J.K., and Gardea, A. (2007). Postharvest hot air treatment effects on the antioxidant system in stored mature-green tomatoes. *Postharvest Biology and Technology*, 44, 107–115.

Yam, K.L., Takhisto, P.T., and Miltz, J. (2005). Intelligent packaging: Concepts and application. *Journal of Food Science*, 70, R1–R10.

Yamaguchi, S., Yoshikawa, T., Ikeda, S., and Ninomiya, T. (1970). Studies on the taste of some sweet substances Part I. Measurement of the relative sweetness. *Agricultural and Biological Chemistry*, 34, 181–186.

Yang, S.F., and Hoffman, N.E. (1984). Ethylene biosynthesis and its regulation in higher plants. *Annual Review of Plant Physiology*, 35, 155–189.

Yao, H., Tian, S., and Wang, Y. (2004). Sodium bicarbonate enhances biocontrol efficacy of yeasts on fungal spoilage of pears. *International Journal of Food Microbiology*, 93, 297–304.

Yeum, K.J., Russle, R.M., Krinsky, N.I., and Aldini, G. (2004). Biomarkers of antioxidant capacity in the hydrophilic and lipophilic compartments of human plasma. *Archives of Biochemistry and Biophysics*, 430, 97–103.

Yoo, S.D., Cho, Y., and Sheen, J. (2009). Emerging connections in the ethylene signalling network. *Trends in Plant Sciences*, 14, 270–279.

Yuen, C.M.C. (1994). Calcium and fruit storage potential. *Australian Quarterly International Agricultural Research*, 50, 218–227.

Zapata, P.J., Guillén, F., Martínez-Romero, D., Castillo, S., Valero, D., and Serrano, M. (2008). Use of alginate or zein as edible coatings to delay postharvest ripening process and to maintain tomato (*Solanum lycopersicon* Mill) quality. *Journal of the Science of Food and Agriculture*, 88, 1287–1293.

Zhang, H., Wang, S., Huang, X., Dong, Y., and Zheng, X. (2008). Integrated control of postharvest blue old decay of pears with hot water treatment and *Rhodotorula glutinis*. *Postharvest Biology and Technology*, 49, 308–313.

Zhou, C.-H., Xu, C.-J., Sun, C.-D., Li, X., and Chen, K.S. (2007). Carotenoids in white- and red-fleshed loquat fruits. *Journal of Agricultural and Food Chemistry*, 55, 7822–7830.

Zhu, H.L., Zhu, B.Z., Fu, D.Q., Xie, Y.H., Hao, Y.L., and Luo, Y.B. (2005). Role of ethylene in the biosynthetic pathways of aroma volatiles in ripening fruit. *Russian Journal of Plant Physiology*, 52, 691–695.

Zingg, J.M. (2007). Vitamin E: An overview of major research directions. *Molecular Aspects of Medicine*, 28, 400–422.

Ziosi, V., Bregoli, A.M., Bonghi, C., Fossati, T., Biondi, S., Costa, G., and Torrigiani, P. (2006). Transcription of ethylene perception and biosynthesis genes is altered by putrescine, spermidine and aminoethoxyvinylglycine (AVG) during ripening in peach fruit (*Prunus persica*). *New Phytologist*, 172, 229–238.

Zoumas-Morse, C., Rock, C.L., Quintana, E.L., Neuhouser, M.L., Gerner, E.W., and Meyskens, F.L. (2007). Development of a polyamine database for assessing dietary intake. *Journal of the American Dietetic Association*, 107, 1024–1027.

Zuzunaga, M., Serrano, M., Martínez-Romero, D., Valero, D., and Riquelme, F. (2001). Comparative study of two plum (*Prunus salicina* Lindl.) cultivars during growth and ripening. *Food Science and Technology International*, 7, 123–130.

Index

B

C

D

E

F

G

L

M

P